FOURTH EDITION

PHILOSOPHY

and SEX

FOURTH EDITION

PHILOSOPHY
and SEX

ADULTERY • MONOGAMY • FEMINISM •

RAPE • SAME-SEX MARRIAGE • ABORTION •

PROMISCUITY • PERVERSION

EDITED BY
ROBERT B. BAKER and
KATHLEEN J. WININGER

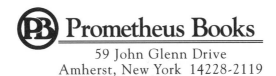 Prometheus Books

59 John Glenn Drive
Amherst, New York 14228-2119

Published 2009 by Prometheus Books

Inquiries should be addressed to
Prometheus Books
59 John Glenn Drive
Amherst, New York 14228–2119
VOICE: 716–691–0133, ext. 210
FAX: 716–691–0137
WWW.PROMETHEUSBOOKS.COM

13 12 11 10 09   5 4 3 2 1

Library of Congress Cataloging-in-Publication Data

Philosophy and sex / edited by Robert B. Baker, Kathleen J. Wininger. — 4th ed.
      p. cm.
    Includes bibliographical references.
    ISBN 1–59102–609–9 (pbk. : alk. paper)
    1. Sexual ethics. 2. Sex customs. 3. Marriage. 4. Moral conditions. I. Baker, Robert, 1937– II. Wininger, Kathleen J.

HQ32.P5 2009
306.701—dc22

                                                            2009017699

To our children and grandchildren

CONTENTS

7

PART 2. GENDER, SEXUALITY, AND PERVERSION

PART 3. DESIRE, PORNOGRAPHY, AND RAPE

PREFACE

L ike any compilation, this one owes many debts of thanks. We would like to thank the contributors, especially those who wrote or rewrote papers for this volume, and family and friends who sacrificed to allow us to produce this new edition. In particular we would like to acknowledge the assistance of Kathryn Leary, Aramis Lopez, Christina Dibiase, Heidi Record, and Brenda McGovern. A special thank you to our kind, long-suffering editor, Steven L. Mitchell, whose publication plans were disrupted by delays in the latest manuscript. Finally, we would like to express our gratitude to Deborah Elliston, who graciously acknowledged that while the spirit of her late father, Frederick Elliston, lives on in this book, the present edition no longer bears his imprint. We are pleased to acknowledge some of Deborah Elliston's own work in anthropology and sexuality in the selection "To Cut or Not to Cut."

Robert B. Baker,
Union College & Union Graduate College—
Mount Sinai School of Medicine Bioethics Program

Kathleen J. Wininger,
University of Southern Maine

INTRODUCTION TO
THE FOURTH EDITION

It was the best of times, it was the worst of times, it was the age of wisdom, it was the age of foolishness, it was the epoch of belief, it was the epoch of incredulity, it was the season of Light, it was the season of Darkness, it was the spring of hope, it was the winter of despair, we had everything before us, we had nothing before us. . . .

Charles Dickens, *A Tale of Two Cities*

Charles Dickens published these words in 1859 to introduce readers to a revolution of a previous century. They seem appropriate to introduce twenty-first-century readers to the 1970s context in which the first edition of this book was published. America was undergoing a radical transformation. The disempowered and disenfranchised—African Americans and other minorities like homosexuals and women—were finding their voice, voicing their views, and demanding change. However, the ivory-towered world of Anglo-American philosophy was professionally aloof. The received construction of moral philosophy could not properly offer insight or even commentary. At that time philosophical ethics was construed as metaethics, that is, the epistemological, ontological, and semantic analysis of moral discourse and knowledge claims. This construction relegated moral philosophy to the role of logic umpire and left moral philosophers speechless about real-world moral issues in a world that sought their insights. A generation of philosophers broke with professional shibboleths and began to pronounce upon and debate the issues of the day. In the process, they developed alternative conceptions of moral philosophy and the role of philosophers.

The editors of the first edition of this book, Bob Baker and Fred Elliston, belong to that generation. The first edition was conceived when Elliston walked into Baker's Union College office in search of teaching material for a course he was offering, called "Sex and Society." Baker, ever a "piler" and seldom a "filer," pointed to a motley stack of manuscripts decked out in the carbon-copy-gray, ditto-blue, and mimeograph-black hues characteristic of copies in pre-photocopier 1970. These "samizdat" manuscripts had been circulated by philosophers who wrote about sexual issues in spite of the knowledge that the subject was considered unsuitable for philosophical reflection by the received philosophy of the day.

Although unpublishable and undiscussable in formal philosophical fora, the manuscripts were nonetheless circulated, debated, dissected at professional conventions, albeit always in corridors and coffee shops, never from the podium. The common thread running through these motley—then unpublishable— manuscripts was that they converted the personal into the philosophical and formally broached issues of sex, sexuality, and gender considered undiscussable in official philosophical circles. It was philosophy written from the heart, analyzed from the head, circulated, read, and reread because of philosophers' personal investment in the issues.

After Elliston perused the stack of manuscripts from Baker's office, he turned to Baker and said, "I know a publisher who will put these into print." Three years later, in 1975, with the backing of Paul Kurtz and Prometheus Books, the first edition of contemporary English-language essays on philosophy and sex was published. Resonating with defiance, the cover of the first edition paraded its previously unspeakable, unprintable, unpublishable, "unprofessional" subject matter in bright neon-colored words displayed against a black background— "abortion," "adultery," "feminism," "homosexuality," "monogamy," "perversion," "promiscuity." Philosophy of sex had come out of the closet. No one knew how the profession would receive it. As it turned out, *Philosophy and Sex* had innumerable kindred spirits. It proved to be part of a generational reconception of moral philosophy that came to be known initially as the applied ethics movement and then, more simply, as "applied ethics."

The expression "applied ethics" is something of a misnomer. Many works of applied ethics actually do what the expression indicates: they apply an ethical precept, principle, theory, or some mode of ethical analysis to a practical moral issue. Thus the selection from the English philosopher Jeremy Bentham (1748–1832), the founder of the modern utilitarian moral philosophy, directly applies the principle of utility (act so as to produce the greatest happiness for the greatest number) to the question of criminalizing homosexual intercourse. John Scott Gray's chapter, aptly titled, "Rawls's Principle of Justice as Fairness and Its Application to the Issue of Same-Sex Marriage," is a paradigm case of applying an ethical principle—in this case the principle of justice as fairness as articulated by the Harvard philosopher John Rawls (1921–2002)—to the issue of same-sex marriage. Baker's "'Pricks' and 'Chicks': A Plea for 'Persons,'" on the other hand, applies techniques of philosophical analysis to uncover everyday conceptions of male-female relationships.

Nonetheless most of the papers in this book do not directly "apply" a principle of moral philosophy to an issue, nor do they apply some technique of philosophical analysis. Some are even written by non-philosophers, like Alicia Ouellette, the Albany Law School professor who was lead counsel on the law professors' amicus curiae brief in support of the forty-four same-sex couples who sought the right to marry in New York State. Yet a moral perspective informs Ouellette's paper, even though it does not apply techniques or principles of moral philosophy to specific issues in any literal sense. As the inclusion of this paper suggests, in current usage "applied ethics" is a catch-all phrase used to designate ethical dimensions of occupations, professions, and of everyday life. The issues covered range from animal rights, to bioethics, business ethics, cyberethics, engineering ethics, environmental ethics, to nanoethics and neuroethics, and, of course, to issues involving sex and gender.

The first two editions of *Philosophy and Sex* originated because the editors and the publisher strove to create a place to publish the previously unpublishable manuscripts of philosophers delving into questions of philosophy and sex. Although success of the applied ethics movement has changed the publishing environment, we reprint the introduction to the first edition of the book because it captures something of the spirit of this book's original purpose and because it presents a still useful history of philosophical writings on sex. The other original purpose of the book was to offer a collection of teachable philosophical materials for courses on philosophy and sex. As the number of venues publishing philosophical analyses of sex, gender, and sexuality increased, this became the primary purpose of later editions of the book.

After the untimely death of Fredrick Elliston (1945–1987), Baker's former Union College colleague, Kathleen J. Wininger, a philosopher interested in feminism and African philosophy, as well as a Nietzsche expert, undertook the role of co-editor. The third and fourth editions bear her imprint as the volume broadens to considered female sexual desire, trans- and inter-sexual issues, and the history of sexuality theory. Following the spirit of philosophy and the present age, and the specific interest of Wininger in African philosophy, this fourth edition of

Philosophy and Sex is more global, and provides perspectives from outside the Western world. Three contributions from South Africa—including an essay by Archbishop Desmond Tutu, comparing homophobia to apartheid, condemning both as crimes against humanity—add a global perspective to the volume.

The editors have divided this fourth edition of *Philosophy and Sex* into three parts. The first part deals with issues of love, marriage, and reproduction. As in earlier editions, this section opens with a debate on the nature of love between the Canadian-born Jewish feminist Shulamith Firestone, author of the classic feminist work *The Dialectic of Sex* (1970), and the late Robert Solomon (1942–2007), an American existentialist and philosopher of love and other emotions. There follow selections from Augustine (354–430) and Thomas Aquinas (1225–1274) and a more recent statement by Pope Paul VI (1897–1978) that characterize, define, and defend the Christian view of celibacy, sexuality, sexual intercourse, and reproduction—including contraception and abortion. Offering a more secular perspective on abortion is a set of essays by the distinguished philosophers Judith Jarvis Thomson and Frances Myrna Kamm. These are followed by reflections on spinsterhood (the state of being female, unmarried, and of a certain age), marriage, fidelity, and adultery. The section closes with a series of essays on same-sex marriage.

The Christian conception of sex represented by Augustine, Aquinas, and Paul VI—discussed at length in the introduction to the first edition—defined the function of sexual intercourse, drew the boundaries of sexuality, and cast gender roles. Deviations from these constructions were condemned as perverse by religion, law, and medicine. Part 2 of the book deals with the language and conceptual framework of these constructions and the treatment of intersexuals and others who fall outside of them. Part 3 turns to reflections on the darker side of sexuality, including its connection to domination, violence, and violation. The volume focuses introspectively on a discussion of the historical construction of sexuality and homosexuality.

Three and one-half decades ago, when this collection was first sent to the publisher, in Britain, the 1957 Wolfenden Report first led to the decriminalization of homosexuality. A July 28, 1969, police raid on a gay bar in New York City, the Stonewall Inn, led to the so-called Stonewall Riots, which date the birth of the gay rights movement in the United States. Just five years earlier, in 1964, the Civil Rights Act officially gave American females equal rights with American males and prohibited discrimination in employment. The first edition of *Philosophy and Sex* collected philosophical essays written within the context of these events. In the most recent edition, the debate on these issues has globalized as philosophers from Africa to America debate the wisdom of legally recognizing same-sex marriage, and discuss the issues confronting physicians the world over as they decide how best to respond to intersexual infants. As it has in the past, the current edition seeks to document the current debate, even as it preserves for students and non-philosophers the classic works in the older literature.

Robert B. Baker,
Philosophy and Bioethics,
Union College & Union Graduate College—
Mount Sinai School of Medicine Bioethics Program

Kathleen J. Wininger,
Philosophy & Women and Gender Studies,
University of Southern Maine

Part 1.

LOVE, MARRIAGE, AND REPRODUCTION

1.

LOVE

A Feminist Critique

Shulamith Firestone

book on radical feminism that did not deal with love would be a political failure. For love, perhaps even more than childbearing, is the pivot of women's oppression today. I realize this has frightening implications: Do we want to get rid of love?

The panic felt at any threat to love is a good clue to its political significance. Another sign that love is central to any analysis of women or sex psychology is its omission from culture itself, its relegation to "personal life." (And whoever heard of logic in the bedroom?) Yes, it is portrayed in novels, even metaphysics, but in them it is described, or better, recreated, not analyzed. Love has never been *understood* though it may have been fully *experienced* and that experience communicated.

There is reason for this absence of analysis: *Women and Love are underpinnings. Examine them and you threaten the very structure of culture.*

The tired question "What were women doing while men created masterpieces?" deserves more than the obvious reply: Women were barred from culture, exploited in their role of mother. Or its reverse: Women had no need for paintings since they created children. Love is tied to culture in much deeper ways than that. Men were thinking, writing, and creating, because women were pouring their energy into those men; women are not creating culture because they are preoccupied with love.

That women live for love and men for work is a truism. Freud was the first to attempt to ground this dichotomy in the individual psyche: the male child, sexually rejected by the first person in his attention, his mother, "sublimates" his "libido"—his reservoir of sexual (life) energies—into long-term projects, in the hope of gaining love in a more generalized form; thus he displaces his need for love into a need for recognition. This process does not occur as much in the female: most women never stop seeking direct warmth and approval.

There is also much truth in the clichés that "behind every man there is a woman," and that "women are the power behind [read: voltage in] the throne." (Male) culture was built on the love of women, and at their expense. Women provided the substance of those male masterpieces; and for millennia they have done the work, and suffered the costs, of one-way emotional relationships the benefits of which went to men and to the work of men. So if women are a parasitical class living off, and at the margins of, the male economy, the reverse too is true: *(Male) culture was (and is) parasitical, feeding on the emotional strength of women without reciprocity.*

Moreover, we tend to forget that this culture is not universal, but rather sectarian, presenting only half the spectrum. The very structure of culture itself, as we shall see, is saturated with the sexual polarity, as well as being in every degree run by, for, and in the interests of male society. But while the male half is termed all of culture, men have not forgotten there is a female "emotional" half: They live it on the sly. As the result of their battle to reject the female in themselves . . . they are unable to take love seriously as a cultural matter; but they can't do without it altogether. Love is the underbelly of (male) culture just as love is the weak spot of every man, bent on proving his virility in that large male world of "travel and adventure." Women have always known how men need love, and how they deny this need. Perhaps this explains the peculiar contempt women so universally feel for men ("men are so dumb"), for they can see their men are posturing in the outside world.

I.

How does this phenomenon "love" operate? Contrary to popular opinion, love is not altruistic. The initial attraction is based on curious admiration (more often today, envy and resentment) for the self-possession, the integrated unity, of the other and a wish to become part of this Self in some way (today, read: intrude or take over), to become important to that psychic balance. The self-containment of the other creates desire (read: a challenge); admiration (envy) of the other becomes a wish to incorporate (possess) its qualities. A clash of selves follows in which the individual attempts to fight off the growing hold over him of the other. Love is the final opening up to (or, surrender to the dominion of) the other. The lover demonstrates to the beloved how he himself would like to be treated. ("I tried so hard to make him fall in love with me that I fell in love with him myself.") Thus love is the height of selfishness: the self attempts to enrich itself through the absorption of another being. Love is being psychically wide-open to another. It is a situation of total emotional vulnerability. Therefore it must be not only the incorporation of the other, but an *exchange* of selves. Anything short of a mutual exchange will hurt one or the other party.

There is nothing inherently destructive about this process. A little healthy selfishness would be a refreshing change. Love between two equals would be an enrichment; each enlarging himself through the other: instead of being one, locked in the cell of himself with only his own experience and view, he could participate in the existence of another—an extra window on the world. This accounts for the bliss that successful lovers experience: Lovers are temporarily freed from the burden of isolation that every individual bears.

But bliss in love is seldom the case: For every successful contemporary love experience, for every short period of enrichment, there are ten destructive love experiences, post-love "downs" of much longer duration—often resulting in the destruction of the individual, or at least an emotional cynicism that makes it difficult or impossible ever to love again. Why should this be so, if it is not actually inherent in the love process itself?

Let's talk about love in its destructive pulse—and why it gets that way, referring . . . to the work of Theodore Reik. Reik's concrete observation brings him closer than many better minds to understanding the *process* of "falling in love," but he is off insofar as he confuses love as it exists in our present society with love itself. He notes that love is a reaction formation, a cycle of envy, hostility, and possessiveness: he sees that it is preceded by dissatisfaction with oneself, a yearning for something better, created by a discrepancy between the ego and the ego-ideal; that the bliss love produces is due to the resolution of this tension by the substitution, in place of one's own ego-ideal, of the other; and finally that love fades "because the other can't live up to your high ego-ideal any more than you could, and the judgment will be the harsher the higher are the claims on oneself." Thus in Reik's view love wears down just as it wound up: Dissatisfaction with oneself (whoever heard of falling in love the week one is leaving for Europe?) leads to astonishment at the other person's self-containment; to envy;

to hostility; to possessive love; and back again through exactly the same process. This is the love process *today*. But why must it be this way?

Many, for example Denis de Rougemont in *Love in the Western World*, have tried to draw a distinction between romantic "falling in love" with its "false reciprocity which disguises a twin narcissism" (the Pagan Eros) and an unselfish love for the other person as that person really is (the Christian Agape). De Rougemont attributes the morbid passion of Tristan and Iseult (romantic love) to a vulgarization of specific mystical and religious currents in Western civilization.

I believe instead that *love is essentially a simple phenomenon—unless it has become complicated, corrupted, or obstructed by an unequal balance of power*. We have seen that love demands a mutual vulnerability or it turns destructive: the destructive effects of love occur only in a context of inequality. But if, as we have seen, (biological) inequality has always remained a constant, existing to varying degrees, then it is understandable that "romantic love" would develop. . . .

How does the sex class system based on the unequal power distribution of the biological family affect love between the sexes? In discussing Freudianism, we have gone into the psychic structuring of the individual within the family and how this organization of personality must be different for the male and the female because of their very different relationships to the mother. At present the insular interdependency of the mother/child relationship forces both male and female children into anxiety about losing the mother's love, on which they depend for physical survival. When later (Erich Fromm notwithstanding) the child learns that the mother's love is conditional, to be rewarded the child in return for approved behavior (that is, behavior in line with the mother's own values and personal ego gratification—for she is free to mold the child "creatively," however she happens to define that), the child's anxiety turns into desperation. This, coinciding with the sexual rejection of the male child by the mother, causes, as we have seen, a schizophrenia in the boy between the emotional and the physical, and in the girl, the mother's rejection, occurring for different reasons, produces an insecurity about her identity in general, creating a lifelong need for approval. (Later her lover replaces her father as a grantor of the necessary surrogate identity—she sees everything through his eyes.) Here originates the hunger for love that later sends both sexes searching in one person after the other for a state of ego security. But because of the early rejection, to the degree that it occurred, the male will be terrified of committing himself, of "opening up" and then being smashed. . . . To the degree that a woman is like his mother, the incest taboo operates to restrain his total sexual/emotional commitment; for him to feel safely the kind of total response he first felt for his mother, which was rejected, he must degrade this woman so as to distinguish her from the mother. This behavior reproduced on a larger scale explains many cultural phenomena, including perhaps the ideal love-worship of chivalric times, the forerunner of modern romanticism.

Romantic idealization is partially responsible, at least on the part of men, for a peculiar characteristic of "falling" in love: the change takes place in the lover almost independently of the character of the love object. Occasionally the lover, though beside himself, sees with another rational part of his faculties that, objectively speaking, the one he loves isn't worth all this blind devotion; but he is helpless to act on this, "a slave to love." More often he fools himself entirely. But others can see what is happening ("How on earth he could love her is beyond me!"). This idealization occurs much less frequently on the part of women, as is borne out by Reik's clinical studies. A man must idealize one woman over the rest in order to justify his descent to a lower caste. Women have no such reason to idealize men—in fact, when one's life depends on one's ability to "psych" men out, such idealization may actually be dangerous—though a fear of male power in general may carry over into relationships with individual men, appearing to be the same phenomenon. But though women know to be inauthentic, this male "falling in love," all women, in one way or another, require proof of it from men before they can allow themselves to love (genuinely, in their case) in return. For this idealization process acts to artificially equalize the two parties, a minimum precondition for the development of an uncorrupted love—we have seen that love requires a mutual vulnerability that is impossible to achieve in an unequal power situation. *Thus "falling in love" is no more than the process of alteration of male vision—through idealization, mystification, glorification—that renders void the woman's class inferiority.*

However, the woman knows that this idealization, which she works so hard to produce, is a lie, and that it is only a matter of time before he "sees through her." Her life is a hell, vacillating between an all-consuming need for male love and approval to raise her from her class subjection, to persistent feelings of inauthenticity when she does achieve his love. Thus her whole identity hangs in the balance of her love life. She is allowed to love herself only if a man finds her worthy of love.

But if we could eliminate the political context of love between the sexes, would we not have some degree of idealization remaining in the love process itself? I think so. For the process occurs in the same manner whoever the love choice: the lover "opens up" to the other. Because of this fusion of egos, in which each sees and cares about the other as a new self, the beauty/character of the beloved, perhaps hidden to outsiders under layers of defenses, is revealed. "I wonder what she sees in him," then, means not only, "She is a fool, blinded with romanticism," but, "Her love has lent her x-ray vision. Perhaps we are missing something." (Note that this phrase is most commonly used about women. The equivalent phrase about *men's* slavery to love is more often something like, "She has him wrapped around her finger," she has him so "snowed" that he is the last one to see through her.) Increased sensitivity to the real, if hidden, values in the other, however, is not "blindness" or "idealization," but is, in fact, deeper vision. It is only the *false* idealization we have described above that is responsible for the destruction. Thus it is not the process of love itself that is at fault, but its *political*, i.e., unequal *power* context: the who, why, when and where of it is what makes it now such a holocaust.

II

But abstractions about love are only one more symptom of its diseased state. (As one female patient of Reik so astutely put it, "Men take love either too seriously or not seriously enough.") Let's look at it more concretely, as we now experience it in its corrupted form. Once again we shall quote from the Reikian Confessional. For if Reik's work has any value it is where he might least suspect, i.e., in his trivial feminine urge to "gossip." Here he is, justifying himself (one supposes his Superego is troubling him):

> A has-been like myself must always be somewhere and working on something. Why should I not occupy myself with those small questions that are not often posed and yet perhaps can be answered? The "petites questions" have a legitimate place beside the great and fundamental problems of psychoanalysis.
>
> It takes moral courage to write about certain things, as for example about a game that little girls play in the intervals between classes. Is such a theme really worthy of a *serious* psychoanalyst who has passed his 77th year? (Italics mine)

And he reminds himself:

> But in psychoanalysis there are no unimportant thoughts; there are only thoughts that pretend to be unimportant in order not to be told.

Thus he rationalizes what in fact may be the only valuable contribution of his work. Here are his patients of both sexes speaking for themselves about their love lives:

WOMEN:

> Later on he called me a sweet girl . . . I didn't answer . . . what could I say . . . but I knew I was not a sweet girl at all and that he sees me as someone I'm not.

No man can love a girl the way a girl loves a man.

I can go a long time without sex, but not without love.

It's like H_2O instead of water.

I sometimes think that all men are sex-crazy and sex-starved. All they can think about when they are with a girl is going to bed with her. Have I nothing to offer this man but this body?

I took off my dress and my bra and stretched myself out on his bed and waited. For an instant I thought of myself as an animal of sacrifice on the altar.

I don't understand the feelings of men. My husband has me. Why does he need other women? What have they got that I haven't got?

Believe me, if all wives whose husbands had affairs left them, we would only have divorced women in this country.

After my husband had quite a few affairs, I flirted with the fantasy of taking a lover. Why not? What's sauce for the gander is sauce for the goose. . . . But I was stupid as a goose: I didn't have it in me to have an extramarital affair.

I asked several people whether men also sometimes cry themselves to sleep. I don't believe it.

MEN (for further illustration, see *Screw*):

It's not true that only the external appearance of a woman matters. The under-wear is also important.

It's not difficult to make it with a girl. What's difficult is to make an end of it.

The girl asked me whether I cared for her mind. I was tempted to answer I cared more for her behind.

"Are you going already?" she said when she opened her eyes. It was a bedroom cliché whether I left after an hour or after two days.

Perhaps it's necessary to fool the woman and to pretend you love her. But why should I fool myself?

When she is sick, she turns me off. But when I'm sick she feels sorry for me and is more affectionate than usual.

It is not enough for my wife that I have to hear her talking all the time—blah, blah, blah. She also expects me to hear what she is saying.

Simone de Beauvoir said it: "The word love has by no means the same sense for both sexes, and this is one cause of the serious misunderstandings which divide them." Above I have illustrated some of the traditional differences between men and women in love that come up so frequently in parlor discussions of the "double standard," where it is generally agreed: That women are monogamous, better at loving, possessive, "clinging," more interested in (highly involved) "relationships" than in sex per se, and they confuse affection with sexual desire. That men are interested in nothing but a screw (Wham, bam, thank you Ma'am!), or else romanticize the woman ridiculously; that once sure of her, they become notorious philanderers, never satisfied; that they mistake sex for emotion. All this bears out what we have discussed—the difference in the psychosexual organizations of the two sexes, determined by the first relationship to the mother.

I draw three conclusions based on these differences:

1. That men can't love. (Male hormones? Women traditionally expect and accept an emotional invalidism in men that they would find intolerable in a woman.)
2. That women's "clinging" behavior is necessitated by their objective social situation.
3. That this situation has not changed significantly from what it ever was.

Men can't love. We have seen why it is that men have difficulty loving and that while men may love, they usually "fall in love"—with their own projected image. Most often they are pounding down a woman's door one day, and thoroughly disillusioned with her the next; but it is rare for women to leave men, and then it is usually for more than ample reason.

It is dangerous to feel sorry for one's oppressor—women are especially prone to this failing—but I am tempted to do it in this case. Being unable to love is hell. This is the way it proceeds: as soon as the man feels any pressure from the other partner to commit himself, he panics and may react in one of several ways:

He may rush out and screw ten other women to prove that the first woman has no hold over him. If she accepts this, he may continue to see her on this basis. The other women verify his (false) freedom; periodic arguments about them keep his panic at bay. But the women are paper tigers, for nothing very deep could be happening with them anyway; he is balancing them against each other so that none of them can get much of him. Many smart women, recognizing this to be only a safety valve on their man's anxiety, give him "a long leash." For the real issue under all the fights about other women is that the man is unable to commit himself.

1. He may consistently exhibit unpredictable behavior, standing her up frequently, being indefinite about the next date, telling her that "my work comes first," or offering a variety of other excuses. That is, though he senses her anxiety, he refuses to reassure her in any way, or even to recognize her anxiety as legitimate. For he *needs* her anxiety as a steady reminder that he is still free, that the door is not entirely closed.

2. When he is forced into (an uneasy) commitment, he makes her pay for it: by ogling other women in her presence, by comparing her unfavorably to past girlfriends or movie stars, by snide reminders in front of his friends that she is his "ball and chain," by calling her a "nag," a "bitch," "a shrew," or by suggesting that if he were only a bachelor he would be a lot better off. His ambivalence about women's "inferiority" comes out: by being committed to one, he has somehow made the hated female identification, which he now must repeatedly deny if he is to maintain his self-respect in the (male) community. This steady derogation is not entirely put on: for in fact every other girl suddenly does look a lot better, he can't help feeling he has missed something—and, naturally, his woman is to blame. For he has never given up the search for the ideal; she has forced him to resign from it. Probably he will go to his grave feeling cheated, never realizing that there isn't much difference between one woman and the other, that it is the loving that *creates* the difference.

3. There are many variations of straining at the bit. Many men go from one casual thing to another, getting out every time it begins to get hot. And yet to live without love in the end proves intolerable to men just as it does to women. The question that remains for every normal male is, then, *how do I get someone to love me without her demanding an equal commitment in return?*

Women's "clinging" behavior is required by the objective social situation. The female *response* to such a situation of male hysteria at any prospect of mutual commitment was the development of subtle methods of manipulation, to force as much commitment as *could* be forced from men. Over the centuries strategies have been devised, tested, and passed on from mother to daughter in secret tête-à-têtes, passed around at "kaffee-klatsches" ("I never understand what it is women spend so much time talking about!"), or, in recent times, via the telephone. These are not trivial gossip sessions at all (as women prefer men to believe), but desperate strategies for survival. More real brilliance goes into one-hour coed telephone dialogue about men than into that same coed's four years of college study, or for that matter, than into most male political maneuvers. It is no wonder, then, that even the few women without "family obligations" always arrive exhausted at the starting line of any serious endeavor. It takes one's major energy for the best portion of one's creative years to "make a good catch," and a good part of the rest of one's life to "hold" that catch. ("To be in love can be a full-time job for a woman, like that of a profession for a man.") Women who choose to drop out of this race are choosing a life without love, something that, as we have seen, most *men* don't have the courage to do.

But unfortunately The Manhunt is characterized by an emotional urgency beyond this simple desire for return commitment. It is compounded by the very class reality that produced the male inability to love in the first place. In a male-run society that defines women as an inferior and parasitical class, a woman who does not achieve male approval in some form is doomed. To legitimate her existence, a woman must be *more* than woman, she must continually search for an out from her inferior definition;[1] and men are the only ones in a position to bestow on her this state of grace. But because the woman is rarely allowed to realize herself through activity in the larger (male) society—and when she is, she is seldom granted the recognition she deserves—it becomes easier to try for the recognition of one man than of many; and in fact this is exactly the choice most women make. Thus once more the phenomenon of love, good in itself, is corrupted by its class context: women must have love not only for healthy reasons but actually to validate their existence.

In addition, the continued *economic* dependence of women makes a situation of healthy love between equals impossible. Women today still live under a system of patronage: With few exceptions, they have the choice, not between either freedom or marriage, but between being either public or private property. Women who merge with a member of the ruling class can at least hope that some of his privilege will, so to speak, rub off. But women without men are in the same situation as orphans: they are a helpless sub-class lacking the protection of the powerful. This is the antithesis of freedom when they are still (negatively) defined by a class situation: for now they are in a situation of *magnified* vulnerability. To participate in one's subjection by choosing one's master often gives the illusion of free choice; but in reality a woman is never free to choose love without external motivations. For her at the present time, the two things, love and status, must remain inextricably intertwined.

Now assuming that a woman does not lose sight of these fundamental factors of her condition when she loves, she will never be able to love gratuitously, but only in exchange for security:

1) the emotional security which, we have seen, she is justified in demanding.
2) the emotional identity which she should be able to find through work and recognition, but which she is denied—thus forcing her to seek her definition through a man.

3) the economic class security that, in this society, is attached to her ability to "hook" a man.

Two of these three demands are invalid as conditions of "love," but are imposed on it, weighing it down.

Thus, in their precarious political situation, women can't afford the luxury of spontaneous love. It is much too dangerous. The love and approval of men is all-important. To love thoughtlessly, before one has ensured return commitment, would endanger that approval. Here is Reik:

> It finally became clear during psychoanalysis that the patient was afraid that if she should show a man she loved him, he would consider her inferior and leave her.

For once a woman plunges in emotionally, she will be helpless to play the necessary games: her love would come first, demanding expression. To pretend a coolness she does not feel, *then*, would be too painful, and further, it would be pointless: she would be cutting off her nose to spite her face, for freedom to love is what she was aiming for. But in order to guarantee such a commitment, she *must* restrain her emotions, she *must* play games. For, as we have seen, men do not commit themselves to mutual openness and vulnerability until they are forced to.

How does she then go about forcing this commitment from the male? One of her most potent weapons is sex—she can work him up to a state of physical torment with a variety of games: by denying his need, by teasing it, by giving and taking it back, by jealousy, and so forth. A woman under analysis wonders why:

> There are few women who never ask themselves on certain occasions, "How hard should I make it for a man?" I think no man is troubled with questions of this kind. He perhaps asks himself only, "When will she give in?"

Men are right when they complain that women lack discrimination, that they seldom love a man for his individual traits but rather for what he has to offer (his class), that they are calculating, that they use sex to gain other ends, etc. For in fact women are in no position to love freely. If a woman is lucky enough to find "a decent guy" to love her and support her, she is doing well—and usually will be grateful enough to return his love. About the only discrimination women *are* able to exercise is the choice between the men who have chosen them, or a playing off of one male—one power, against the other. But *provoking* a man's interest, and *snaring* his commitment once he has expressed that interest, is not exactly self-determination.

Now what happens after she has finally hooked her man, after he has fallen in love with her and will do anything? She has a new set of problems. Now she can release the vise, open her net, and examine what she has caught. Usually she is disappointed. It is nothing she would have bothered with were *she* a man. It is usually way below her level. (Check this out sometime: Talk to a few of those mousy wives.) "He may be a poor thing, but at least I've got a man of my own" is usually more the way she feels. But at least now she can drop her act. For the first time it is safe to love—now she must try like hell to catch up to him emotionally, to really mean what she has pretended all along. Often she is troubled by worries that he will find her out. She feels like an impostor. She is haunted by fears that he doesn't love the "real" her—and usually she is right. ("She wanted to marry a man with whom she could be as bitchy as she really is.")

This is just about when she discovers that love and marriage mean a different thing for a male than they do for her: Though men in general believe women in general to be inferior, every man has reserved a special place in his mind for the one woman he will elevate above the rest by virtue of association with himself. Until now the woman, out in the cold, begged for his approval, dying to clamber onto this clean, well-lighted place. But once there, she realizes that she was elevated above other women not in recognition of her real value, but only because she matched nicely his store-bought pedestal. Probably he doesn't even know who she is (if indeed by this time she herself knows). He has let her in not because he genuinely loved her, but only because she played so well into his preconceived fantasies. Though she knew his love to be false, since she herself engineered it, she can't help feeling contempt for him. But she is afraid, at first, to reveal her true self, for then perhaps even that false love would go. And finally she understands that for him, too, marriage had all kinds of motivations that had nothing to do with love. She was merely the one closest to his fantasy image: she has been named Most Versatile Actress for the multi-role of Alter Ego, Mother of My Children, Housekeeper, Cook, and Companion—in *his* play. She has been bought to fill an empty space in his life; but her life is nothing.

So she has not saved herself from being like other women. She is lifted out of that class only because she now is an appendage of a member of the master class; and he cannot associate with her unless he raises her status. But she has not been freed, she has been promoted to "house-nigger," she has been elevated only to be used in a different way. She feels cheated. She has gotten not love and recognition, but possessorship and control. This is when she is transformed from Blushing Bride to Bitch; a change that, no matter how universal and predictable, still leaves the individual husband perplexed. ("You're not the girl I married.")

The situation of women has not changed significantly from what it ever was. For the past fifty years women have been in a double bind about love: under the guise of a "sexual revolution," presumed to have occurred ("Oh, c'mon Baby, where have you *been?* Haven't you heard of the sexual revolution?"), women have been persuaded to shed their armor. The modern woman is in horror of being thought a bitch, where her grandmother expected that to happen as the natural course of things. Men, too, in her grandmother's time, expected that any self-respecting woman would keep *them* waiting, would play all the right games without shame: a woman who did not guard her own interests in this way was not respected. It was out in the open.

But the rhetoric of the sexual revolution, if it brought no improvements for women, proved to have great value for men. By convincing women that the usual female games and demands were despicable, unfair, prudish, old-fashioned, puritanical, and self-destructive, a new reservoir of available females was created to expand the tight supply of goods available for traditional sexual exploitation, disarming women of even the little protection they had so painfully acquired. Women today dare not make the old demands for fear of having a whole new vocabulary, designed just for this purpose, hurled at them: "fucked up," "ball-breaker," "cockteaser," "a real drag," "a bad trip"—to be a "groovy chick" is the ideal.

Even now many women know what's up and avoid the trap, preferring to be called names rather than be cheated out of the little they can hope for from men (for it is still true that even the hippest want an "old lady" who is relatively unused). But more and more women are sucked into the trap, only to find out too late, and bitterly, that the traditional female games had a point; they are shocked to catch themselves at thirty complaining in a vocabulary dangerously close to the old I've-been-used-men-are-wolves-they're-all-bastards variety. Eventually they are forced to acknowledge the old wives' truth: a fair and generous woman is (at best) respected, but seldom loved. Here is a description, still valid today, of the "emancipated" woman—in this case a Greenwich Village artist of the thirties—from *Mosquitoes*, an early Faulkner novel:

> She had always had trouble with her men . . . Sooner or later they always ran out on her . . . Men she recognized as having potentialities all passed through a violent but temporary period of interest which ceased as abruptly as it began, without leaving even the lingering threads of mutually remembered incidence, like those brief thunderstorms of August that threaten and dissolve for no apparent reason without producing any rain.
>
> At times she speculated with almost masculine detachment on the reason for this. She always tried to keep their relationships on the plane which the men themselves seemed to prefer—certainly no woman would, and few women could, demand less of their men than she did. She never made arbitrary demands on their time, never caused them to wait for her nor to see her home

at inconvenient hours, never made them fetch and carry for her; she fed them and flattered herself that she was a good listener. And yet—She thought of the women she knew; how all of them had at least one obviously entranced male; she thought *of* the women she had observed; how they seemed to acquire a man at will, and if he failed to stay acquired, how readily they replaced him.

Women of high ideals who believed emancipation possible, women who tried desperately to rid themselves of feminine "hang-ups," to cultivate what they believed to be the greater directness, honesty, and generosity of men, were badly fooled. They found that no one appreciated their intelligent conversation, their high aspirations, their great sacrifices to avoid developing the personalities of their mothers. For much as men were glad to enjoy their wit, their style, their sex, and their candlelight suppers, they always ended up marrying The Bitch, and then, to top it all off, came back to complain of what a horror she was. "Emancipated" women found out that the honesty, generosity, and camaraderie of men was a lie: men were all too glad to use them and then sell them out, in the name of *true* friendship. ("I respect and like you a great deal, but let's be reasonable . . ." And then there are the men who take her out to discuss Simone de Beauvoir, leaving their wives at home with the diapers.) "Emancipated" women found out that men were far from "good guys" to be emulated; they found out that by imitating male sexual patterns (the roving eye, the search for the ideal, the emphasis on physical attraction, etc.), they were not only achieving liberation, they were falling into something much worse than what they had given up. They were *imitating*. And they had inoculated themselves with a sickness that had not even sprung from their own psyches. They found that their new "cool" was shallow and meaningless, that their emotions were drying up behind it, that they were aging and becoming decadent: they feared they were losing their ability to love. They had gained nothing by imitating men: shallowness and callowness, and they were not so good at it either, because somewhere inside it still went against the grain.

Thus women who had decided not to marry because they were wise enough to look around and see where it led found that it was marry or nothing. Men gave their commitment only for a price: share (shoulder) his life, stand on his pedestal, become his appendage, or else. Or else—be consigned forever to that limbo of "chicks" who mean nothing, or at least not what mother meant. Be the "other woman" the rest of one's life, used to provoke his wife, prove his virility and/or his independence, discussed by his friends as his latest "interesting" conquest. (For even if she had given up those terms and what they stood for, no male had.) Yes, love means an entirely different thing to men than to women: it means ownership and control; it means jealousy, where he never exhibited it before—when she might have wanted him to (who cares if she is broke or raped until she officially belongs to him: then he is a raging dynamo, a veritable cyclone, because his property, his ego extension has been threatened); it means a growing lack of interest, coupled with a roving eye. Who needs it?

Sadly, women do. Here are Reik's patients once more:

> She sometimes has delusions of not being persecuted by men anymore. At those times of her nonpersecution mania she is very depressed.

And:

> All men are selfish, brutal and inconsiderate—and I wish I could find one.

We have seen that a woman needs love, first, for its natural enriching function, and second, for social and economic reasons which have nothing to do with love. To deny her need is to put herself in an extra-vulnerable spot socially and economically, as well as to destroy her emotional equilibrium, which, unlike most men's, is basically healthy. Are men worth that? Decidedly no. Most women feel that to do such tailspins for a man would be to add insult to injury. They go on as before, making the best of a bad situation. If it gets *too* bad, they head for a (male) shrink:

> A young woman patient was once asked during a psychoanalytic consultation whether she preferred to see a man or woman psychoanalyst. Without the slightest hesitation she said, "A woman psychoanalyst because I am too eager for the approval of a man."

NOTE

1. Thus the peculiar situation that women never object to the insulting of women as a class, *as long as* they individually are excepted. The worst insult for a woman is that she is "just like a woman," i.e., no better; the highest compliment that she has the brains, talent, dignity, or strength of a man. In fact, like every member of an oppressed class, she herself participates in the insulting of others like herself, hoping thereby to make it obvious that *she* as an individual is above their behavior. Thus women as a class are set against each other ["Divide and Conquer"], the "other woman" believing that the wife is a "bitch" who "doesn't understand him," and the wife believing that the other woman is an "opportunist" who is "taking advantage" of him—while the culprit himself sneaks away free.

2.

LOVE AND FEMINISM

Robert C. Solomon

"Love. Being in love. Yuck!" Val poured more wine . . . "I mean, it's one of those things they've erected, a bunch of nonsense erected—and that's the crucial word—into truth by a bunch of intelligent *men*—*another* crucial word. What the particular nonsense is, isn't particularly important. What's important is why they do it."
—Marilyn French, *The Women's Room*

Is romantic love—the perennial obsession of the Western world—unfair to women, perhaps even a systematic form of rape? So it has been charged.

The charge itself is simple and persuasive. It begins with a fact, that some (many? most? almost all?) women are unhappy and unfulfilled; the fact suggests a hypothesis, that the cause of this unhappiness is the promise of romantic love, which will turn household chores into meaningful and significant acts of devotion, which will transform the biological pains and daily difficulties of having babies into cosmic events, which is said to last "forever" but normally lasts but a few months or years, followed by a lifetime in which to dwell on one's wasted opportunities. The hypothesis in turn implies a theory: that romantic love is neither "natural" nor "divine," as the (male) poets have always insisted, but rather a cultural invention, created by men for the subjugation of women.

Adapted from *Love: Emotion, Myth & Metaphor* (Doubleday-Anchor, 1981)

It is, when spelled out, an extremely persuasive polemic, far more so than the murky and pious praise of love and lessons on our alleged "need for love" that have been the topic of so many predominantly male theoreticians and theologians from Plato and St. Paul to Rollo May. But it is a polemic with a tragic double bind, one that is also evident in *The Women's Room* and in the work of other authors from Virginia Woolf to Doris Lessing. In its simplest formulation, it is the feeling that love is a lie but nevertheless one cannot live without it.

A double bind is not a question of mere addiction, a romantic habit that we would like to break but cannot; it is rather an impossible confusion in which we both accept and at the same time reject an utterly absurd ideal of love. What I would like to do here is attack this ideal, and to suggest that we can continue to honor a more reasonable notion of romantic love, not in spite of or even in addition to but as a presupposition of feminism. The latter, I would argue, depends largely upon the former.

The "dump love" argument begins with the realization that romantic love, which has so often been promised to women (by men), is an illusion, a fraud, a myth. It does not, as promised, change one's life once and for all or turn the drudgery of housework into joy, much less forever. But not only that: It is the myth itself that has this as its ulterior motive; it is an illusion whose deconstruction reveals a political purpose. Love was invented by men, as an instrument of a kind of culture—which might be summarized as "capitalist"—in order to "keep women in their place," or in any case isolated and dependent on men, and if not happy then at least hopeful of love and complacent about their socially inferior but infinitely useful occupations. By preaching that love is always good and desirable, it is charged, men have convinced at least most women that love is more important than politics and power, thus limiting the competition to themselves. By teaching that love is "everything," men have convinced many women that it is also worth any sacrifice, and like generals in their luxurious tents behind the battle lines, they have succeeded in getting others to make the sacrifices without having to make them themselves. Within the realm of love itself, men have created an image of the "feminine," such that the virtues a woman finds or creates in herself for the sake of love are directly at odds with the virtues required for success in the world: soft, yielding, quiet, accepting versus hard, aggressive, outspoken and critical. A man can be sexy in pursuit of his career; a woman is sexy despite or in contrast to hers (unless, of course, sex is her career). For a woman, to be in love is to be submissive, and therefore disadvantaged and powerless within the relationship, second-class and degraded. If the lover or husband also insists on praising her effusely, worshipping the ground she walks on or putting her "on a pedestal," that is just so much worse, for he is disguising the fact that she is becoming the willing victim in her own political oppression even while being worshiped.

This is not the smirking cynicism of neo-Freudian male reductionist "love is nothing but . . ." theorists like Philip Slater who argue that "romantic love is a scarcity mechanism . . . whose only function is to transmute that which is plentiful [i.e., sex] into that which is in short supply. Although romantic love always verges on the ridiculous, Western peoples and Americans in particular have shown an impressive tendency to take it seriously."[1] The argument that is so well-presented in *The Women's Room* represents the personal outrage and bitter disappointment of a million or more women, only some of whom would identify themselves as "feminists" and few of whom would be able to articulate the precise mechanism by which they have been systematically shut out of power or what all of this has to do with love. But that means it is an argument to be taken especially seriously, for it is not just an academic theory that is at stake.

Now to begin with, there is much here that is no longer controversial, no longer deniable:

1. Much of what we believe about love is demonstrably false or hopelessly obscure, mere mythology and pious illusion—men merely masturbating with the archaic concept of *eros*.
2. Love is not "everything"; nor is it "the answer"; it is not always good or desirable. Sometimes, and for some people, it is simply stupid.
3. Love provides private compensation for public impotence or anonymity. Indeed, it is the very essence of love that it allows us to play roles and feel "special" in our personal relationships even when—especially when—we feel overburdened or underappreciated in our jobs or in our social roles.
4. Love is a cultural creation, the product of a male-dominated society, and so, we may reasonably suppose, "erected by men," presumably not to their own disadvantage. Indeed, our current conception of romantic love is largely a literary creation, from Plato and the Bible, from the medieval poets to Shakespeare and the Brownings. On the other hand, romantic love is unknown and would be considered ludicrous in many societies around the world.
5. Love consists of personal roles, which more often than not, cast the women into the more submissive and subservient position. There cannot be any argument against the claim that the promise of love, at least, has long been used against women, by way of compensation for political impotence, as an excuse to keep them in the home (and away from the public positions of power) and as a ready rationalization for social inequities in everything from politics ("women are too emotional") to changing diapers ("women are naturally better at that sort of thing").

Indeed there can be no objection to the charge that the "feminine" role in love makes it difficult for a woman to be both romantically desirable and successful in the male-dominated world of money and power.

So what is left of love to defend?

What does not follow is the conclusion that love itself is exploitative, a source of inequity or an obstacle to equality between the sexes. The fact that much of what we believe about love is illusion does not mean that love itself is illusion, nor does it follow from the fact that love is a cultural artifact that it is simply artificial, a "fiction" or a manipulative ploy. It does not follow from the fact that it was (probably) invented by men that love is disadvantageous to women (a man may have invented the wheel and the toothbrush too). It does not follow from the fact that romantic love is often used to reinforce submissive and subservient female roles that those roles are intrinsic to romantic love as such.

If, as the feminist argument charges, romantic love *required* in its structure a division into distinctively male and female roles, strictly corresponding to what has traditionally been called "masculinity" and "femininity," then I would agree that love and the love world constitute archaic emotional structures that we would be better off leaving behind us. But if, as I will argue, romantic roles are fundamentally sex-neutral and presuppose a significant degree of equality, then the much-abused neo-Victorian crypto-caveman scenario of macho "me-Tarzan" and passive-submissive, lovingly house-cleaning Jane is not at all a paradigm of love but at most one of its many historical curiosities—like Quasimodo and Esmerelda.

Looking back at the history of romantic love, it is no doubt true that it was "erected," in part by men, in order to fill a need in a certain kind of society, but this does not warrant the leap into the antagonistic and somewhat paranoid conclusion that the need could only have been the suppression of women. Indeed, if we look back to Plato, we find that at least one classical author of love introduced *eros* not as a weapon against women but rather as a relationship between males and between men and the gods; eros simply excluded women or at least dismissed the love of women as "vulgar" and "inferior." Reading Aristophanes, on the other hand, gives a very different impression: relations between men and women, even 2,500 years before birth control, were not that different from today. There were the same battles for power, the same charges and countercharges, with women getting the upper hand as often as men.[2]

If we follow the scholars and locate the origins of romantic love more properly in the chivalric spirit of twelfth-century France, however, we get a very different picture again; what we find is that romantic (or "courtly") love was indeed the invention of wandering free-agent knights and their poetic brethren the troubadours, but it was not at all an instrument of female oppression. Quite the contrary; courtly love quite literally placed women (often married, their husbands off to the Crusades) on pedestals, but thereby freed them from their strict identities in terms of their families, marriages, and household duties. We may now look at the "reduction" of women to their physical appearance and attractiveness as "dehumanizing," a denial of the *person*, but at its origins this celebration of individual attractiveness and personality was the first step in the individualization of women, the recognition that a woman was something more than a household convenience, an object for inter-family barter—a mother, mistress, and, literally, a possession.

It is often argued, nowadays, that romantic love is essentially an invention of capitalism, a creation of industrialized society. This is by any measure not true. Shakespeare described a fully developed conception of romantic love well over a century before the Industrial Revolution in England. It has been argued (by Linda Nicholson, for example) that the breakdown of feudalism and the origins of a market-based society gave rise to the breakdown as well as the old religious view of women as "creatures before God" and began our current capitalist insistence on evaluating people according to what they are "good for." But the truth seems to be rather that under feudalism women were evaluated and considered "worth something" only according to what they were "good for," and it is with the rise of a less regimented society that individual identity—as opposed to mere market value— came to mean anything at all. It is true, for example, as Shulamith Firestone argued in her *Dialectic of Sex*, that romantic love became more important with industrialization, but her Marxist urge to equate sexism with capitalism ignores the historical facts: that romantic love and our current conception of the feminine predates capitalism in any guise by several centuries, and that the parallel, in any case, is not with capitalism or industrialism, but with the idea of individualism. Romantic love became possible with the severing of "natural" ties between a person and his or her family, the historical drama of a society of individuals—wandering knights and poets and abandoned wives and daughters—finding themselves for the first time required to make commitments rather than merely recognize predetermined allegiances, free to "devote" themselves to a master or mistress of their choice, and no longer locked into a rigid structure of arranged marriages and obligations. Because these "natural" ties were broken, love became not only desirable, but a need.

Love is indeed a cultural invention, created by males perhaps, but certainly to the advantage and also with the cooperation of women. Love is a cultural creation, but it is not, therefore, either arbitrary or easily dispensable. Romantic love is our primary mode of forming intimate relationships in a society in which we are all systematically uprooted and sent away from our families and communities. Though love is not the only way of achieving intimacy (friendship certainly deserves mention here), it is eminently successful in doing so. This is as true for men as for women. So it is not in the purpose or original design of romantic love that we are going to find the origins of its use against women.

LOVE AND POWER

A distinction of fundamental importance in recent literature about sexual identity has been marked out between *sex* (that is, male and female) and gender (that is, masculine and feminine). Sex is essentially a biological category, though what we *make* out of sexual differences is a matter of culture, no matter how they may be tied to history or biology by habit or some very suspiciously self-serving arguments. (Women are "naturally" this or that because of the mating habits of some species of fish.) Romantic love is from its very origins neutral to sex; homosexual and lesbian love is just as much romantic love as unkinky, heterosexual love.

But what about gender roles? What would become of our romantic literature without *her* soft and dutiful gaze, waiting for *him* to return from the battle and give her a hard and possessive embrace? But who cares? In our non-warrior society, in which the day's battle is more than likely a screaming telephone battle with the local tax office, we can switch the above pronouns all that we want, delete as well the adjectives "soft" and "hard," dispense with the roles as well as the sexes. Yet it is part of the history of romantic love, and so part of the "dump love" argument as well, that masculine and feminine gender roles are, if not essential, at least central to love.

Years ago, in one of the more virulent classics of the genre, Firestone argued in her *Dialectic of Sex* that it is precisely the "liberation of women from their biology," not now but several generations ago, that brought about the distinctively male invention of romantic love:

Romantic love developed in opposition to the liberation of women from their biology. . . . Male supremacy must shore itself up with artificial institutions or exaggerations of previous institutions.[3]

Romantic role models, she argues, the gender distinctions of "masculine" and "feminine," are developed *in place of* the no longer essential distinction between male and female. Gender depends not on nature but on culture; thus the question, for what purpose, and for whose benefit, has gender been created? The answer is not long forthcoming.

Romanticism is a cultural tool of male power to keep women from knowing their condition. It is especially needed—and therefore strongest—in Western countries with the highest rate of industrialization.[4]

Romantic love is thus to be understood in terms of *power*, and so viewed, the main difference between masculine and feminine gender roles becomes obvious. The argument, interestingly enough, is traced to Freud. Freud is usually considered the nemesis of feminism, but Firestone rightly credits him "as having grasped the crucial problem of modern life, sexuality."[5] But where Freud takes sexuality to be a psychobiological problem, Firestone sees it as a political problem. Where Freud mysteriously talks about the powers of the libido, Firestone talks concretely about *power* itself. And where Freud talks murkily and unconvincingly about penis envy and castration fears, Firestone substitutes the tangible fact of family power relationships, the all-powerful father and the privileged sons.[6] Penis envy becomes privilege envy, and Firestone quite plausibly suggests that the young girl who is said to envy her brother's curious genitalia is more likely feeling deprived because she is not allowed to play her brother's rough-and-tumble games. With this switch on Freud, the theory can begin: romantic love is the extension of this power-game into adult life, a more subtle way of depriving women of "male" roles and at the same time flattering her as a "lady." Promise her anything, but offer her only love.

What Firestone is arguing, from Freud, is what Freud and many neo-Freudians prefer to ignore: the institutional nature of romantic love and its functional role, not only in the individual psyche and the family but in the power structure of society as a whole. According to Firestone's argument, now that female sexuality as such is of much less importance for survival, the institution of romantic love serves the function of introducing femininity as a matter of emotional significance, as a way of continuing archaic male-dominated institutions and power structures. Femininity, in a word, is *impotency*. Masculinity is *potency*. To reinforce the roles, femininity is isolated in the home, while masculinity gathers further power in the marketplace. Women, in turn, find themselves seeking approval—the test of success in their feminine roles—entirely from men, while men gain their support and approval as well in a variety of friendships and business or professional relationships. The power relations thus become self-perpetuating.

The isolation of women and the exclusively male-dominated world of power are starting to break down extremely quickly on any reasonable historical scale, and this changes at least one of the key connections between romantic love, gender identity, and power. Much of the power that was once the exclusive domain of males had to do not only with the fact that they had power, but with their variable sources of recognition and approval as well. Men were not solely dependent on women for their sense of self-esteem as women were upon men. But now, as women aggressively find friendships and alliances for themselves even to the extent that a current popular argument maintains that *only* women are even *capable* of friendship—and as women are beginning to find professional, political, and other sources of self-esteem, this source of power is becoming open to them as well. Thus, in this sense, it has become evident that it is not romantic love or gender roles as such that determine one major traditional source of asymmetrical female dependency, but an entirely distinct set of inequities which might be summarized as unequal access to approval and self-esteem. This isolation of women is now at an end, once and for all, I would argue. Even the reactionary countermovement, the "total woman" syndrome, has the ironic outcome of helping to bring about the public visibility of women speakers and "women's issues," thus destroying this sense of isolation. Romantic love, consequently, no longer remains a woman's sole source of self-esteem, a burden that, in any case, no single emotion could ever be expected to sustain.

ROMANTIC ROLES: BEYOND ANDROGYNY, TOO

Are romantic roles themselves oppressive? If by "romantic roles" one means gender roles—masculine and feminine—the answer is yes. For a woman, if being in love meant accepting a position of subservience and passivity, if being romantically attractive meant being quiet, unaggressive, and apparently helpless, then I doubt that I could argue in favor of romantic love at all. But the truth of the matter seems to be that these roles are not so automatically involved in male-female love as our cheaper novels and more reactionary politicians would suggest. Indeed, love tends to destroy these stereotypes rather than reinforce them, and in theory as well as in practice the concepts of femininity and masculinity ought to be rejected, not only in the public sphere, where they put the woman to a serious disadvantage, but in the personal sphere as well, where they still tend to turn even the best relationships into one-role, one-plot, television-like situation comedies, or worse.

There are at least three ways of overcoming sexual stereotypes. Two of them have become popularly known under the camp word "androgyny." The word is often confused with "bisexual," which is only one of its variations, but in any case, I tend to agree with Mary Daly when she writes that "'androgyny' makes me think of Farrah Fawcett and John Travolta Scotch-taped together." The first form of androgyny (or "androgynism") insists that masculine and feminine characteristics exist together in everyone, and so it is unnecessary, the argument goes, for each individual to feel that he or she should develop only one set of sex-bound characteristics. In the public sphere, the argument is appealing, since what it says, in effect, is that everyone has the same potential and so should have the same opportunities. Its effect, in other words, is to deny the difference between men and women and to provide a single ideal of rights and potential for all, which leads one author, Joyce Trebilcot, to call it "monoandrogynism."[7] In the personal sphere, however, the same view leads logically to the idea of bisexuality; if we each have essentially the same masculine and feminine characteristics, then it would follow that we each also have the same masculine and feminine desires. This sounds like Freud's well-known bisexuality argument, but it isn't. For Freud, this was a sexual matter, a fact about biology; for the monoandrogynist, it is a matter of cultural potential, not biology at all. But here, too, we see a problem with this simple view; as a theory about *potentials*, it slips too easily between the idea that the various roles that we call "masculine" and "feminine" *can* be developed in everyone (whether or not they should be) and the idea that these roles are *already* lurking somewhere inside of us, waiting to be developed. But, alas, in our society, only one of the roles ever is, thus frustrating the other. The recognition of the cultural origins of these roles ought to lead us not to the view that they are "there in everybody" but to the more radical conclusion that they are unnecessary, unreal—they do not exist except in so far as we *will* them.

The second form of androgyny is more radical in just this sense; it denies the simple duality between masculinity and femininity and emphasizes the wide variety of gender roles, including any number of combinations of the two "pure" extremes. In effect, this breaks down the extremes while refocusing our attention on particular traits and roles rather than on the monolithic extremes, and opens up the possibility of a large variety of roles that are, traditionally speaking, neither masculine nor feminine. (Because of its pluralism, Trebilcot calls this "polyandrogynism.")

But this second form of androgyny or androgynism suggests a third possibility, which escapes the man-woman etymological orientation of "androgyny" by dismissing masculinity and femininity as roles, particularly where romantic love is involved. What we have been allowing without comment for too long is the idea that these two roles define, if not all, at least a large part of our romantic tradition. In fact, they had no place in Plato; there the crucial distinction was one of age and experience, the lover as teacher, the beloved as pupil. The notion of masculine-feminine may have played a significant part in courtly love, but the notions of chivalry and attractiveness were a matter of historical context, and not necessarily essential to the concept of love as such. As one looks at the structure of romantic love—apart from the grade "B" novels—divisions according to sex and gender have had a very small part to play, even where sex itself is concerned. Indeed, romantic love consists of roles, private roles that are only occasionally or coincidentally played out in public. But the point now to be made once and for all is that few of these roles have anything to do with sex or gender, and insofar as they do, it is not *because* they are male or female or masculine or feminine roles, but only because they contain roles that are usually associated with sex and gender, such as domination and submissiveness, aggressiveness and passivity. But what happens in love is that these roles are continuously redefined, and whatever might be expected on the masculine-feminine model, what we actually do in love is something quite different. Indeed, this leads to the unexpected conclusion that masculinity and femininity are, in fact, *public* roles, and not private, and that love requires the overcoming of these roles rather than the realization of them. Femininity is a show, not an expression, and trying to be "feminine" in bed or in love is more like trying to be a comedian or a prima donna rather than a lover. Indeed, as soon as one begins to list the huge gamut of roles through which we are intimate with one another, not only the thousand varieties of sex that need have nothing to do with gender, but cooking, talking, walking, dancing, looking, scratching, fighting, driving cross country, feeding the squirrels, confessing, celebrating, crying, laughing, knowingly nodding to each other in a room full of people, sharing the events of the day, consoling one another in defeat, studying Spanish, staying in bed on Sunday, reading the funnies, bitching about the weather, whispering and occasionally whimpering—the emphasis that is so stressed on a single set of asymmetrical roles, "masculine and feminine," becomes more than embarrassing. Indeed, people who are too caught up in their "masculine" and "feminine" roles are inevitably, after the initial attraction, disappointing lovers. This has nothing to do with sexism, but only with boredom. How can you build your life around a one-act actor? Or perhaps, in some cases, a movie poster?

Beyond sex and gender means beyond *androgyny too*, beyond that one-dimensional set of man-woman identities that too many bad movies and sadomasochistic Freudian fantasies have set out for us. Love is a multiplex of personal roles of all kinds, which are being continuously redefined and reenacted and which need have nothing to do with sex or with those simple stereotypes of gender. In fact, to think of love in terms of masculinity and femininity is like having a conversation in which each party is allowed to say just one sentence. At most, one can expect a predictable performance, instead of the "anything goes" exhilaration of love.

Romantic love, unlike many other emotions and other forms of love, *requires* equality. It may be, as Stendhal argued a century ago, that love creates rather than discovers equals; and it may also be that within the bounds of equality love divides into unequal roles, into domination and submission, for example, with sado-masochism as its extreme. But it is absolutely crucial to this emotion that one sees the other as an equal, which is not to deny either that it is possible for one person to love more than the other (which is not a question of the nature of love) or that there are other emotions, distinct from romantic love, that sometimes borrow its promiscuous name (adoration, feeling motherly or fatherly, fear, and simple possessiveness). Indeed, in a still class-ridden and unequal society, romantic love is our favorite if not most effective political equalizer. Cinderella moves from maid to princess not only in the eyes of her prince but in the eyes of the law, too, whether or not she lives thereby "happily ever after." King Edward VIII found it necessary to lower his social status to match that of the woman he loved, and with a perverse twist of this perception, Firestone argues in *Dialectic of Sex* that men "fall in love (with women) to justify their descent into a lower caste." But what is *equality*, in a relationship?

"Equality" is one of those political glow-words with very little determinate content, like "liberty." One gives it a content by giving it a context, for example—equal work time, or equal say in an issue, equal responsibility for some specific activity or equal power. What counts as equality in a particular relationship may indeed be quite different from what counts as equality in another. The equality that is the precondition for love only consists in the demand that social differences do not matter, that both lovers are mutually willing to take up the various personal and private roles that make up intimacy. But as the notion of equality starts to become more "objective" and more concerned with social rather than personal status, once the private is measured by public criteria, the tacitly accepted roles within the relationship tend to be shattered. The quasi-political self-consciousness that replaces them undermines the intimacy of love. What was once a relationship now becomes a "partnership," which may well be more efficient, even a model of fairness and success in "having worked it out," but it isn't love. It is too dominated by foreign and critical observers, external measurements and publicly defined if nominally private roles. It was a problem that many of us had with women's liberation in the sixties (though that is by no means the only ideology that has that consequence; sex books and our modern therapeutic attitudes towards sex can do the same thing). The demands may all be completely reasonable. They may indeed force a relationship to conform with some more general and "objective" form of equity. But what is too often sacrificed is love, for love is not objective, not negotiable, not a "partnership." None of which is to say, let me quickly add, that love itself is inherently, "objectively" unequal, or that what inequality there may be necessarily gives the woman the disadvantage, or that our idea of "women's roles" cannot be changed, or that romantic love and feminism are incompatible. To the contrary, they even presuppose one another. But the problem that defies ideology and one-sided "consciousness raising" by its very nature is to bring these demands—if they must be demands rather than shared ideals—into the relationship itself. As a set of demands or ideals imposed from the outside, "equality" becomes antithetical to, rather than the precondition for, love.

The division between the public and the personal, and the quite different concerns for equality of the sexes in the public sphere (equal pay for equal work, equal access to jobs and careers, equal rights and responsibilities under the law) on the one hand and the sense of equality that is the precondition for intimacy on the other, have been commonly confused by both feminist theorists and anti-feminists alike. Firestone is just one of the many theorists who have argued that romantic love and "the relegation of love to the personal" is part and parcel of the manipulative ploy to "keep women in their place" and to rationalize, even idealize, their class inferiority. But love is by its very nature personal, and if it isolates women in romantic relationships, it isolates men in exactly the same way. That is what we mean by a "personal" relationship. The mistake is to think that the *overemphasis* on the personal, which is foisted upon women, to the exclusion of public roles and interests, is a feature of romantic love itself, and that the indefensible inequality in the public sphere necessarily has its counterpart in the personal sphere as well. But these are quite distinct, and to treat them together as a single problem may mean blurring the very different strategies that are required to encounter each of them.

A more vicious version of the same confusion has given birth to the outlandish conception of the "total woman," who is in fact a medieval woman, more at home in Khomeini's Persia than contemporary America. The strategy of these anti-feminists is to systematically confuse questions about intimacy and personal relationships with questions about equality and public life. *Whatever* one says about the private, romantic, and family roles to which women have become accustomed (which is misleadingly described as their "natural" roles), nothing follows about the public roles or abilities or ambitions of women in society, in which sex and gender considerations simply drop out of the picture, or ought to. It is simply false, where public criteria are concerned, that "men and women are different by nature," since nature has nothing to do with most public functions (given, that is, that we no longer inherit our leaders through their birthright) and sex, in any case, is irrelevant to our roles. But in the personal sphere, questions of sex do indeed arise, but not of necessity, much less "by nature." They arise because we choose to make sex—and heterosexuality specifically—the basis of our most intimate relationships. But it is not difficult to find cultures in which sexual relationships are perfunctory, and other encounters—with friends or fellow workers or soldiers—are far more intimate and "meaningful." One need only look again at Plato to appreciate the power of love in which the difference in the sexes plays no part whatever. It is what we *make* of the sexes and sex that determines the roles in our personal relationships, and it is here that the slippery argument from the historical *public* place of women in certain kinds of roles, to an inference about what is "natural," and to a conclusion about the properly submissive and subservient place of women in love is particularly vicious. There is nothing "natural" about public roles, and there is nothing "natural" about personal roles either. Our roles in romance are in every case personally determined, if on the basis of public instruction, and the kinds of roles one chooses to play with one's lover cannot be dictated a priori. To say that a woman *ought* to be submissive, and also to say that she ought not, is nothing less than a kind of emotional fascism, a way of dismissing and degrading huge numbers of women who find that their personal preferences do not match up to the latest official line. "The totalitarian woman" might be a better designation for the conservative tendency to confuse questions about public equality with questions about personal roles; but the tendency to confuse the demand for social equality with an authoritarian attack on love is to be found on the other side as well. Romantic love *requires* equality, and to deny this or to enforce it from the outside is the denial of love as well.

Yet, it would be absurd to deny that one's personal self-image and one's public, social image are related and affect each other. So what does this mean about equality in love? First of all, that it is aided immensely by social-political-economic equality. Whatever truth may be in the argument that women have always wielded "the *real* power" at home, there is no question that status in public and status at home are mutually supportive. But more crucial to the argument here is the fact that equality in personal relationships is essential to seeing oneself as equal in social relationships as well, in part because we (unlike most people of the world) tend to take our personal identities as more real ("more myself") than our public identities. If love is an emotion *requiring* that we see one another as equals, it is therefore an important tool for equality in the public sphere as well.

But what does "equality" mean in relations? It does not mean "being the same." It does not exclude all sorts of asymmetrical and uneven roles and relationships, including the absolute domination of one person by the other. It does not require, as such, the equal division of housework or "bread earning" tasks, though these have become rather routine expectations (whether or not routinely fulfilled). Equality in love essentially means a mutually-agreed upon indeterminacy, more or less free from social strictures and limitations (short of violence and illegality, sometimes), a sense of reformulation in which one's self-images and personal roles and identity are up for grabs, in negotiation with one other person, in which there are no preordained roles or predestined status relationships, including, particularly, those which are traditionally labeled "masculine" and "feminine." Indeed, it is the heart of love that it involves the breakdown of these television stereotypes and an openness to change and mutual reevaluation which is available in very few of our experiences. It is not yet political equality (or "liberation") and equality in love is no guarantee that the public demand will be successful. But it is a self-effacing error, and an unrealistic demand for most women besides, that the demand for political equality *preclude* romantic love (with men). The latter is and has often been a means to the former.

Love and Illusion

The central argument of *The Women's Room* is an anti-romantic version of an old argument in philosophy that is usually called "the argument from illusion." It is the fallacious but persuasive inference from the fact that one is sometimes fooled to the paranoid supposition that one might always be deceived. Quite a few years ago, Firestone exploited this argument by attacking what she called "idealization": the fact that women tend to imagine their lovers with virtues they never had, and in return men mock-worship women, which Firestone says is an effective substitution for physical abuse—and the result is the same. (How this is so is never quite clear.) What is so obvious in Firestone is the double bind asymmetry itself: men idealize women and thereby exploit them, women idealize men and are therefore exploited. Idealization and the argument from illusion also enter into the work of a new spokesperson for the "dump love" movement, Jill Tweedie (*In the Name of Love*), who argues that love is a pair of "rose colored glasses" that when removed . . . reveal "that what was taken to be precious is simply a bare dull pebble, like any other." But the most spectacular description of idealization as illusion is in *The Women's Room* itself, as Val describes with exquisite irony the bloated idealization of love, followed by its inevitable collapse:

> Okay. Love is one of those things you think is supposed to happen, is a fact of life, and if it doesn't happen to you, you feel cheated. You're walking around feeling rotten, you know, because it's never happened to you. So one day you meet this guy, right? And, ZING! He is gorgeous! It doesn't matter what he's doing. He may be making a point in a debate, he may be chopping up concrete on a city street, with his shirt off and his back tanned. It doesn't matter. Even if you've met him before and not thought much about him, at some moment you look at him and everything you've thought about him before goes straight out of your head. You never really saw him before! You realize that in a split second! You never saw how totally gorgeous he was![8]

Val, the narrator, then proceeds in almost obscene detail to describe his wonderful arms, his sensual mouth, his pithy intelligence, the desperation with which one wants him, and so on, for several salivating pages.

> Then one day, the unthinkable happens. You are sitting together at the breakfast table and you're a little hung over, and you look across at beloved, beautiful golden beloved, and beloved opens his lovely rosebud mouth showing his glistening white teeth, and beloved says something stupid. Your whole body stops midstream: your temperature drops. Beloved has never said anything stupid before. You turn and look at him; you're sure you misheard. You ask him to repeat. And he does . . .

Thus, the doubt begins, but that's only the start, and soon you see that he is *always* saying stupid things—and suddenly you see that he's skinny, or flabby, or fat. His teeth are crooked, his toenails are dirty, and he farts in bed. So on now in the other direction. The initial idealizations were all *falsehoods.* Now you see you've been had:

> And you hate yourself for having deluded yourself about him (you tell yourself it was HIM you were deluded about—not love), and you hate him for having believed your delusions, and you feel guilty and responsible and you try, slowly, to disengage. But now, just try to get rid of him! He clutches, he clings, he doesn't understand. How could you want to separate from a deity?

Love always involves idealization, and, indeed, idealization, like hallucination and flattery, can be abused to deceive either oneself or a lover. But the problem with the argument is that it flatly fails to make the distinction between innocent fantasy and celebration on the one hand and self-deception and illusion on the other. All emotions, not only love, are blind (that is, myopic) in that they see what they want to see, emphasize what they want to emphasize, celebrate what they want to celebrate. Without that element of enthusiasm, birthdays and anniversaries would be just another day, life would be grey, and even family and friends would be reduced to social security numbers and vital statistics. *All* values are idealizations in this sense; all hopes and plans are fantasies, and even day-dreams are, in one sense, false. Yes, we do disappoint one another (women as well as men, though this would never be known from *The Women's Room*), but to infer from this that our fantasies are fraudulent, much less that love is itself an illusion, is a piece of painful self-deception.

> Except for her [Camille's] passion for Bernard, she is tough and fun. Don't ask what it is about Bernard that makes her so adore him. It is not Bernard, but love itself. She believes in love, goes on believing in it against all odds. Therefore, Bernard is a little bored. It is boring to be adored. At thirty-eight, she should be tough and fun, not adoring. When he leaves her, a month or two from now, she will contemplate suicide. Whereas, if she had been able to bring herself to stop believing in love, she would have been tough and fun and he would have adored her forever. Which would have bored her. She then would have had to be the one to tell him to clear out. It is a choice to give one pause?[9]

The genius of *The Women's Room*—perhaps as opposed to *The Dialectic of Sex*—is in its descriptions, presented for the most part in a flat matter-of-fact familiarity that leaves many people who reject the tone of the book incapable of saying what is wrong with it. But the first thing to see about the above illustration, and a hundred others like it, is its unwarranted one-sidedness. French tells us that the dilemma is symmetrical, that it is the same for Bernard as for Camille, but Bernard remains a mere name for us; the problem is all Camille's. It has been said that French is unsympathetic to her male characters, but this isn't true. She *has* no male characters, no men with problems and paradoxes themselves, just cardboard figures who periodically fall down on, blow away from, or on occasion confess to their disappointed female lovers. But French, unlike Firestone, for example, doesn't put the blame on men. She blames love itself, and idealization is the key to love.

The Women's Room is built on a brutal dichotomy, between an overidealized and impossible form of love—expecting love to be everything: instant happiness, creativity, undying devotion, adoring and being adored "forever"—and the disillusioning facts of our lives: that love doesn't last, that love isn't everything, that one can be in love and still be unhappy, suffer from writer's block, feel insecure and inadequate. But what remains intact is the ideal itself, unattainable, a bitter disappointment and a cruel promise. What we do not get, unfortunately, is a less pregnant but still desirable promise of love that is more in tune with experience, and thus not so prone to disillusionment.

The refrain of *The Women's Room*, "but of course, she would not think of blaming love," should have been about blaming certain ideas we have about love, not love itself. The danger of confusing love with illusion is more than the personal unhappiness it causes: its cost also includes creating a serious obstacle in the public fight for women's equality. Even if one assumes that the battle for equality will entail antagonism with men on a public level, it is sheer folly, and also unnecessary, to carry that antagonism into intimate relationships which, despite certain utopian hopes and radical experiments to the contrary, may well be indispensable in our society, at least for the present and the foreseeable future. But the argument goes beyond this, too: for if, as I have argued, romantic love actually *requires* a sense of equality, then love provides, rather than works against, the ideal of feminism. Historically, romantic love (and Christian love, too) was a powerful force in breaking down the old hierarchies and roles. Today, that conception is still at work, in spite of the continuing overemphasis on sex and gender roles and despite the fact that too many feminists see love as the problem, instead of as part of the solution. Indeed, here as elsewhere in politics, projecting one's personal disappointments into the world as cynical "realism" is not the way to win adherents. Romantic love between men and women, from its very inception, has always been the primary vehicle of personal and, consequently, social equality. It has always been "feminist" in its temperament, whatever the mythologies that have sometimes been imposed on top of it. Romantic love and feminism are neither incompatible nor antagonistic; in fact, I would argue that, for the present at least, they should not try to do without one another.

Notes

1. Philip Slater, *The Pursuit of Loneliness: American Culture at the Breaking Point* (Boston: Beacon Press, 1970), p. 8.

2. In *Euripides at Bay*, for example, as well as in Aristophanes' best-known play, *Lysistrata.*

3. Shulamith Firestone, *The Dialectic of Sex: The Case for Feminist Revolution* (New York: Morrow, 1970), p. 165.

4. Ibid., p. 166.

5. Ibid., p. 49.

6. Ibid., p. 53.

7. Joyce Trebilcot, "Two Forms of Androgynism," in *Feminism and Philosophy* by Vetterling-Braggin, Elliston, and English, eds. (Totowa, NJ: Littlefield Adams, 1977), pp. 70–78.

8. Marilyn French, *The Women's Room* (New York: Summit Books, 1977), p. 362.

9. Ibid., pp. 210–11.

3.

SEXUAL LUST AND ORIGINAL SIN

Augustine

St. Augustine's City of God and the Christian Doctrine

Chapter 15.—Of the Justice of the Punishment with Which Our First Parents Were Visited for Their Disobedience.

Therefore, because the sin was a despising of the authority of God,—who had created man; who had made him in His own image; who had set him above the other animals; who had placed him in Paradise; who had enriched him with abundance of every kind and of safety; who had laid upon him neither many, nor great, nor difficult commandments, but, in order to make a wholesome obedience easy to him, had given him a single very brief and very light precept by which He reminded that creature whose service was to be free that He was Lord,—it was just that condemnation followed, and condemnation such that man, who by keeping the commandments should have been spiritual even in his flesh, became fleshly even in his spirit; and as in his pride he had sought to be his own satisfaction, God in His justice abandoned him to himself, not to live in the absolute independence he affected, but instead of the liberty he desired, to live

Augustine, "Sexual Lust and Original Sin," St. Augustin's City of God and Christian Doctrine. Schaff, Philip (1819–1893) New York: Christian Literature Publishing Co., 1890 Rights: Public Domain.

dissatisfied with himself in a hard and miserable bondage to him to whom by sinning he had yielded himself, doomed in spite of himself to die in body as he had willingly become dead in spirit, condemned even to eternal death (had not the grace of God delivered him) because he had forsaken eternal life. Whoever thinks such punishment either excessive or unjust shows his inability to measure the great iniquity of sinning where sin might so easily have been avoided. For as Abraham's obedience is with justice pronounced to be great, because the thing commanded, to kill his son, was very difficult, so in Paradise the disobedience was the greater, because the difficulty of that which was commanded was imperceptible. And as the obedience of the second Man was the more laudable because He became obedient even "unto death,"[1] so the disobedience of the first man was the more detestable because he became disobedient even unto death. For where the penalty annexed to disobedience is great, and the thing commanded by the Creator is easy, who can sufficiently estimate how great a wickedness it is, in a matter so easy, not to obey the authority of so great a power, even when that power deters with so terrible a penalty?

In short, to say all in a word, what but disobedience was the punishment of disobedience in that sin? For what else is man's misery but his own disobedience to himself, so that in consequence of his not being willing to do what he could do, he now wills to do what he cannot? For though he could not do all things in Paradise before he sinned, yet he wished to do only what he could do, and therefore he could do all things he wished. But now, as we recognize in his offspring, and as divine Scripture testifies, "Man is like to vanity."[2] For who can count how many things he wishes which he cannot do, so long as he is disobedient to himself, that is, so long as his mind and his flesh do not obey his will? For in spite of himself his mind is both frequently disturbed, and his flesh suffers, and grows old, and dies; and in spite of ourselves we suffer whatever else we suffer, and which we would not suffer if our nature absolutely and in all its parts obeyed our will. But is it not the infirmities of the flesh which hamper it in its service? Yet what does it matter *how* its service is hampered, so long as the fact remains, that by the just retribution of the sovereign God whom we refused to be subject to and serve, our flesh, which was subjected to us, now torments us by insubordination, although our disobedience brought trouble on ourselves, not upon God? For He is not in need of our service as we of our body's; and therefore what we did was no punishment to Him, but what we receive is so to us. And the pains which are called bodily are pains of the soul in and from the body. For what pain or desire can the flesh feel by itself and without the soul? But when the flesh is said to desire or to suffer, it is meant, as we have explained, that the man does so, or some part of the soul which is affected by the sensation of the flesh, whether a harsh sensation causing pain, or gentle, causing pleasure. But pain in the flesh is only a discomfort of the soul arising from the flesh, and a kind of shrinking from its suffering, as the pain of the soul which is called sadness is a shrinking from those things which have happened to us in spite of ourselves. But sadness is frequently preceded by fear, which is itself in the soul, not in the flesh; while bodily pain is not preceded by any kind of fear of the flesh, which can be felt in the flesh before the pain. But pleasure is preceded by a certain appetite which is felt in the flesh like a craving, as hunger and thirst and that generative appetite which is most commonly identified with the name "lust," though this is the generic word for all desires. For anger itself was defined by the ancients as nothing else than the lust of revenge;[3] although sometimes a man is angry even at inanimate objects which cannot feel his vengeance, as when one breaks a pen, or crushes a quill that writes badly. Yet even this, though less reasonable, is in its way a lust of revenge, and is, so to speak, a mysterious kind of shadow of [the great law of] retribution, that they who do evil should suffer evil. There is therefore a lust for revenge, which is called anger; there is a lust of money, which goes by the name of avarice; there is a lust of conquering, no matter by what means, which is called opinionativeness; there is a lust of applause, which is named boasting. There are many and various lusts, of which some have names of their own, while others have not. For who could readily give a name to the lust of ruling, which yet has a powerful influence in the soul of tyrants, as civil wars bear witness?

Chapter 16.—Of the Evil of Lust,—A Word Which, Though Applicable to Many Vices, is Specially Appropriated to Sexual Uncleanness.

Although, therefore, lust may have many objects, yet when no object is specified, the word lust usually suggests to the mind the lustful excitement of the organs of generation. And this lust not only takes possession of the whole body and outward members, but also makes itself felt within, and moves the whole man with a passion in which mental emotion is mingled with bodily appetite, so that the pleasure which results is the greatest of all bodily pleasures. So possessing indeed is this pleasure, that at the moment of time in which it is consummated, all mental activity is suspended. What friend of wisdom and holy joys, who, being married, but knowing, as the apostle says, "how to possess his vessel in sanctification and honor, not in the disease of desire, as the Gentiles who know not God,"[4] would not prefer, if this were possible, to beget children without this lust, so that in this function of begetting offspring the members created for this purpose should not be stimulated by the heat of lust, but should be actuated by his volition, in the same way as his other members serve him for their respective ends? But even those who delight in this pleasure are not moved to it at their own will, whether they confine themselves to lawful or transgress to unlawful pleasures; but sometimes this lust importunes them in spite of themselves, and sometimes fails them when they desire to feel it, so that though lust rages in the mind, it stirs not in the body. Thus, strangely enough, this emotion not only fails to obey the legitimate desire to beget offspring, but also refuses to serve lascivious lust; and though it often opposes its whole combined energy to the soul that resists it, sometimes also it is divided against itself, and while it moves the soul, leaves the body unmoved.

Chapter 17.—Of the Nakedness of Our First Parents, Which They Saw After Their Base and Shameful Sin.

Justly is shame very specially connected with this lust; justly, too, these members themselves, being moved and restrained not at our will, but by a certain independent autocracy, so to speak, are called "shameful." Their condition was different before sin. For as it is written, "They were naked and were not ashamed,"[5]—not that their nakedness was unknown to them, but because nakedness was not yet shameful, because not yet did lust move those members without the will's consent; not yet did the flesh by its disobedience testify against the disobedience of man. For they were not created blind, as the unenlightened vulgar fancy;[6] for Adam saw the animals to whom he gave names, and of Eve we read, "The woman saw that the tree was good for food, and that it was pleasant to the eyes."[7]

Their eyes, therefore were open, but were not open to this, that is to say, were not observant so as to recognize what was conferred upon them by the garment of grace, for they had no consciousness of their members warring against their will. But when they were stripped of this grace,[8] that their disobedience might be punished by fit retribution, there began in the movement of their bodily members a shameless novelty which made nakedness indecent: it at once made them observant and made them ashamed. And therefore, after they violated God's command by open transgression, it is written: "And the eyes of them both were opened, and they knew that they were naked; and they sewed fig leaves together, and made themselves aprons."[9]

> "The eyes of them both were opened," not to see, for already they saw, but to discern between the good they had lost and the evil into which they had fallen. And therefore also the tree itself which they were forbidden to touch was called the tree of the knowledge of good and evil from this circumstance, that if they ate of it, it would impart to them this knowledge. For the discomfort of sickness reveals the pleasure of health. "They knew," therefore, "that they were naked,"—

naked of that grace which prevented them from being ashamed of bodily nakedness while the law of sin offered no resistance to their mind. And thus they obtained a knowledge which they would have lived in blissful ignorance of, had they, in trustful obedience to God, declined to commit that offence which involved them in the experience of the hurtful effects of unfaithfulness and disobedience. And therefore, being ashamed of the disobedience of their own flesh, which witnessed to their disobedience while it punished it, "they sewed fig leaves together, and made themselves aprons," that is, cinctures for their privy parts; for some interpreters have rendered the word by *succinctoria*. *Campestria* is, indeed, a Latin word, but it is used of the drawers or aprons used for a similar purpose by the young men who stripped for exercise in the *campus*; hence those who were so girt were commonly called *campestrati*. Shame modestly covered that which lust disobediently moved in opposition to the will, which was thus punished for its own disobedience. Consequently all nations, being propagated from that one stock, have so strong an instinct to cover the shameful parts, that some barbarians do not uncover them even in the bath, but wash with their drawers on. In the dark solitudes of India also, though some philosophers go naked, and are therefore called gymnosophists, yet they make an exception in the case of these members and cover them.

Chapter 18.—Of the Shame Which Attends All Sexual Intercourse.

Lust requires for its consummation darkness and secrecy; and this not only when unlawful intercourse is desired, but even such fornication as the earthly city has legalized. Where there is no fear of punishment, these permitted pleasures still shrink from the public eye. Even where provision is made for this lust, secrecy also is provided; and while lust found it easy to remove the prohibitions of law, shamelessness found it impossible to lay aside the veil of retirement. For even shameless men call this shameful; and though they love the pleasure, dare not display it. What! does not even conjugal intercourse, sanctioned as it is by law for the propagation of children, legitimate and honorable though it be, does it not seek retirement from every eye? Before the bridegroom fondles his bride, does he not exclude the attendants, and even the paranymphs, and such friends as the closest ties have admitted to the bridal chamber? The greatest master of Roman eloquence says, that all right actions wish to be set in the light, i.e., desire to be known. This right action, however, has such a desire to be known, that yet it blushes to be seen. Who does not know what passes between husband and wife that children may be born? Is it not for this purpose that wives are married with such ceremony? And yet, when this well-understood act is gone about for the procreation of children, not even the children themselves, who may already have been born to them, are suffered to be witnesses. This right action seeks the light, in so far as it seeks to be known, but yet dreads being seen. And why so, if not because that which is by nature fitting and decent is so done as to be accompanied with a shame-begetting penalty of sin?

Chapter 19.—That It is Now Necessary, as It Was Not Before Man Sinned, to Bridle Anger and Lust by the Restraining Influence of Wisdom.

Hence it is that even the philosophers who have approximated to the truth have avowed that anger and lust are vicious mental emotions, because, even when exercised towards objects which wisdom does not prohibit, they are moved in an ungoverned and inordinate manner, and consequently need the regulation of mind and reason. And they assert that this third part of the mind is posted as it were in a kind of citadel, to give rule to these other parts, so that, while it rules and they serve, man's righteousness is preserved without a breach.[10]

These parts, then, which they acknowledge to be vicious even in a wise and temperate man, so that the mind, by its composing and restraining influence, must bridle and recall them from those objects towards which they are unlawfully moved, and give them access to those which the law of wisdom sanctions,—that anger, e.g., may be allowed for the enforcement of a just authority, and lust for the duty of propagating offspring,—these parts, I say, were not vicious in Paradise before sin, for they were never moved in opposition to a holy will towards any object from which it was necessary that they should be withheld by the restraining bridle of reason. For though now they are moved in this way, and are regulated by a bridling and restraining power, which those who live temperately, justly, and godly exercise, sometimes with ease, and sometimes with greater difficulty, this is not the sound health of nature, but the weakness which results from sin. And how is it that shame does not hide the acts and words dictated by anger or other emotions, as it covers the motions of lust, unless because the members of the body which we employ for accomplishing them are moved, not by the emotions themselves, but by the authority of the consenting will? For he who in his anger rails at or even strikes some one, could not do so were not his tongue and hand moved by the authority of the will, as also they are moved when there is no anger. But the organs of generation are so subjected to the rule of lust, that they have no motion but what it communicates. It is this we are ashamed of; it is this which blushingly hides from the eyes of onlookers. And rather will a man endure a crowd of witnesses when he is unjustly venting his anger on some one, than the eye of one man when he innocently copulates with his wife.

Chapter 20.—Of the Foolish Beastliness of the Cynics.

It is this which those canine or cynic[11] philosophers have overlooked, when they have, in violation of the modest instincts of men, boastfully proclaimed their unclean and shameless opinion, worthy indeed of dogs, viz., that as the matrimonial act is legitimate, no one should be ashamed to perform it openly, in the street or in any public place. Instinctive shame has overborne this wild fancy. For though it is related[12] that Diogenes once dared to put his opinion in practice, under the impression that his sect would be all the more famous if his egregious shamelessness were deeply graven in the memory of mankind, yet this example was not afterwards followed. Shame had more influence with them, to make them blush before men, than error to make them affect a resemblance to dogs. And possibly, even in the case of Diogenes, and those who did imitate him, there was but an appearance and pretence of copulation, and not the reality. Even at this day there are still Cynic philosophers to be seen; for these are Cynics who are not content with being clad in the *pallium*, but also carry a club; yet no one of them dares to do this that we speak of. If they did, they would be spat upon, not to say stoned, by the mob. Human nature, then, is without doubt ashamed of this lust; and justly so, for the insubordination of these members, and their defiance of the will, are the clear testimony of the punishment of man's first sin. And it was fitting that this should appear specially in those parts by which is generated that nature which has been altered for the worse by that first and great sin,—that sin from whose evil connection no one can escape, unless God's grace expiate in him individually that which was perpetrated to the destruction of all in common, when all were in one man, and which was avenged by God's justice.

Chapter 21.—That Man's Transgression Did Not Annul the Blessing of Fecundity Pronounced Upon Man Before He Sinned But Infected It with the Disease of Lust.

Far be it, then, from us to suppose that our first parents in Paradise felt that lust which caused them afterwards to blush and hide their nakedness, or that by its means they should have fulfilled the benediction of God, "Increase and multiply and replenish the earth;"[13] for it was after sin that lust began. It was after sin that our nature, having lost the power it had over the whole body, but not having lost all shame, perceived, noticed, blushed at, and covered it. But that blessing upon marriage, which encouraged them to increase and multiply and replenish the earth, though it continued even after they had sinned, was yet given before they sinned, in order that the procreation of children might be recognized as part of the glory of marriage, and not of the punishment of sin. But now, men being ignorant of the blessedness of Paradise, suppose that children could not have been begotten there in any other way than they know them to be begotten now, i.e., by lust, at which even honorable marriage blushes; some not simply rejecting, but sceptically deriding the divine Scriptures, in which we read that our first parents, after they sinned, were ashamed of their nakedness, and covered it; while others, though they accept and honor Scripture, yet conceive that this expression, "Increase and multiply," refers not to carnal fecundity, because a similar expression is used of the soul in the words, "Thou wilt multiply me with strength in my soul;"[14] and so, too, in the words which follow in Genesis, "And replenish the earth, and subdue it," they understand by the earth the body which the soul fills with its presence, and which it rules over when it is multiplied in strength. And they hold that children could no more then than now be begotten without lust, which, after sin, was kindled, observed, blushed for, and covered; and even that children would not have been born in Paradise, but only outside of it, as in fact it turned out. For it was after they were expelled from it that they came together to beget children, and begot them.

Chapter 22.—Of the Conjugal Union as It Was Originally Instituted and Blessed by God.

But we, for our part, have no manner of doubt that to increase and multiply and replenish the earth in virtue of the blessing of God, is a gift of marriage as God instituted it from the beginning before man sinned, when He created them male and female,—in other words, two sexes manifestly distinct. And it was this work of God on which His blessing was pronounced. For no sooner had Scripture said, "Male and female created He them,"[15] than it immediately continues, "And God blessed them, and God said unto them, Increase, and multiply, and replenish the earth, and subdue it," etc. And though all these things may not unsuitably be interpreted in a spiritual sense, yet "male and female" cannot be understood of two things in one man, as if there were in him one thing which rules, another which is ruled; but it is quite clear that they were created male and female, with bodies of different sexes, for the very purpose of begetting offspring, and so increasing, multiplying, and replenishing the earth; and it is great folly to oppose so plain a fact. It was not of the spirit which commands and the body which obeys, nor of the rational soul which rules and the irrational desire which is ruled, nor of the contemplative virtue which is supreme and the active which is subject, nor of the understanding of the mind and the sense of the body, but plainly of the matrimonial union by which the sexes are mutually bound together, that our Lord, when asked whether it were lawful for any cause to put away one's wife (for on account of the hardness of the hearts of the Israelites

Moses permitted a bill of divorcement to be given), answered and said, "Have ye not read that He which made them at the beginning made them male and female, and said, For this cause shall a man leave father and mother, and shall cleave to his wife, and they twain shall be one flesh? Wherefore they are no more twain, but one flesh. What, therefore, God hath joined together, let not man put asunder."[16] It is certain, then, that from the first men were created, as we see and know them to be now, of two sexes, male and female, and that they are called one, either on account of the matrimonial union, or on account of the origin of the woman, who was created from the side of the man. And it is by this original example, which God Himself instituted, that the apostle admonishes all husbands to love their own wives in particular.[17]

Chapter 23.—Whether Generation Should Have Taken Place Even in Paradise Had Man Not Sinned, or Whether There Should Have Been Any Contention There Between Chastity and Lust.

But he who says that there should have been neither copulation nor generation but for sin, virtually says that man's sin was necessary to complete the number of the saints. For if these two by not sinning should have continued to live alone, because, as is supposed, they could not have begotten children had they not sinned, then certainly sin was necessary in order that there might be not only two but many righteous men. And if this cannot be maintained without absurdity, we must rather believe that the number of the saints fit to complete this most blessed city would have been as great though no one had sinned, as it is now that the grace of God gathers its citizens out of the multitude of sinners, so long as the children of this world generate and are generated.[18]

And therefore that marriage, worthy of the happiness of Paradise, should have had desirable fruit without the shame of lust, had there been no sin. But how that could be, there is now no example to teach us. Nevertheless, it ought not to seem incredible that one member might serve the will without lust then, since so many serve it now. Do we now move our feet and hands when we will to do the things we would by means of these members? Do we meet with no resistance in them, but perceive that they are ready servants of the will, both in our own case and in that of others, and especially of artisans employed in mechanical operations, by which the weakness and clumsiness of nature become, through industrious exercise, wonderfully dexterous? And shall we not believe that, like as all those members obediently serve the will, so also should the members have discharged the function of generation, though lust, the award of disobedience, had been awanting? Did not Cicero, in discussing the difference of governments in his

De Republica, adopt a simile from human nature, and say that we command our bodily members as children, they are so obedient; but that the vicious parts of the soul must be treated as slaves, and be coerced with a more stringent authority? And no doubt, in the order of nature, the soul is more excellent than the body; and yet the soul commands the body more easily than itself. Nevertheless this lust, of which we at present speak, is the more shameful on this account, because the soul is therein neither master of itself, so as not to lust at all, nor of the body, so as to keep the members under the control of the will; for if they were thus ruled, there should be no shame. But now the soul is ashamed that the body, which by nature is inferior and subject to it, should resist its authority. For in the resistance experienced by the soul in the other emotions there is less shame, because the resistance is from itself, and thus, when it is conquered by itself, itself is the conqueror, although the conquest is inordinate and vicious, because accomplished by those parts of the soul which ought to be subject to reason, yet, being accomplished by its own parts and energies, the conquest is, as I say, its own. For when the soul conquers itself to a due subordination, so that its unreasonable motions are controlled by reason, while it again is subject to God, this is a conquest virtuous and praiseworthy. Yet there is less shame when the soul is resisted by its own vicious parts than when its will and order are resisted by the body, which is distinct from and inferior to it, and dependent on it for life itself.

But so long as the will retains under its authority the other members, without which the members excited by lust to resist the will cannot accomplish what they seek, chastity is preserved, and the delight of sin foregone. And certainly, had not culpable disobedience been visited with penal disobedience, the marriage of Paradise should have been ignorant of this struggle and rebellion, this quarrel between will and lust, that the will may be satisfied and lust restrained, but those members, like all the rest, should have obeyed the will. The field of generation[19] should have been sown by the organ created for this purpose, as the earth is sown by the hand. And whereas now, as we essay to investigate this subject more exactly, modesty hinders us, and compels us to ask pardon of chaste ears, there would have been no cause to do so, but we could have discoursed freely, and without fear of seeming obscene, upon all those points which occur to one who meditates on the subject. There would not have been even words which could be called obscene, but all that might be said of these members would have been as pure as what is said of the other parts of the body. Whoever, then, comes to the perusal of these pages with unchaste mind, let him blame his disposition, not his nature; let him brand the actings of his own impurity, not the words which necessity forces us to use, and for which every pure and pious reader or hearer will very readily pardon me, while I expose the folly of that scepticism which argues solely on the ground of its own experience, and has no faith in anything beyond. He who is not scandalized at the apostle's censure of the horrible wickedness of the women who "changed the natural use into that which is against nature,"[20] will read all this without being shocked, especially as we are not, like Paul, citing and censuring a damnable uncleanness, but are explaining, so far as we can, human generation, while with Paul we avoid all obscenity of language.

NOTES

1. Phil. 2:8.
2. Ps. 144:4.
3. Cicero, Tusc. Quaest. 3:6 and 4:9. So Aristotle.
4. 1 Thess. 4:4.
5. Gen. 2:25.
6. Gen. 3:7.—(See *De Genesi ad lit.* ii. 40). An error which arose from the words, "The eyes of them both were opened."
7. Gen. 3:6.
8. (This doctrine and phraseology of Augustine being important in connection with his whole theory of the fall, we give some parallel passages to show that the words are not used at random: *De Genesi ad lit.* 11:41; *De Corrept. et Gratia* 11:31; and especially *Cont. Julian.* 4:82.)
9. Gen. 3:7.
10. See Plato's *Republic*, book iv.
11. The one word being the Latin form, the other the Greek, of the same adjective.
12. By Diogenes Laertius, 4:69, and Cicero, *De Offic.* 1:41.
13. Gen. 1:28.
14. Ps. 138:3.
15. Gen. 1:27, 28.
16. Matt. 19:4, 5.
17. Eph. 5:25.
18. Luke 10:34.
19. See Virgil, *Georg.* 2:136.
20. Rom. 1:26.

4.

OF THE REASON FOR WHICH SIMPLE FORNICATION IS A SIN BY DIVINE LAW, AND OF THE NATURAL INSTITUTION OF MARRIAGE

Thomas Aquinas

Hence appears the folly of those who say that simple fornication is not a sin.[1] For they say: Given a woman free from a husband, and under no control of father or any other person, if any one approaches her with her consent, he does her no wrong, because she is pleased so to act, and has the disposal of her own person: nor does he do any wrong to another, for she is under no one's control: therefore there appears no sin. Nor does it seem to be a sufficient answer to say that she wrongs God, for God is not offended by us except by what we do against our own good (Chap. CXXI[2]):[3] but it does not appear that this conduct is against man's good: hence no wrong seems to be done to God thereby. In like manner also it does not appear a sufficient answer, that wrong is thereby done to one's neighbour, who is scandalised: for sometimes a neighbour is scandalised by what of itself is not a sin, in which case the sin is only incidental: but the question is not whether fornication is a sin incidentally, but whether it is a sin ordinarily and in itself.

We must seek a solution from what has been said before: for it has been said (Chap. XVI[4], LXIV[5]) that God has care of everything according to that which is

From *Summa Contra Gentiles*: Book Three by St. Thomas Aquinas, translated by Venon K. Bourke. Translation copyright 1956 by Doubleday, a division of Bantam Doubleday Dell Publishing Group, Inc. Used by permission of Doubleday, a division of Bantam Doubleday Dell Publishing Group, Inc.

good for it. Now it is good for everything to gain its end, and evil for it to be diverted from its due end. But as in the whole so also in the parts, our study should be that every part of man and every act of his may attain its due end. Now though the *semen* is superfluous for the preservation of the individual, yet it is necessary to him for the propagation of the species: while other excretions, such as excrement, urine, sweat, and the like, are needful for no further purpose: hence the only good that comes to man of them is by their removal from the body. But that is not the object in the emission of the *semen*, but rather the profit of generation, to which the union of the sexes is directed. But in vain would be the generation of man unless due nurture followed, without which the offspring generated could not endure. The emission of the *semen* then ought to be so directed as that both the proper generation may ensue and the education of the offspring be secured.

Hence it is clear that every emission of the *semen* is contrary to the good of man, which takes place in a way whereby generation is impossible; and if this is done on purpose, it must be a sin. I mean a way in which generation is impossible in itself as is the case in every emission of the *semen* without the natural union of male and female: wherefore such sins are called "sins against nature." But if it is by accident that generation cannot follow from the emission of the *semen*, the act is not against nature on that account, nor is it sinful; the case of the woman being barren would be a case in point.

Likewise it must be against the good of man for the *semen* to be emitted under conditions which, allowing generation to ensue, nevertheless bar the due education of the offspring. We observe that in those animals, dogs for instance, in which the female by herself suffices for the rearing of the offspring, the male and female stay no time together after the performance of the sexual act. But with all animals in which the female by herself does not suffice for the rearing of the offspring, male and female dwell together after the sexual act so long as is necessary for the rearing and training of the offspring. This appears in birds, whose young are incapable of finding their own food immediately they are hatched: for since the bird does not suckle her young with milk, according to the provision made by nature in quadrupeds, but has to seek food abroad for her young, and therefore keep them warm in the period of feeding, the female could not do this duty all alone by herself: hence divine providence has put in the male a natural instinct or standing by the female for the rearing of the brood. Now in the human species the female is clearly insufficient of herself for the rearing of the offspring, since the need of human life makes many demands, which cannot be met by one parent alone. Hence the fitness of human life requires man to stand by woman after the sexual act is done, and not to go off at once and form connections with any one he meets, as is the way with fornicators. Nor is this reasoning traversed by the fact of some particular woman having wealth and power enough to nourish her offspring all by herself: for in human acts the line of natural rectitude is not drawn to suit the accidental variety of the individual, but the properties common to the whole species.[6]

A further consideration is, that in the human species the young need not only bodily nutrition, as animals do, but also the training of the soul. Other animals have their natural instincts (*suas prudentias*) to provide for themselves: but man lives by reason, which [read *quam*] takes the experience of a long time to arrive at discretion. Hence children need instruction by the confirmed experience of their parents: nor are they capable of such instruction as soon as they are born, but after a long time, the time in fact taken to arrive at the years of discretion. For this instruction again a long time is needed; and then moreover, because of the assaults of passion, whereby the judgement of prudence is thwarted, there is need not of instruction only, but also of repression. For this purpose the woman by herself is not competent, but at this point especially there is requisite the concurrence of the man, in whom there is at once reason more perfect to instruct, and force more potent to chastise. Therefore in the human race the advancement of the young in good must last, not for a short time, as in birds, but for a long period of life. Hence, whereas it is necessary in all animals for the male to stand by the female for such time as the father's concurrence is requisite for bringing up of the progeny, it is natural for man to be tied to the society of one fixed woman for a long period, not a short one. This social tie we call marriage. Marriage then is natural to man, and an irregular connection outside of marriage is contrary to the good of man; and therefore fornication must be sinful.

Nor yet should it be counted a slight sin for one to procure the emission of the *semen* irrespective of the due purpose of generation and rearing of issue, on the pretence that it is a slight sin, or no sin at all, to apply any part of one's body to another use than that to which it is naturally ordained, as if, for example, one were to walk on his hands, or do with his feet something that ought to be done with his hands. The answer is that by such inordinate applications as those mentioned the good of man is not greatly injured: but the inordinate emission of the *semen* is repugnant to the good of nature, which is the conservation of the species.[7] Hence, after the sin of murder, whereby a human nature already in actual existence is destroyed, this sort of sin seems to hold the second place, whereby the generation of human nature is precluded.

The above assertions are confirmed by divine authority. The unlawfulness of any emission of *semen*, upon which offspring cannot be consequent, is evident from such texts as these: *Thou shalt not lie with mankind as with womankind: Thou shalt not lie with any beast* (Levit. xviii, 22, 23); *Nor the effeminate, nor sodomites, shall possess the kingdom of God* (1 Cor. vi, 10). The unlawfulness of fornication and of all connection with any other woman than one's own wife is clear from Deut. xxiii, 17: *There shall be no whore among the daughters of Israel, nor whoremonger among the sons of Israel: Keep thyself from all fornication, and beyond thine own wife suffer not the charge of knowing another* (Job. iv, 13); *Fly fornication* (1 Cor. vi, 18).

Hereby is refuted the error of those who say that there is no more sin in the emission of the *semen* than in the ejection of other superfluous products from the body.

That Marriage ought to be Indissoluble

Looking at the matter rightly, one must see that the aforesaid reasons not only argue a long duration for that natural human partnership of male and female, which we call marriage, but further imply that the partnership ought to be lifelong.

1. Property is a means to the preservation of human life. And because natural life cannot be preserved in one and the same person of the father living on for all time, nature arranges for its preservation by the son succeeding his father in likeness of species: wherefore it is appropriate that the son should succeed his father in his property. It is natural therefore that the father's interest in his son should continue to the end of his life, and that father and mother should dwell together to the end.[8]

2. Woman is taken into partnership with man for the need of childbearing: therefore when the fertility and beauty of woman ceases, there is a bar against her being taken up by another man. If then a man, taking a woman to wife in the time of her youth, when beauty and fertility wait upon her, could send her away when she was advanced in years, he would do the woman harm, contrary to natural equity.

3. It is manifestly absurd for the woman to be able to send away the man, seeing that woman is naturally subject to the rule of man, and it is not in the power of a subject to run away from control. It being then against the order of nature for the woman to be allowed to desert the man, if the man were allowed to desert the woman, the partnership of man and woman would not be on fair terms, but would be a sort of slavery on the woman's side.

4. Men show a natural anxiety to be sure of their own offspring; and whatever stands in the way of that assurance runs counter to the natural instinct of the race. But if the man could send away the woman, or the woman the man, and form a connection with another, certainty as to parentage would be difficult, when a woman had intercourse first with one man and then with another.

5. The greater the love, the more need for it to be firm and lasting. But the

love of man and woman is counted strongest of all; seeing that they are united, not only in the union of the sexes, which even among beasts makes a sweet partnership, but also for the sharing in common of all domestic life, as a sign whereof a man leaves even father and mother for the sake of his wife (Gen. ii, 24). It is fitting therefore for marriage to be quite indissoluble.

6. Of natural acts, generation alone is directed to the good of (the specific) nature: for eating and the separation from the body of other excretions concern the individual, but generation has to do with the preservation of the species. Hence, as law is instituted for the common good, the function of procreation ought to be regulated by laws divine and human. Now the laws laid down ought to proceed on the basis of the dictate of nature (*ex naturali instinctu*), if they are human laws, as in the exact sciences every human discovery takes its origin from principles naturally known: but if they are divine laws, they not only develop the dictate of nature, but also make up the deficiency of what nature dictates, as dogmas divinely revealed surpass the capacity of natural reason. Since then there is in the human species a natural exigency for the union of male and female to be one and indivisible, such unity and indissolubility must needs be ordained by human law. To that ordinance the divine law adds a supernatural reason, derived from the significancy of marriage as a type of the inseparable union of Christ with His Church, which is one as He is one.[9] Thus then irregularities in the act of generation are not only contrary to the dictate of nature, but are also transgressions of laws divine and human:[10] hence on this account any irregular behaviour in this matter is even a greater sin than in the matter of taking food or the like. But since all other factors in human life should be subordinate to that which is the best thing in man, it follows that the union of male and female must be regulated by law, not from the mere point of view of procreation, as in other animals, but also with an eye to good manners, or manners conformable to right reason, as well for man as an individual, as also for man as a member of a household or family, or again as a member of civil society. Thus understood, good manners involve the indissolubility of the union of male and female: for they will love one another with greater fidelity, when they know that they are indissolubly united: each partner will take greater care of the things of the house, reflecting that they are to remain permanently in possession of the same things: occasions of quarrels are removed, that might otherwise arise between the husband and the wife's relations, if the husband were to divorce his wife; and thus affinity becomes a firmer bond of amity: also occasions of adultery are cut off, occasions which would readily offer themselves, if husband could divorce his wife, or wife her husband.[11]

Hence it is said: *But I say to you that whoever putteth away his wife, except for fornication, and marrieth another, committeth adultery; and he that marrieth her that is put away, committeth adultery* (Matt. xix, 9): *But to them that are united in marriage, it is not I that give commandment, but the Lord, that the wife depart not from her husband* (1 Cor. vii, 10).

Divorce was reckoned an impropriety also among the ancient Romans, of whom Valerius Maximus (*De memor. dictis*, II, 1) relates that they believed that the marriage tie ought not to be broken off even for barrenness.[12]

Hereby the custom is banned of putting away wives, which however in the Old Law was permitted to the Jews for their hardness of heart, because they were prone to the killing of their wives: so the less evil was permitted to keep out the greater.

NOTES

1. Fornication is said to be "simple," when neither of the parties is married.—There is plain speaking in this chapter, but it contains "a godly and wholesome doctrine, and necessary for our times." There would be less sin, if there were a little more plain speaking to persons under temptation. http://maritain.nd.edu/jmc/etext/gc3_122a.htm.

2. http://www.ccel.org/ccel/aquinas/gentiles.vi.xcvi.html#vi.xcvi-p1.1.

3. His saying should be noted by all moralists. It means that ethics must stand on rational, and not on mere theological grounds. The theological argument should supervene upon the ethical, and complete its force: but ethics are not theology, as air is not sunlight.

4. http://www.ccel.org/ccel/aquinas/gentiles.vi.xiii.html#vi.xiii-p1.1.

5. http://maritain.nd.edu/jmc/etext/gc3_64.htm.

6. This is the scholastic form of the principle of general consequences. http://www.ccel.org/ccel/aquinas/gentiles.vi.xcvii.html.

7. In any community in which the inordinate practice here mentioned is carried on without scruple or remorse, the race is sure to suffer for it. Historians do not dwell on this unsavoury topic: but the inordination in question was the ruin of the Greek race, politically, socially, and physically.

8. If the family is a good thing, and family property a good thing, divorce must be an evil thing, as dissolving the family. http://www.ccel.org/ccel/aquinas/gentiles.vi.xcviii.html.

9. Eph. v, 22–33. See *Ethics and Natural Law*, p. 276: *Political and Moral Essays*, pp. 287–289. http://www.ccel.org/ccel/aquinas/gentiles.vi.xcviii.html.

10. This distinction between the dictate (or exigency) of nature, and the divine law, answering to what Cardinal Newman calls "the critical and the judicial function of conscience" (*Grammar of Assent*, pp. 102–107), is of the first importance in the theory of morals. I have endeavoured to bring it out elsewhere: *Ethics and Natural Law*, pp. 109–25. St. Thomas speaks of the "divine law" as known in the Jewish and Christian revelation. In a "state of pure nature," without revelation, we should have had to argue a priori that God must have willed to ratify the exigences of human nature and natural reason, and com-

mand their observance. What those exigences of nature are, see chap. CXXIX. http://www
.ccel.org/ccel/aquinas/gentiles.vi.xcviii.html.

11. Carried down to our own time, St. Thomas's words come to this, that to make
adultery a legal ground of divorce is to set a premium on adultery. http://www.ccel.org/
ccel/aquinas/gentiles.vi.xcviii.html.

12. In the Latin editions this remark appears in the next chapter. I have restored it
to the chapter to which it evidently belongs. I know of no historical evidence to show that
the Jews were "prone to the killing of their wives." http://www.ccel.org/ccel/aquinas/
gentiles.vi.xcviii.html.

5.

HUMANAE VITAE

Pope Paul VI

THE TRANSMISSION OF LIFE

1. The most serious duty of transmitting human life, for which married persons are the free and responsible collaborators of God the Creator, has always been a source of great joys to them, even if sometimes accompanied by not a few difficulties and by distress.

At all times the fulfillment of this duty has posed grave problems to the conscience of married persons, but, with the recent evolution of society, changes have taken place that give rise to new questions which the Church could *not* ignore, having to do with a matter which so closely touches upon the life and happiness of men. . . . [Sections 2–6 have been deleted from this selection.]

"Declaration on Sexual Ethics," from the Encyclical Letter "Human Vitae" of Pope Paul VI. By permission of the Pontifical Council for Social Communications.

Doctrinal Principles

A Total Vision of Man

7. The problem of birth, like every other problem regarding human life, is to be considered, beyond partial perspectives—whether of the biological or psychological, demographic or sociological orders—in the light of an integral vision of man and of his vocation, not only his natural and earthly, but also his supernatural and eternal vocation. And since, in the attempts to justify artificial methods of birth control, many have appealed to the demands both of conjugal love and of "responsible parenthood," it is good to state very precisely the true concept of these two great realities of married life, referring principally to what was recently set forth in this regard, and in a highly authoritative form, by the Second Vatican Council in its pastoral constitution *Gaudium et Spes*.

Conjugal Love

8. Conjugal love reveals its true nature and nobility when it is considered in its supreme origin, God, who is love,[1] "the Father, from whom every family in heaven and on earth is named."[2]

Marriage is not, then, the effect of chance or the product of evolution of unconscious natural forces; it is the wise institution of the Creator to realize in mankind His design of love. By means of the reciprocal personal gift of self, proper and exclusive to them, husband and wife tend towards the communion of their beings in view of mutual personal perfection, to collaborate with God in the generation and education of new lives.

For baptized persons, moreover, marriage invests the dignity of a sacramental sign of grace, inasmuch as it represents the union of Christ and of the Church.

Its Characteristics

9. Under this light, there clearly appear the characteristic marks and demands of conjugal love, and it is of supreme importance to have an exact idea of these.

This love is first of all fully human, that is to say, of the senses and of the spirit at the same time. It is not, then, a simple transport of instinct and sentiment, but also, and principally, an act of the free will, intended to endure and to grow by means of the joys and sorrows of daily life, in such a way that husband and wife become only one heart and one only soul, and together attain their human perfection.

Then, this love is total, that is to say, it is a very special form of personal friendship, in which husband and wife generously share everything, without undue reservations or selfish calculations. Whoever truly loves his marriage partner loves not only for what he receives, but for the partner's self, rejoicing that he can enrich his partner with the gift of himself.

Again, this love is faithful and exclusive until death. Thus, in fact, do bride and groom conceive it to be on the day when they freely and in full awareness assume the duty of the marriage bond. A fidelity, this, which can sometimes be difficult, but is always possible, always noble and meritorious, as no one can deny. The example of so many married persons down through the centuries shows, not only that fidelity is according to the nature of marriage, but also that it is a source of profound and lasting happiness and, finally, this love is fecund for it is not exhausted by the communion between husband and wife, but is destined to continue, raising up new lives. Marriage and conjugal love are by their nature ordained toward the begetting and educating of children. Children are really the supreme gift of marriage and contribute very substantially to the welfare of their parents.[3]

Responsible Parenthood

10. Hence conjugal love requires in husband and wife an awareness of their mission of "responsible parenthood," which today is rightly much insisted upon, and which also must be exactly understood. Consequently it is to be considered under different aspects which are legitimate and connected with one another.

In relation to the biological processes, responsible parenthood means the knowledge and respect of their functions; human intellect discovers in the power of giving life biological laws which are part of the human person.[4]

In relation to the tendencies of instinct or passion, responsible parenthood means that necessary dominion which reason and will must exercise over them.

In relation to physical, economic, psychological and social conditions, responsible parenthood is exercised, either by the deliberate and generous decision to raise a large family, or by the decision, made for grave motives and with due respect for the moral law, to avoid for the time being, or even for an indeterminate period, a new birth.

Responsible parenthood also and above all implies a more profound relationship to the objective moral order established by God, of which a right conscience is the faithful interpreter. The responsible exercise of parenthood implies, therefore, that husband and wife recognize fully their own duties towards God, towards themselves, towards the family and towards society, in a correct hierarchy of values. In the task of transmitting life, therefore, they are not free to proceed completely at will, as if they could determine in a wholly autonomous way the honest path to follow; but they must conform their activity to the creative intention of God, expressed in the very nature of marriage and of its acts, and manifested by the constant teaching of the Church.[5]

Respect for the Nature and Purpose of the Marriage Act

11. These acts, by which husband and wife are united in chaste intimacy, and by means of which human life is transmitted, are, as the Council recalled, "noble and worthy,"[6] and they do not cease to be lawful if, for causes independent of the will of husband and wife, they are foreseen to be infecund, since they always remain ordained towards expressing and consolidating their union. In fact, as experience bears witness, not every conjugal act is followed by a new life. God has wisely disposed natural laws and rhythms of fecundity which, of themselves, cause a separation in the succession of births. Nonetheless the Church, calling men back to the observance of the norms of the natural law, as interpreted by their constant doctrine, teaches that each and every marriage act (*quilibet matrimonii usus*) must remain open to the transmission of life.[7]

Two Inseparable Aspects: Union and Procreation

12. That teaching, often set forth by the magisterium, is founded upon the inseparable connection, willed by God and unable to be broken by man on his own initiative, between the two meanings of the conjugal act: the unitive meaning and the procreative meaning. Indeed, by its intimate structure, the conjugal act, while most closely uniting husband and wife, empowers them to generate new lives, according to laws inscribed in the very being of man and of woman. By safeguarding both these essential aspects, unitive and procreative, the conjugal act preserves in its fullness the sense of true mutual love and its ordination towards man's most high calling to parenthood. We believe that the men of our day are particularly capable of seizing the deeply reasonable and human character of this fundamental principle.

Faithfulness to God's Design

13. It is in fact justly observed that a conjugal act imposed upon one's partner without regard for his or her condition and lawful desires is not a true act of love, and therefore denies an exigency of right moral order in the relationships between husband and wife. Hence, one who reflects well must also recognize that a reciprocal act of love, which jeopardizes the responsibility to transmit life

which God the Creator, according to particular laws, inserted therein is in contradiction with the design constitutive of marriage, and with the will of the Author of life. To use this divine gift destroying, even if only partially, its meaning and its purpose is to contradict the nature both of man and of woman and of their most intimate relationship, and therefore, it is to contradict also the plan of God and His will. On the other hand, to make use of the gift of conjugal love while respecting the laws of the generative process means to acknowledge oneself not to be the arbiter of the sources of human life, but rather the minister of the design established by the Creator. In fact, just as man does not have unlimited dominion over his body in general, so also, with particular reason, he has no such dominion over his generative faculties as such, because of their intrinsic ordination towards raising up life, of which God is the principle. "Human life is sacred," Pope John XXIII recalled; "from its very inception it reveals the creating hand of God."[8]

Illicit Ways of Regulating Birth

14. In conformity with these landmarks in the human and Christian vision of marriage, we must once again declare that the direct interruption of the generative process already begun, and, above all, directly willed and procured abortion, even if for therapeutic reasons, are to be absolutely excluded as licit means of regulating birth.[9]

Equally to be excluded, as the teaching authority of the Church has frequently declared, is direct sterilization, whether perpetual or temporary, whether of the man or of the woman.[10] Similarly excluded is every action which, either in anticipation of the conjugal act, or in its accomplishment, or in the development of its natural consequences, proposes, whether as an end or as a means, to render procreation impossible.[11]

To justify conjugal acts made intentionally infecund, one cannot invoke as valid reasons the lesser evil, or the fact that such acts would constitute a whole together with the fecund acts already performed or to follow later, and hence would share in one and the same moral goodness. In truth, if it is sometimes licit to tolerate a lesser evil in order to avoid a greater evil or to promote a greater good,[12] it is not licit, even for the gravest reasons, to do evil so that good may follow therefrom,[13] that is, to make into the object of a positive act of the will something which is intrinsically disordered, and hence unworthy of the human person, even when the intention is to safeguard or promote individual, family, or social well-being. Consequently it is an error to think that a conjugal act which is deliberately made infecund and so is intrinsically dishonest could be made honest and right by the ensemble of a fecund conjugal life.

Licitness of Therapeutic Means

15. The Church, on the contrary, does not at all consider illicit the use of those therapeutic means truly necessary to cure diseases of the organism, even if an impediment to procreation, which may be foreseen, should result therefrom, provided such impediment is not, for whatever motive, directly willed.[14]

Licitness of Resource to Infecund Periods

16. To this teaching of the Church on conjugal morals, the objection is made today . . . that it is the prerogative of the human intellect to dominate the energies offered by irrational nature and to orientate them towards an end conformable to the good of man. Now, some may ask: in the present case, is it not reasonable in many circumstances to have recourse to artificial birth control if, thereby, we secure the harmony and peace of the family, and better conditions for the education of the children already born? To this question it is necessary to reply with clarity: the Church is the first to praise and recommend the intervention of intelligence in a function which so closely associates the rational creature with his Creator; but she affirms that this must be done with respect for the order established by God.

If, then, there are serious motives to space out births, which derive from the physical or psychological condition of husband and wife, or from external conditions, the Church teaches that it is then licit to take into account the natural rhythms immanent in the generative functions, for the use of marriage in the infecund periods only, and in this way to regulate birth without offending the moral principles which have been recalled earlier.[15]

The Church is consistent with herself when she considers recourse to the infecund periods to be licit, while at the same time condemning, as being always illicit, the use of means directly contrary to fecundation, even if such use is inspired by reasons which may appear honest and serious. In reality, there are essential differences between the two cases; in the former, the married couple make legitimate use of a natural disposition; in the latter, they impede the development of natural processes. It is true that, in the one and the other case, the married couple are in agreement in the positive will of avoiding children for plausible reasons, seeking the certainty that offspring will not arrive; but it is also true that only in the former case are they able to renounce the use of marriage in the fecund periods when, for just motives, procreation is not desirable, while making use of it during infecund periods to manifest their affection and to safeguard their mutual fidelity. By so doing, they give proof of a truly and integrally honest love.

Grave Consequences of Methods of Artificial Birth Control

17. Upright men can even better convince themselves of the solid grounds on which the teaching of the Church in this field is based, if they care to reflect upon the consequences of methods of artificial birth control. Let them consider, first of all, how wide and easy a road would thus be opened up towards conjugal infidelity and the general lowering of morality. Not much experience is needed in order to know human weakness, and to understand that men—especially the young, who are so vulnerable on this point—have need of encouragement to be faithful to the moral law, so that they must not be offered some easy means of eluding its observance. It is also to be feared that the man, growing used to the employment of anticonceptive practices, may finally lose respect for the woman and, no longer caring for her physical and psychological equilibrium, may come to the point of considering her as a mere instrument of selfish enjoyment, and no longer as his respected and beloved companion.

Let it be considered also that a dangerous weapon would thus be placed in the hands of those public authorities who take no heed of moral exigencies. Who could blame a government for applying to the solution of the problems of the community those means acknowledged to be licit for married couples in the solution of a family problem? Who will stop rulers from favoring, from even imposing upon their peoples, if they were to consider it necessary, the method of contraception which they judge to be most efficacious? In such a way men, wishing to avoid individual, family, or social difficulties encountered in the observance of the divine law, would reach the point of placing at the mercy of the intervention of public authorities the most personal and most reserved sector of conjugal intimacy.

Consequently, if the mission of generating life is not to be exposed to the arbitrary will of men, one must necessarily recognize insurmountable limits to the possibility of man's domination over his own body and its functions; limits which no man, whether a private individual or one invested with authority, may licitly surpass. And such limits cannot be determined otherwise than by the respect due to the integrity of the human organism and its functions, according to the principles recalled earlier, and also according to the correct understanding of the "principle of totality" illustrated by our predecessor Pope Pius XII.[16] . . . [Sections 18–20 have been deleted from this selection.]

Pastoral Directives

Mastery of Self

21. The honest practice of regulation of birth demands first of all that husband and wife acquire and possess solid convictions concerning the true values of life and of the family, and that they tend towards securing perfect self-mastery. To dominate instinct by means of one's reason and free will undoubtedly requires ascetical practices, so that the affective manifestations of conjugal life may observe the correct order, in particular with regard to the observance of periodic continence. Yet this discipline which is proper to the purity of married couples, far from harming conjugal love, rather confers on it a higher human value. It demands continual effort yet, thanks to its beneficent influence, husband and wife fully develop their personalities, being enriched with spiritual values. Such discipline bestows upon family life fruits of serenity and peace, and facilitates the solution of other problems; it favors attention for one's partner, helps both parties to drive out selfishness, the enemy of true love; and deepens their sense of responsibility. By its means, parents acquire the capacity of having a deeper and more efficacious influence in the education of their offspring; little children and youths grow up with a just appraisal of human values, and in the serene and harmonious development of their spiritual and sensitive faculties.

Creating an Atmosphere Favorable to Chastity

22. On this occasion, we wish to draw the attention of educators, and of all who perform duties of responsibility in regard to the common good of human society, to the need of creating an atmosphere favorable to education in chastity, that is, to the triumph of healthy liberty over license by means of respect for the moral order.

Everything in the modern media of social communications which leads to sense excitation and unbridled habits, as well as every form of pornography and licentious performances, must arouse the frank and unanimous reaction of all those who are solicitous for the progress of civilization and the defense of the common good of the human spirit. Vainly would one seek to justify such depravation with the pretext of artistic or scientific exigencies,[17] or to deduce an argument from the freedom allowed in this sector by the public authorities.

Appeal to Public Authorities

23. To Rulers, who are those principally responsible for the common good, and who can do so much to safeguard moral customs, we say: Do not allow the

morality of your peoples to be degraded; do not permit that by legal means practices contrary to the natural and divine law be introduced into that fundamental cell, the family. Quite other is the way in which public authorities can and must contribute to the solution of the demographic problem: namely, the way of a provident policy for the family, of a wise education of peoples in respect of moral law and the liberty of citizens.

We are well aware of the serious difficulties experienced by public authorities in this regard, especially in the developing countries. To their legitimate preoccupations we devoted our encyclical letter *Populorum Progressio*. But with our predecessor Pope John XXIII, we repeat: No solution to these difficulties is acceptable "which does violence to man's essential dignity" and is based only on an utterly materialistic conception of man himself and of his life. The only possible solution to this question is one which envisages the social and economic progress both of individuals and of the whole of human society, and which respects and promotes true human values.[18] Neither can one, without grave injustice, consider divine providence to be responsible for what depends, instead, on a lack of wisdom in government, on an insufficient sense of social justice, on selfish monopolization, or again on blameworthy indolence in confronting the efforts and the sacrifices necessary to ensure the raising of living standards of a people and of all its sons.[19]

May all responsible public authorities—as some are already doing so laudably—generously revive their efforts. And may mutual aid between all the members of the great human family never cease to grow. This is an almost limitless field which thus opens up to the activity of the great international organizations.

NOTES

1. Cf. I John 4:8.

2. Cf. Eph. 3:15.

3. Cf. II Vatican Council, Pastoral Constitution *Gaudium et Spes*, no. 50.

4. Cf. St. Thomas, *Summa Theologica*, I–II, q. 94, art. 2.

5. Cf. Pastoral Constitution *Gaudium et Spes*, nos. 50, 51.

6. Ibid., no. 49.

7. Cf. Pius XI, encyclical *Casti Connubii*, in AAS XXII (1930), p. 560; Pius XII, in AAS XLIII (1951), p. 843.

8. Cf. John XXIII, encyclical *Mater et Magistra*, in MS LIII (1961), p. 447.

9. Cf. *Catechismus Romanus Concilii Tridentini*, part 2, chap. 8; Pius XI, encyclical *Casti Connubii*, in MS XXII (1930), pp. 562–64; Pius XII, *Discorsi e Radiomessaggi*, VI (1944), pp. 191–92; MS XLIII (1951), pp. 842–43, 857–59; John XXIII, encyclical *Pacem in Terris*, April 11, 1963, in AAS LV (1963), pp. 259–60; *Gaudium et Spes*, no. 51.

10. Cf. Pius XI, encyclical *Casti Connubii*, in AAS XXII (1930), p. 565; decree of the Holy Office, February 22, 1940, in AAS L (1958), pp. 734–35.

11. Cf. *Catechismus Romanus Concilii Tridentini*, part 2, chap. 8; Pius XI, encyclical *Casti Connubii*, in MS XXII (1930), pp. 559–61; Pius XII, MS XLIII (1951), p. 843; MS L (1958), pp. 734–35; John XXIII, encyclical *Mater et Magistra*, in MS LIII (1961), p. 447.

12. Cf. Pius XII, alloc. to the National Congress of the Union of Catholic Jurists, December 6, 1953, in MS XLV (1953), pp. 798–99.

13. Cf. Rom. 3:8.

14. Cf. Pius XII, alloc. to Congress of the Italian Association of Urology, October 8, 1953, in MS XLV (1953), pp. 674–75; MS L (1958), pp. 734–35.

15. Cf. Pius XII, MS XLIII (1951), p. 846.

16. Cf. MS XLV (1953), pp. 674–75; MS XLVIII (1956), pp. 461–62.

17. Cf. II Vatican Council, decree *Inter Mirifica*, On the Instruments of Social Communication, nos. 6–7.

18. Cf. encyclical *Mater et Magistra* in AAS LIII (1961), p. 447.

19. Cf. encyclical *Populorum Progressio*, nos. 48–55.

6.

A DEFENSE OF ABORTION

Judith Jarvis Thomson

Most opposition to abortion relies on the premise that the fetus is a human being, a person, from the moment of conception.[1] The premise is argued for, but, as I think, not well. Take, for example, the most common argument. We are asked to notice that the development of a human being from conception through birth into childhood is continuous; then it is said that to draw a line, to choose a point in this development and say "before this point the thing is not a person, after this point it is a person" is to make an arbitrary choice, a choice for which in the nature of things no good reason can be given. It is concluded that the fetus is, or that we had better say it is, a person from the moment of conception. But this conclusion does not follow. Similar things might be said about the development of an acorn into an oak tree, and it does not follow that acorns are oak trees, or that we had better say they are. Arguments of this form are sometimes called "slippery-slope arguments"—the phrase is perhaps self-explanatory—and it is dismaying that opponents of abortion rely on them so heavily and uncritically.

I am inclined to agree, however, that the prospects for "drawing a line" in the development of the fetus look dim. I am inclined to think also that we shall prob-

Judith Jarvis Thomson, "A Defense of Abortion," first published in *Philosophy & Public Affairs* 1, no. 1. Copyright © 1971 by Princeton University Press. Reprinted by permission of Princeton University Press.

ably have to agree that the fetus has already become a human person well before birth. Indeed, it comes as a surprise when one first learns how early in its life the fetus begins to acquire human characteristics. By the tenth week, for example, it already has a face, arms and legs, fingers and toes; it has internal organs, and brain activity is detectable.[2] On the other hand, I think that the premise is false, that the fetus is not a person from the moment of conception. A newly fertilized ovum, a newly implanted clump of cells, is no more a person than an acorn is an oak tree. But I shall not discuss any of this. For it seems to me to be of greater interest to ask what happens if, for the sake of argument, we allow the premise. How, precisely, are we supposed to get from there to the conclusion that abortion is morally impermissible? Opponents of abortion commonly spend most of their time establishing that the fetus is a person, and hardly any time explaining the step from there to the impermissibility of abortion. Perhaps they think the step too simple and obvious to require much comment. Or perhaps they are simply being economical in argument. Many of those who defend abortion rely on the premise that the fetus is not a person, but only a bit of tissue that will become a person at birth; and why pay out more arguments than you have to? Whatever the explanation, I suggest that the step they take is neither easy nor obvious, that it calls for closer examination than it is commonly given, and that when we do give it this closer examination we shall feel inclined to reject it.

I propose, then, that we grant that the fetus is a person from the moment of conception. How does the argument go from here? Something like this, I take it. Every person has a right to life. So the fetus has a right to life. No doubt the mother has a right to decide what shall happen in and to her body; everyone would grant that. But surely a person's right to life is stronger and more stringent than the mother's right to decide what happens in and to her body, and so out-weighs it. So the fetus may not be killed; an abortion may not be performed.

It sounds plausible. But now let me ask you to imagine this. You wake up in the morning and find yourself back to back in bed with an unconscious famous violinist. He has been found to have a fatal kidney ailment, and the Society of Music Lovers has canvassed all the available medical records and found that you alone have the right blood type to help. They have therefore kidnapped you, and last night the violinist's circulatory system was plugged into yours so that your kidneys could be used to extract poisons from his blood as well as your own. The director of the hospital now tells you: "Look, we're sorry the Society of Music Lovers did this to you—we would never have permitted it if we had known. But still, they did it and the violinist now is plugged into you. To unplug you would be to kill him. But never mind, it's only for nine months. By then he will have recovered from his ailment and can safely be unplugged from you." Is it morally incumbent on you to accede to this situation? No doubt it would be very nice of you if you did, a great kindness. But do you *have* to accede to it? What if it were not nine months but nine years? Or longer still? What if the director of the hospital said: "Tough luck, I agree, but you've now got to stay in bed, with the violinist plugged into you, for the rest of your life. Because remember this: All persons have a right to life, and violinists are persons. Granted you have a right to decide what happens in and to your body, but a person's right to life outweighs your right to decide what happens in and to your body. So you cannot ever be unplugged from him." I imagine you would regard this as outrageous, which suggests that something really is wrong with that plausible-sounding argument that was mentioned previously.

In this case, of course, you were kidnapped; you did not volunteer for the operation that plugged the violinist into your kidneys. Can those who oppose abortion on the grounds I mentioned make an exception for a pregnancy due to rape? Certainly. They can say that persons have a right to life only if they did not come into existence because of rape; or they can say that all persons have a right to life, but that some have less of a right to life than others, in particular, that those who came into existence because of rape have less. But these statements have a rather unpleasant sound. Surely the question of whether one has a right to life at all, or how much of a right one has, should not turn on the question of whether or not one is the product of a rape. And in fact the people who oppose abortion on the ground I mentioned do not make this distinction, and hence do not make an exception in case of rape.

Nor do they make an exception for a case in which the mother has to spend the nine months of her pregnancy in bed. They would agree that that would be a great pity and hard on the mother, but would insist all the same that all persons have a right to life; and that the fetus is a person. I suspect, in fact, that they would not make an exception for a case in which, miraculously enough, the pregnancy went on for nine years, or even for the rest of the mother's life.

Some would not even make an exception for a case in which continuation of the pregnancy is likely to shorten the mother's life; they regard abortion as impermissible even to save the mother's life. Such cases are nowadays very rare, and many opponents of abortion do not accept this extreme view. All the same, it is a good place to begin: a number of points of interest come out in respect to it.

1. Let us call the view that abortion is impermissible even to save the mother's life "the extreme view." I want to suggest, first, that it does not issue from the argument I mentioned earlier without the addition of some fairly powerful premises. Suppose a woman has become pregnant, and now learns that she has a cardiac condition such that she will die if she carries the baby to term. What may be done for her? The fetus, being a person, has a right to life; but as the mother is a person too, so has she a right to life. Presumably they have an equal

right to life. How is it supposed to come out that an abortion may not be performed? If mother and child have an equal right to life, should not we perhaps flip a coin? Or should we add to the mother's right to life her right to decide what happens in and to her body, which everybody seems to be ready to grant—the sum of her rights now outweighing the fetus' right to life?

The most familiar argument here is the following. We are told that performing the abortion would be directly killing[3] the child, whereas doing nothing would not be killing the mother, but only letting her die. Moreover; in killing the child, one would be killing an innocent person, for the child has committed no crime and is not aiming at his mother's death. And then there are a variety of ways in which this argument might be continued. (1) As directly killing an innocent person is always and absolutely impermissible, an abortion may not be performed. Or, (2) as directly killing an innocent person is murder, and murder is always and absolutely impermissible, an abortion may not be performed.[4] Or, (3) as one's duty to refrain from directly killing an innocent person is more stringent than one's duty to keep a person from dying, an abortion may not be performed. Or, (4) if one's only options are directly killing an innocent person or letting a person die, one must prefer letting the person die, and thus an abortion may not be performed.[5]

Some people seem to have thought that these are not further premises that must be added if the conclusion is to be reached, but that they follow from the very fact that an innocent person has a right to life.[6] But this seems to me a mistake, and perhaps the simplest way to show this is to point out that while we must certainly grant that innocent persons have a right to life, the theses in arguments 1 through 4 are all false. Take argument 2 for example. If directly killing an innocent person is murder, and thus is impermissible, then the mother's directly killing the innocent person inside her is murder, and thus is impermissible. But it cannot seriously be thought to be murder if the mother performs an abortion on herself to save her life. It cannot seriously be said that she *must* refrain, that she *must* sit passively by and wait for her death. Let us look again at the case of you and the violinist. There you are, in bed with the violinist, and the director of the hospital says to you: "It's all most distressing, and I deeply sympathize, but you see this is putting an additional strain on your kidneys, and you'll be dead within the month. But you *have* to stay where you are all the same, because unplugging you would be directly killing an innocent violinist, and that's murder, and that's impermissible." If anything in the world is true, it is that you do not commit murder, you do not do what is impermissible, if you reach around to your back and unplug yourself from that violinist to save your life.

The main focus of attention in writings on abortion has been on what a third party may or may not do in answer to a request from a woman for an abortion. This is in a way understandable. Things being as they are, there is not much a woman can safely do to abort herself. So the question asked is, What may a third party do? And what the mother may do, if it is mentioned at all, is deduced, almost as an afterthought, from what it is concluded that a third party may do. But it seems to me that to treat the matter in this way is to refuse to grant to the mother that very status of person that is so firmly insisted on for the fetus. For we cannot simply read off what a person may do from what a third party may do. Suppose you find yourself trapped in a tiny house with a growing child—I mean a very tiny house, and a rapidly growing child; you are already up against the wall of the house and in a few minutes you'll be crushed to death. The child, on the other hand, will not be crushed to death; if nothing is done to stop him from growing he will be hurt, but in the end he will simply burst open the house and walk out a free man. Now I could well understand it if a bystander were to say: "There's nothing we can do for you. We cannot choose between your life and his, we cannot be the ones to decide who is to live, we cannot intervene." But it cannot be concluded that you too can do nothing, that you cannot attack the child to save your life. However innocent the child may be, you do not have to wait passively while it crushes you to death. Perhaps a pregnant woman is vaguely felt to have the status of a house, which we do not allow the right of self-defense But if the woman houses the child, it should be remembered that she is a person who houses it.

I should perhaps pause to say explicitly that I am not claiming that people have a right to do anything whatever to save their lives. I think, rather, that there are drastic limits to the right of self-defense. If someone threatens you with death unless you torture someone else to death, I think you have not the right, even to save your life, to do so. But the case under consideration here is very different. In our case there are only two people involved, one whose life is threatened, and one who threatens it. Both are innocent: the one who is threatened is not threatened because of any fault; the one who threatens does not threaten because of any fault. For this reason we may feel that we bystanders cannot intervene. But the person threatened can.

In sum, a woman surely can defend her life against the threat to it posed by the unborn child, even if doing so involves its death. And this shows not merely that the theses in arguments 1 through 4 are false; it shows also that the extreme view of abortion is false, and so we need not canvass any other possible ways of arriving at it from the argument I mentioned at the outset.

2. The extreme view could of course be weakened to say that while abortion is permissible to save the mother's life, it may not be performed by a third party, but only by the mother herself. But this cannot be right either. For what we have to keep in mind is that the mother and the unborn child are not like two tenants

in a small house that has, by an unfortunate mistake, been rented to both: the mother *owns* the house. The fact that she does adds to the offensiveness of deducing that the mother can do nothing from the supposition that third parties can do nothing. But it does more than this; it also casts a bright light on the supposition that third parties can do nothing. Certainly it lets us see that a third party who says "I cannot choose between you" is fooling himself if he thinks this is impartiality. If Jones has found and fastened on a certain coat that he needs to keep himself from freezing but that Smith also needs to keep from freezing, then it is not impartiality that says "I cannot choose between you" when Smith owns the coat. Women have said again and again, "This body is my body!" and they have reason to feel angry, reason to feel that it has been like shouting into the wind. Smith, after all, is hardly likely to bless us if we say to him: "Of course it's your coat; anybody would grant that it is. But no one may choose between you and Jones who is to have it."

We should really ask what it is that says "no one may choose" in the face of the fact that the body that houses the child is the mother's body. It may be simply a failure to appreciate this fact. But it may be something more interesting, namely the sense that one has a right to refuse to lay hands on people, even where it would be just and fair to do so, even where justice seems to require that somebody do so. Thus justice might call for somebody to get Smith's coat back from Jones, and yet you have a right to refuse to be the one to lay hands on Jones, a right to refuse to do physical violence to him. This, I think, must be granted. But then what should be said is not "no one may choose," but only "*I* cannot choose"—indeed not even this, but rather "*I* will not act," leaving it open that somebody else can or should, in particular that anyone in a position of authority, with the job of securing people's rights, both can and should. So this is no difficulty. I have not been arguing that any given third party must accede to the mother's request that he perform an abortion to save her life, but only that he may.

I suppose that in some views of human life the mother's body is only on loan to her, the loan not being one that gives her any prior claim to it. One who held this view might well think it impartiality to say, "I cannot choose." But I shall simply ignore this possibility. My own view is that if a human being has any just, prior claim to anything at all, he has a just, prior claim to his own body. And perhaps this need not be argued for here anyway, since, as I mentioned, the arguments against abortion we are looking at do grant that the woman has a right to decide what happens in and to her body.

But although they do grant it, I have tried to show that they do not take seriously what is done in granting it. I suggest the same thing will reappear even more clearly when we turn away from cases in which the mother's life is at stake and attend, as I propose we now do, to the vastly more common cases in which a woman wants an abortion for some less weighty reason than preserving her own life.

3. Where the mother's life is not at stake the argument I mentioned at the outset seems to have a much stronger pull. "Everyone has a right to life, so the unborn person has a right to life." And isn't the child's right to life weightier than anything other than the mother's own right to life, which she might put forward as ground for an abortion?

This argument treats the right to life as if it were unproblematic. It is not, and this seems to me to be precisely the source of the mistake.

For we should now, at long last, ask what it comes to, to have a right to life. In some views having a right to life includes having a right to be given at least the bare minimum one needs for continued life. But suppose that what in fact *is* the bare minimum a man needs for continued life is something he has no right at all to be given? If I am sick unto death, and the only thing that will save my life is the touch of Henry Fonda's cool hand on my fevered brow, then all the same, I have no right to be given the touch of Henry Fonda's cool hand on my fevered brow. It would be frightfully nice of him to fly in from the West Coast to provide it. It would be less nice, though no doubt well meant, if my friends flew to the West Coast and carried Henry Fonda back with them. But I have no right at all against anybody that he should do this for me. Or again, to return to the story I told earlier, the fact that for continued life the violinist needs the continued use of your kidneys does not establish that he has a right to be given the continued use of your kidneys. He certainly has no right against you that *you* should give him continued use of your kidneys. For nobody has any right to use your kidneys unless you give him such a right; and nobody has the right against you that you shall give him this right. If you do allow him to go on using your kidneys, this is a kindness on your part, and not something he can claim from you as his due. Nor has he any right against anybody else that they should give him continued use of your kidneys. Certainly he had no right against the Society of Music Lovers that they should plug him into you in the first place. And if you now start to unplug yourself, having learned that you will otherwise have to spend nine years in bed with him, there is nobody in the world who must try to prevent you, in order to see to it that he is given something he has a right to be given.

Some people are rather stricter about the right to life. In their view it does not include the right to be given anything, but amounts to, and only to, the right not to be killed by anybody. But here a related difficulty arises. If everybody is to refrain from killing the violinist, then everybody must refrain from doing a great many different sorts of things. Everybody must refrain from slitting his throat, everybody must refrain from shooting him—and everybody must refrain from unplugging you from him. But does he have a right against everybody that they shall refrain from unplugging you from him? To refrain from doing this is to allow him to continue to use your kidneys. It could be argued that he has a right against us that we should allow him to continue to use your kidneys. That is, while he had no right against us that we should give him the use of your kidneys, it might be argued that he anyway has a right against us that we shall not now intervene and deprive him of the use of your kidneys. I shall come back to third-party interventions later. But certainly the violinist has no right against you that *you* shall allow him to continue to use your kidneys. As I said, if you do allow him to use them, it is a kindness on your part, and not something you owe him.

The difficulty I point to here is not peculiar to the right to life. It reappears in connection with all the other natural rights; and it is something that an adequate account of rights must deal with. For present purposes it is enough just to draw attention to it. But I would stress that I am not arguing that people do not have a right to life—quite the contrary, it seems to me that the primary control we must place on the acceptability of an account of rights is that it should turn out in that account to be a truth that all persons have a right to life. I am arguing only that having a right to life does not guarantee having either a right to be given the use of or a right to be allowed continued use of another person's body—even if one needs it for life itself. So the right to life will not serve the opponents of abortion in the very simple and clear way in which they seem to have thought it would.

4. There is another way to bring out the difficulty. In the most ordinary sort of case, to deprive someone of what he has a right to is to treat him unjustly. Suppose a boy and his small brother are jointly given a box of chocolates for Christmas. If the older boy takes the box and refuses to give his brother any of the chocolates, he is unjust to him, for the brother has been given a right to half of them. But suppose that having learned that otherwise it means nine years in bed with that violinist, you unplug yourself from him. You surely are not being unjust to, him, for you gave him no right to use your kidneys, and no one else can have given him any such right. But we have to notice that in unplugging yourself you are killing him; and violinists, like everybody else, have a right to life, and thus in the view we are considering, the right not to be killed. So here you do what he supposedly has a right that you shall not do, but you do not act unjustly to him in doing it.

The emendation that may be made at this point is this: the right to life consists not in the right not to be killed but rather in the right not to be killed unjustly. This runs a risk of circularity, but never mind: it would enable us to square the fact that the violinist has a right to life with the fact that you do not act unjustly toward him in unplugging yourself, thereby killing him. For if you do not kill him unjustly, you do not violate his right to life, and so it is no wonder you do him no injustice.

But if this emendation is accepted, the gap in the argument against abortion stares us plainly in the face: it is by no means enough to show that the fetus is a person, and to remind us that all persons have a right to life; we need to be shown also that killing the fetus violates its right to life, that is, that abortion is unjust killing. And is it?

I suppose we may take it as a datum that in a case of pregnancy due to rape the mother has not given the unborn person a right to the use of her body for food and shelter. Indeed, in what pregnancy could it be supposed that the mother has given the unborn person such a right? It is not as if there were unborn persons drifting about the world, to whom a woman who wants a child says, "I invite you in."

But it might be argued that there are other ways one can have acquired a right to the use of another person's body than by having been invited to use it by that person. Suppose a woman voluntarily indulges in intercourse, knowing of the chance that it will issue in pregnancy, and then she does become pregnant. Is she not in part responsible for the presence, in fact the very existence, of the unborn person inside her? No doubt she did not invite it in. But doesn't her partial responsibility for its being there itself give it a right to the use of her body?[7] If so, then her aborting it would be more like the boy's taking away the chocolates and less like your unplugging yourself from the violinist—doing so would be depriving it of what it does have a right to, and thus would be doing it an injustice.

And then, too, it might be asked whether or not she can kill it even to save her own life: If she voluntarily called it into existence, how can she now kill it, even in self-defense?

The first thing to be said about this is that it is something new. Opponents of abortion have been so concerned to make out the independence of the fetus, in order to establish that it has a right to life, just as its mother does, that they have tended to overlook the possible support they might gain from making out that the fetus is dependent on the mother, in order to establish that she has a special kind of responsibility for it, a responsibility that gives it rights against her that are not possessed by any independent person—such as an ailing violinist who is a stranger to her.

On the other hand, this argument would give the unborn person a right to its mother's body only if her pregnancy resulted from a voluntary act, undertaken in full knowledge of the chance that a pregnancy might result from it. It would leave out entirely the unborn person whose existence is due to rape, pending the availability of some further argument, then, we would be left with the conclusion that unborn persons whose existence is due to rape have no right to the use of their mothers' bodies, and thus that aborting them is not depriving them of anything they have a right to and hence is not unjust killing.

And we should also notice that it is not at all plain that this argument really does go even as far as it purports to. For there are different kinds of cases, and the details make a difference. If the room is stuffy and I therefore open a window to air it and a burglar climbs in, it would be absurd to say, "Ah, now he can stay; she's given him a right to the use of her house—for she is partially responsible for his presence there, having voluntarily done what enabled him to get in, in full knowledge that there are such things as burglars, and that burglars burgle." It would be still more absurd to say this if I had had bars installed outside my windows precisely to prevent burglars from getting in, and a burglar got in only because of a defect in the bars. It remains equally absurd if we imagine it is not a burglar who climbs in but an innocent person who blunders or falls in. Again, suppose it were like this: people-seeds drift about in the air like pollen, and if you open your windows one may drift in and take root in your carpet or upholstery. You do not want children, so you fix up your windows with fine mesh screens, the very best you can buy. As can happen, however, and on very rare occasions does happen, one of the screens is defective; and a seed drifts in and takes root. Does the person-plant who now develops have a right to the use of your house? Surely not, despite the fact that you voluntarily opened your windows, that you knowingly kept carpets and upholstered furniture, and that you knew that screens were sometimes defective. Someone may argue that you are responsible for its rooting, that it does have a right to your house because, after all, you *could* have lived out your life with bare floors and furniture, or with sealed windows and doors. But this will not do, for by the same token anyone can avoid a pregnancy due to rape by having a hysterectomy, or by never leaving home without a (reliable!) army.

It seems to me that the argument we are looking at can establish at most that there are some cases in which the unborn person has a right to the use of its mother's body, and therefore some cases in which abortion is unjust killing. There is room for much discussion and argument as to precisely which cases, if any, are unjust. But I think we should sidestep this issue and leave it open, for the argument certainly does not establish that all abortion is unjust killing.

5. There is, however, room for yet another argument here. We all surely must grant that there may be cases in which it would be morally indecent to detach a person from your body at the cost of his life. Suppose you learn that what the violinist needs is not nine years of your life but only one hour: all you need do to save his life is to spend one hour in that bed with him. Suppose also that letting him use your kidneys for that one hour would not affect your health in the slightest. Admittedly you were kidnapped. Admittedly you did not give anyone permission to plug him into you. Nevertheless it seems to me plain you *ought* to allow him to use your kidneys for that hour—it would be indecent to refuse.

Again, suppose pregnancy lasted only an hour and constituted no threat to life or health. And suppose that a woman becomes pregnant as a result of rape. Admittedly she did not voluntarily do anything to bring about the existence of a child. Admittedly she did nothing at all that would give the unborn person a right to the use of her body. All the same it might well be said, as in the newly emended violinist story, that she *ought* to allow it to remain for that hour—that it would be indecent of her to refuse.

Now some people are inclined to use the term "right" in such a way that it follows from the fact that you ought to allow a person to use your body for the hour he needs, that he has a right to use your body for the hour he needs, even though he has not been given that right by any person or act. They may say that it follows also that if you refuse you act unjustly toward him. This use of the term is perhaps so common that it cannot be called wrong; nevertheless it seems to me to be an unfortunate loosening of what we would do better to keep a tight rein on. Suppose that the box of chocolates I mentioned earlier had not been given to both boys jointly, but was given only to the older boy. There he sits, stolidly eating his way through the box, his small brother watching enviously. Here we are likely to say: "You ought not to be so mean. You ought to give your brother some of those chocolates." My own view is that it just does not follow from the truth of this that the brother has any right to any of the chocolates. If the boy refuses to give his brother any, he is greedy, stingy, callous—but not unjust. I suppose that the people I have in mind will say it does follow that the brother has a right to some of the chocolates, and thus that the boy does act unjustly if he refuses to give his brother any. But the effect of saying this is to obscure what we should keep distinct, namely the difference between the boy's refusal in this case and the boy's refusal in the earlier case, in which the box was given to both boys jointly, and in which the small brother thus had what was from any point of view clear title to half.

A further objection to so using the term "right," that from the fact that A ought to do a thing for B it follows that B has a right against A that A do it for him, is that it is going to make the question of whether or not a man has a right to a thing turn on how easy it is to provide him with it; and this seems not merely unfortunate but morally unacceptable. Take the case of Henry Fonda again. I said earlier that I had no right to the touch of his cool hand on my fevered brow, even though I needed it to save my life. I said it would be frightfully nice of him to fly in from the West Coast to provide me with it, but that I had no right against him that he should do so. But suppose he isn't on the West Coast. Suppose he has only to walk across the room and place a hand briefly on my brow—and lo, my life is saved. Then surely he ought to do it; it would be indecent to refuse. Is it to be said, "Ah, well, it follows that in this case she has a right to the touch of his hand on her brow, and so it would be an injustice for him to refuse"? So that I have a right to it when it is easy for him to provide it, though no right when it is hard? It's rather a shocking idea that anyone's rights should fade away and disappear as it gets harder and harder to accord them to him.

So my own view is that even though you ought to let the violinist use your kidneys for the one hour he needs, we should not conclude that he has a right to do so; we should say that if you refuse you are, like the boy who owns all the chocolates and will give none away, self-centered and callous—indecent, in fact—but not unjust. And similarly, that even supposing a case in which a woman pregnant due to rape ought to allow the unborn person to use her body for the hour he needs, we should not conclude that he has a right to do so; we should conclude that she is self-centered, callous, indecent, but not unjust, if she refuses. The complaints are no less grave; they are just different. However, there is no need to insist on this point. If anyone does wish to deduce "he has a right" from "you ought," then all the same he must surely grant that there are cases in which it is not morally required of you that you allow that violinist to use your kidneys, and in which he does not have a right to use them, and in which you do not do him an injustice if you refuse. And so also for mother and unborn child. Except in such cases as the unborn person has a right to demand it—and we were leaving open the possibility that there may be such cases—nobody is morally *required* to make large sacrifices, of health, of all other interests and concerns, of all other duties and commitments, for nine years, or even for nine months, in order to keep another person alive.

6. We have in fact to distinguish between two kinds of Samaritans: the Good Samaritan and what we might call the Minimally Decent Samaritan. The story of the Good Samaritan, you will remember, goes like this:

> A certain man went down from Jerusalem to Jericho, and fell among thieves, which stripped him of his raiment, and wounded him, and departed, leaving him half dead.
>
> And by chance there came down a certain priest that way; and when he saw him, he passed by on the other side.
>
> And likewise a Levite, when he was at the place, came and looked on him, and passed by the other side.
>
> But a certain Samaritan, as he journeyed, came where he was; and when he saw him he had compassion on him.
>
> And went to him, and bound up his wounds, pouring in oil and wine, and set him on his own beast, and brought him to an inn, and took care of him.
>
> And on the morrow, when he departed, he took out two pence, and gave them to the host, and said unto him, "Take care of him; and whatsoever thou spendest more, when I come again, I will repay thee." (Luke 10:30–35)

The Good Samaritan went out of his way, at some cost to himself, to help one in need of it. We are not told what the options were, that is, whether or not the priest and the Levite could have helped by doing less than the Good Samaritan did; but assuming they could have, then the fact they did nothing at all shows they were not even Minimally Decent Samaritans, not because they were not Samaritans, but because they were not even minimally decent.

These things are a matter of degree, of course, but there is a difference; it comes out perhaps most clearly in the story of Kitty Genovese, who was murdered while thirty-eight people watched or listened and did nothing at all to help her. A Good Samaritan would have rushed out to give direct assistance against the murderer. Or perhaps we had better allow that it would have been a Splendid Samaritan who did this, on the ground that it would have involved a risk of death for himself. But the thirty-eight people not only did not do this; they did not even trouble to pick up a phone to call the police. Minimally Decent Samaritanism would call for doing at least that, and their not having done so was monstrous.

After telling the story of the Good Samaritan Jesus said, "Go, and do thou likewise." Perhaps he meant that we are morally required to act as the Good Samaritan did. Perhaps he was urging people to do more than is morally required of them. At all events it seems plain that it was not morally required of any of the thirty-eight that he rush out to give direct assistance at the risk of his own life and that it is not morally required of anyone that he give long stretches of his life—nine years or nine months—to sustaining the life of a person who has no special right (we were leaving open the possibility of this) to demand it.

Indeed, with one rather striking class of exceptions, no one in any country in the world is *legally* required to do anywhere near as much as this for anyone else. The class of exceptions is obvious. My main concern here is not the state of the law in respect to abortion, but it is worth drawing attention to the fact that in no state in this country is any man compelled by law to be even a Minimally Decent Samaritan to any person; there is no law under which charges could be brought against the thirty-eight people who stood by while Kitty Genovese died. By contrast, in most states in this country, women are compelled by law to be not merely Minimally Decent Samaritans, but Good Samaritans, to unborn persons inside them. This does not by itself settle anything, because it may well be argued that there should be laws in this country—as there are in many European countries—compelling at least Minimally Decent Samaritanism.[8] But it does show that there is a gross injustice in the existing state of the law. And it shows also that the groups currently working against liberalization of abortion laws, in fact working toward having it declared unconstitutional for a state to permit abortion, had better start working for the adoption of Good Samaritan laws generally, or earn the charge that they are acting in bad faith.

I myself think that Minimally Decent Samaritan laws would be one thing, Good Samaritan laws quite another—and in fact highly improper. But we are not here concerned with the law. What we should ask is not whether anybody should be compelled by law to be a Good Samaritan but whether we must accede to a situation in which somebody is being compelled—by nature, perhaps—to be a Good Samaritan. We have, in other words, to look now at third-party interventions. I have been arguing that no person is morally required to make large sacrifices to sustain the life of another who has no right to demand them, and this even where the sacrifices do not include life itself; we are not morally required to be Good Samaritans, or anyway, Very Good Samaritans, to one another. But what if a man cannot extricate himself from such a situation? What if he appeals to us to extricate him? It seems to me plain that there are cases in which we can, cases in which a Good Samaritan would extricate him. There you are: you were kidnapped, and nine years in bed with the violinist lie ahead of you. You have your own life to lead. You are sorry, but you simply cannot see giving up so much of your life to the sustaining of his. You cannot extricate yourself, and ask us to do so. I should have thought that—in light of his having no right to the use of your body—it was obvious that we do not have to accede to your being forced to give up so much. We can do what you ask. There is no injustice to the violinist in our doing so.

7. Following the lead of the opponents of abortion, I have throughout been speaking of the fetus merely as a person; and what I have been asking is whether or not the argument we began with, which proceeds only from the fetus' being a person, really does establish its conclusion. I have argued that it does not.

But of course there are arguments and arguments, and it may be said that I have simply fastened on the wrong one. It may be said that what is important is not merely the fact that the fetus is a person but that it is a person for whom the woman has a special kind of responsibility issuing from the fact that she is its mother. It might be argued that all my analogies are therefore irrelevant—for you do not have that special kind of responsibility for that violinist and Henry Fonda does not have that special kind of responsibility for me. And our attention might be drawn to the fact that men and women both are compelled by law to provide support for their children.

I have in effect dealt (briefly) with this argument in section 4 above; but a (still briefer) recapitulation now may be in order. Surely we do not have any such "special responsibility" for a person unless we have assumed it, explicitly or implicitly. If a set of parents do not try to prevent pregnancy, do not obtain an abortion, and then at the time of birth of the child do not put it up for adoption but rather take it home with them, then they have assumed responsibility for it, they have given it rights, and they cannot *now* withdraw support from it at the cost of its life because they now find it difficult to go on providing for it. But if they have taken all reasonable precautions against having a child, they do not simply by virtue of their biological relationship to the child who comes into existence have a special responsibility for it. They may wish to assume responsibility for it, or they may not wish to. And I am suggesting that if assuming responsibility for it would require large sacrifices, then they may refuse. A Good Samaritan would not refuse, or, anyway, a Splendid Samaritan would not, if the sacrifices that had to be made were enormous. But then so would a Good Samaritan assume responsibility for that violinist; so would Henry Fonda, if he is a Good Samaritan, fly in from the West Coast and assume responsibility for me.

8. My argument will be found unsatisfactory on two counts by many of those who want to regard abortion as morally permissible. First, while I do argue that abortion is not impermissible, I do not argue that it is always permissible. There may well be cases in which carrying the child to term requires only Minimally Decent Samaritanism of the mother, and this is a standard we must not fall below. I am inclined to think it a merit of my account precisely that it does *not* give a general yes or a general no. It allows for and supports our sense that, for example, a sick and desperately frightened fourteen-year-old schoolgirl, pregnant due to rape, may *of course* choose abortion, and that any law that rules this out is an insane law. And it also allows for and supports our sense that in other cases resort to abortion is even positively indecent. It would be indecent of the woman to request an abortion, and indecent of a doctor to perform it, if she is in her seventh month and wants the abortion just to avoid the nuisance of postponing a trip abroad. The very fact that the arguments I have been drawing attention to treat all cases of abortion, or even all cases of abortion in which the mother's life is not at stake, as morally on a par ought to have made them suspect at the outset.

Second, while I am arguing for the permissibility of abortion in some cases, I am not arguing for the right to secure the death of the unborn child. It is easy to confuse these two things in that up to a certain point in the life of the fetus it is not able to survive outside the mother's body; hence removing it from her body guarantees its death. But they are different in important ways. I have argued that you are not morally required to spend nine months in bed, sustaining the life of the violinist; but to say this is by no means to say that if when you unplug yourself there is a miracle and he survives, you have a right to turn round and slit his throat. You may detach yourself even if this costs him his life; you have no right to be guaranteed his death by some other means if unplugging yourself does not kill him. There are some people who will feel dissatisfied by this feature of my argument. A woman may be utterly devastated by the thought of a child, a bit of herself, put up for adoption and never seen or heard of again. She may therefore want not merely that the child be detached from her but, more, that it die. Some opponents of abortion are inclined to regard this as beneath contempt, thereby showing insensitivity to what is surely a powerful source of despair. All the same, I agree that the desire for the child's death is not one that anybody may gratify, should it turn out to be possible to detach the child alive.

At this place, however, it should be remembered that we have only been pretending throughout that the fetus is a human being from the moment of conception. A very early abortion is surely not the killing of a person and so is not dealt with by anything I have said here.

Notes

1. I am very indebted to James Thomson for discussion, criticism, and many helpful suggestions.

2. Daniel Callahan, *Abortion: Law, Choice, and Morality* (New York: Macmillan, 1970), p. 373. This book gives a fascinating survey of the available information on abortion. The Jewish tradition is surveyed in David M. Feldman, *Birth Control in Jewish Law* (New York: New York University Press, 1968), part 5; the Catholic tradition, in John T. Noonan Jr., "An Almost Absolute Value in History," in *The Morality of Abortion*, ed. John T. Noonan Jr. (Cambridge, MA: Harvard University Press, 1970).

3. The term "direct" in the arguments I refer to is a technical one. Roughly, what is meant by "direct killing" is either killing as an end in itself or killing as a means to some end, for example, the end of saving someone else's life. See note 6 for an example of its use.

4. Cf. *Encyclical Letter of Pope Pius XI on Christian Marriage*, St. Paul Editions (Boston, n.d.), p. 32: "However much we may pity the mother whose health and even life is gravely imperiled in the performance of the duty allotted to her by nature, nevertheless what could ever be a sufficient reason for excusing in any way the direct murder of the innocent? This is precisely what we are dealing with here." Noonan (*The Morality of Abortion*, p. 43) reads this as follows: "What cause can ever avail to excuse in any way the direct killing of the innocent? For it is a question of that."

5. The thesis in argument 4 is in an interesting way weaker than those in 1, 2, and 3: they rule out abortion even in cases in which both mother and child will die if the abortion is not performed. By contrast, one who held the view expressed in 4 could consistently say that one need not prefer letting two persons die to killing one.

6. Cf. the following passage from Pius XII, *Address to the Italian Catholic Society of Midwives*: "The baby in the maternal breast has the right to life immediately from God.— Hence there is no man, no human authority, no science, no medical, eugenic, social, economic or moral 'indication' which can establish or grant a valid juridical ground for a direct deliberate disposition of an innocent human life, that is a disposition which looks to its destruction either as an end or as a means to another end perhaps in itself not illicit.—The baby, still not born, is a man in the same degree and for the same reason as the mother" (quoted in Noonan, *The Morality of Abortion*, p. 45).

7. The need for a discussion of this argument was brought home to me by members of the Society for Ethical and Legal Philosophy, to whom this paper was originally presented.

8. For a discussion of the difficulties involved, and a survey of the European experience with such laws, see *The Good Samaritan and the Law*, ed. James M. Ratcliffe (New York: Peter Smith, 1966).

7.

COMPARING THE OUTPUT CUTOFF ARGUMENT WITH THOMSON'S ARGUMENT

Frances Myrna Kamm

We have already considered one alternative to the output cutoff argument, namely, the self- and assisted-defense argument, as well as these arguments supplemented by the idea of imposing risks. Now we shall see how the output cutoff argument for nonabortion cases compares with Thomson's discussion of nonabortion cases. First we shall summarize her discussion.

BABY IN A HOUSE

Thomson begins by considering a case in which a baby and a woman are in a house together. The baby is expanding so that it will crush the woman unless she or some third party kills it. Thomson believes that the woman may kill the baby in self-defense, presumably even intentionally seeking its death if only that will stop its expansion. But it is not clear, she adds, that a third party may intervene. I have already argued that it is sometimes permissible for third parties to favor the person being threatened, and although there may well be limits on what can

Taken from Frances Myrna Kamm's *Creation and Abortion: A Study in Moral and Legal Philosophy* (Oxford University Press), 1992. By permission of Oxford University Press.

be done to stop innocent threats, third parties may well be able to impose greater losses on these threats than the threats must impose on themselves.

BABY IN A WOMAN'S HOUSE

Thomson then modifies her first case so that the baby and the woman are in a house owned by the woman (owned-house case). Thomson now believes that a third party is permitted to side with the woman and to kill the baby that threatens her life. What is her reasoning? Is it meant to be *additive?* That is, if the threat to the woman's life is not a sufficient loss to make the third party side with her, does the *addition* of the infringement on her property right make the loss to her great enough to kill the baby? But this does not sound right: It is as if we said that we may not kill someone who threatens another's life unless he is also stealing the silverware. Surely it is the loss of life that is significant, not the infringement on property.

I suggest that Thomson's reasoning in this case must be *multiplicative* rather than additive.[1] What she must think is important is that the threat to the woman's life occurs because of the infringement on her property right, that the baby threatens her life by infringing on her property. Something that is hers, and that should serve her interests, is being used against her. (However, is it worse to be shot by one's own gun than by someone else's?) Again, some people may worry whether if the baby does this as an innocent threat, there should not be severe limits on what a third party may do to stop it.

COAT CASE

Thomson introduces a third case in order to defend her claim regarding the owned-house case. In this case, Smith, who would otherwise freeze to death, innocently finds Jones's coat, puts it on, and thereby saves his own life. However, Jones also needs his coat to survive (coat case). In this case, Smith does not impose directly on Jones, but he imposes on something that Jones needs to stay alive. (Should Smith's imposing on Jones's coat be treated any differently from his imposing on Jones's heart?) May a third party take away the coat from Smith and give it to Jones, even though Smith will then die? (This would be a foreseen rather than an intended death and would be the consequence of Smith's not having the coat.) Thomson believes that a third party may take away the coat from Smith.

Besides whether or not she is right, there is the prior question of whether it is appropriate to introduce this case as support for her conclusion in the owned-house case. I believe that Thomson failed to appreciate a crucial difference between the two cases: In the coat case, Smith—who will die if the coat is removed—loses the life-saving benefit of using someone else's property, a benefit relative to the position he would have been in if he had never had use of the property.[2] These factors are not present in the owned-house case: The baby faces no prior threat to its life from which it was rescued by being in the woman's house, and if it is killed, it will be worse off than it would have been had it not been in the woman's house to start with. In addition, there is a direct attack on the baby itself, not just the removal of someone else's property from it.

The argument that can be constructed to permit killing the baby, who will lose the life it would have had quite independently of using the woman's property, is the self- or assisted-defense of someone against a deadly threat. By contrast, the justification for taking the coat away from Smith might be the claim that when two people are in equal need of the use of property that belongs to one of them, a third person may take away this property from the nonowner in order to return it to the owner, even if the nonowner is already using it, if (1) the owner is not obligated to let the nonowner use the property and if the nonowner would have had no right to take it for his own use had he known of the owner's need, (2) if the nonowner will thereby lose only the benefit that he would receive from the use of the property, especially (3) if the nonowner will not then be harmed relative to the opportunities he had before using the coat. (In our case, neither Jones nor his third-party assistant would be harming Smith in regard to his earlier prospects, as they did not originally interfere with Smith's other opportunities. Smith also would not be harmed by anyone else or "by circumstances," as there was no other lifesaving option available. (This contrasts with some cases we have discussed.[3])

VIOLINIST CASE

The justification for taking away the coat from Smith may be compared with the justification for killing the violinist. In the violinist case, unlike the coat case, your life will not be at stake if someone uses your body. Indeed, you stand to lose much less—an imposition on your body but not permanent damage—if the violinist uses your body than he will lose if you do not let him use it. Nevertheless, Thomson's claim is that it is permissible to kill the violinist if this is required in order to remove him.

Even if Thomson's conclusion is correct, are her arguments in defense of it correct? She states that the violinist's right to life does not include the right to use your body merely because he needs it to survive. So it is permissible to allow the violinist to die, and it is wrong to force you to begin letting him use your body, even if all that were at stake for you was nine months' use of your body. Furthermore, she observes, his right to life is not a simple right not to be killed; it is, rather, a right not to be killed unjustly (some killings are not unjust). Why, then, is this killing not unjust? Thomson argues that it is not unjust because *if* it were not permissible to kill the violinist, he would have the right to use your body. But it has been agreed, she says, that he does not have a right to use your body, even to save his life.

We could understand this argument as providing a general way of deciding what efforts or losses we may kill in order to avoid: Whatever efforts or losses we need not suffer in order to save someone's life are efforts or losses we may avoid by killing innocents who are threats to us. Third parties may also defend us against enduring these losses.

Now consider the following objection to this argument: Someone may agree with Thomson that the violinist does not have a right to use your body to save his life but claim that he does have a right to use your body rather than be killed in order to be removed. Thus there is no conflict between not having to do something to save a life and having to do that same thing rather than kill someone.[4] Thomson responds to this conclusion by trying to defend the view that killing someone is not necessarily worse than letting someone die.[5] She does this by considering cases in which killing someone seems not to be morally worse than letting a person die. So if certain losses need not be suffered in order to save a life, she believes, at least sometimes they need not be suffered in order to avoid killing someone.

But this conclusion is problematic. The general claim that killing someone is not morally worse than letting a person die may not be true, even if killing someone in a particular case were no worse than letting someone die in a comparable case.[6] Therefore the general claim that we need not make greater efforts to avoid killing someone than we need make to avoid letting that person die may not be true. If so, we need more than a few cases where a killing is no worse than letting someone die to show that in regard to the violinist, not having to save his life by sharing your body with him proves that you do not have to share your body with him in order to avoid killing him. Further, the general claim that efforts that we need not make to save someone's life are also efforts that we need not make to avoid killing someone does not distinguish between our making efforts instead of threatening someone with death before he threatens us in any way, and our making efforts instead of killing someone who threatens us first. (The latter is what happens in the violinist case.)

In addition, I have already argued that those cases in which we kill someone in order to stop aiding him share a definitional property with letting someone die, and this helps account for these cases' being almost as permissible as letting someone die is. But then Thomson's argument should be supplemented by something like Condition 3, which emphasizes the definitional property of letting someone die: that someone loses life that would be the result of being aided.

If Thomson's argument is not supplemented in this way, her reason for permitting the violinist to be killed will not differentiate between killing him when he uses your body and receives life support, and killing him when he uses your body but does not receive life support. In the latter case we might want to kill the violinist in order to stop making efforts that we need not make in order to save his life, even though our efforts are not now saving his life. Yet it may be that (as I have argued) for efforts of a certain magnitude, it is more difficult to justify causing someone to lose his life that he would have had independently of those efforts than to cause him to lose what he has because of those efforts and would not have had without them.

NOTES

1. Indeed, I believe that this reasoning anticipates Thomson's analyses of the trolley problem, in "The Trolley Problem," *Yale Law Journal* 94 (1985): 1395–1415.

2. However, in connection with the second difference, suppose that someone else would have offered a coat had Smith not already had Jones's on. I do not believe that the fact that if we take away Jones's coat from Smith, Smith would then be worse off than he would have been if he had never had Jones's coat affects whether we may take it away. The reason is that in this case, it is not Jones who offered or is otherwise causally responsible for the use of his coat, and so Jones is not responsible for interfering with other offers that Smith might have had. Furthermore, we are not even attacking what is Smith's (either his body or his property) but are taking away Jones's coat from him.

3. Smith has indeed actively taken the coat, but I am ignoring the fact that he is not a nonactive morally innocent threat.

4. Baruch Brody makes such a counterargument in "Thomson on Abortion," *Philosophy and Public Affairs* 1(1972): 335–40.

5. In Judith Thomson's "Rights and Deaths."

6. A comparable case of letting someone die is one in which all elements in the case of killing someone are present, except killing him. On this general issue, see my "Killing and Letting Die: Methodology and Substance," *Pacific Philosophical Quarterly* (Winter 1983): 297–312.

8.

ON SPINSTERS

Kathleen J. Wininger

And round her house she set
Such a barricade of barb and check
Against mutinous weather
As no mere insurgent man could hope to break
With curse, fist, threat
Or love, either.

"The Spinster" by Sylvia Plath

Whether Bachelor Woman or Spinster Sister, the phenomenon of the unwed woman is catching the public imagination. In the new genres of blogs,[1] chick lit, and Web-based discussion lists, the spinster has had a revival; more interesting still, the revival mirrors confusions that have plagued previous understanding of the older unmarried woman. Depending on the cultural context and the age at which one is assumed to marry, "older" can mean seventeen to seventy. It is interesting that in the twenty-first century this spinster revival is happening in the United States, where the term never had the common usage and legal status that it had in Britain. Yet, the tension between the new "reluctant spinster" and her liberated contemporary, the "bachelor girl," takes us back to views and questions regarding the desirability of marriage for women in other times as well. First, we look at the contemporary trends.

Both the Reluctant Spinster and the Bachelor Girl are now looking for love in the blogosphere. The first spinster is a revival of the stereotypical spinster. Following the cultural norms, she wants but fails to catch and marry a good man; she is the Reluctant Spinster. The Bachelor Girl is usually looked at as the reclaimed spinster of feminist and other libratory historical discourses; this spinster refuses to be defined by cultural pressure, craves autonomy, and is often punished for evading matrimonial norms. The project of her reclamation comes from a suspicion that not every unmarried woman in history is there because she was not chosen for marriage. The spinster can now be seen as sexual, fully human (wanting occupation outside a domestic sphere), and therefore a gender transgressor. She transgresses when she is not reducible to her biological and social function. With a few exceptions,[2] both the Reluctant Spinster and Bachelor Spinster are now assumed to be sexual, looking for both sex and love. Still the presumptive heterosexuality of the spinster can mask a lesbian identity or a commitment to celibacy with no particular orientation designated. Historians have tried to look back and tease out the sexuality of single women of the past. As Dana Luciano explains in "Scouting for Queers," "It isn't always easy to find a lesbian when you're looking for one. This is especially true for those of us who work in historical periods prior to the coming out of the lesbian as an available model of identity."[3] The idea that behind the spinster one can sometimes find the closeted lesbian is reasonable but has been adequately explored in many books and articles.[4] In this essay we will see how the heterosexual norm plays out.

RELUCTANT SPINSTER

The Reluctant Spinster wants to get married, is a reluctant "singleton," to use Bridget Jones's phrase. The blogs of Reluctant Spinsters are socially conservative.[5] This spinster is viewed as a tragic romantic in her struggle. When she does not get married, she is a failure. This is not necessarily her view but how she fits in the cultural landscape. *Sex and the City* is in some ways a prototype for this division, although a more subtle and complex one than the blogs. The unhappy spinsters, like *Sex and the City*'s Charlotte York, are described as having a "a refreshingly optimistic outlook on love and romance. . . . First and foremost, she wanted to get married. She wanted true love. And she wanted her husband to be wealthy, handsome and belong to the social elite." These women are seen as more "romantic" than their "cynical" rivals. A positive spin is put on their pursuit of marriage, especially when the women don't give up the search for romance, love, *and* marriage. As HBO says of its lead character, Carrie Bradshaw, "No one captures the lives of the lovelorn and the love-seeking in New York City." It is a mark of her optimism that "somehow, . . . *she's remained open to the possibility of finding love among the ruins.*"[6] There are many contemporary "chick lit" examples, like Stacey Ballis's *The Spinster Sisters*,[7] books by author Sophie Kinsella, a specialist in the fairytale ending, and blogs like "Ask a Spinster," which features advice columnists whose unrelenting quest for a husband is described as "romantic" at another contemporary spinster Web site, in this case that of another Reluctant Spinster.[8] She also appears in a pre-sexual manifestation in the Internet ephemera as "Celibate in the City,"[9] the intentionally celibate religious virgin looking for the right guy. These are women for whom buying a couch, car, or home can be a symbol of the loss of the belief that a man will come and rescue them from loneliness and their unwed state. So buying a house sometimes represents the death of hope, of rescue from the single state. In the late 1990s one woman was shocked to find that she was a spinster under Illinois law.[10] "Single women face a nasty shock at real estate closings. . . . As they sign the title to a mortgage or deed, many unmarried women learn that, in the eyes of the law, they are spinsters. 'It's not a real flattering term.'" Why is that hope for marriage as a solution to questions of gender identity so real, as real in the late twenty-first century as in previous generations?

BACHELOR GIRL

Bachelor Girls also follow the new definitions of spinsters as fully sexualized but without their eyes on the prize of marriage. In fact, the online Urban Dictionary, where definitions are rated, approves highly of defining the spinster as not necessarily a virgin and as "a woman who is not married, especially a woman who is no longer young and seems unlikely ever to marry. Note: A woman who never enters marriage contract is so smart. '*Spinster means a woman who can stand independently and doesn't need a man for her life.*'"[11] Again a prototype can be found in *Sex and the City*, this time in the character Samantha Jones: "Forget wedding dreams; Samantha takes lust over love any night, and she's proud of it." Miranda Hobbes, another *Sex and the City* girl, "is smart, self-assured and proud of her achievements. . . . she's struggled with her love life and, at times, abandoned the pursuit of love altogether . . . masking her vulnerability with cynicism and self-deprecating humor." Yet HBO's Web site, to narrate her out of competence into reluctant, rather than ambivalent spinsterhood, quotes the character saying, "Do any of you have a completely unremarkable friend or maybe a houseplant I could go to dinner with on Saturday night?" HBO promotes Miranda, the possible Bachelor Girl, into a Reluctant Spinster. The Miranda character, in her intellectual complexity, intelligence, and fear, more resembles Sylvia Plath's spinster of the eponymous poem. An intelligent woman, who, in her concerns about intimacy, protects herself.

The Bachelor Girl, as her name indicates, is more analogous to popular notions of the older (male) bachelor as bon vivant, and fond of good living, although in her case she is perhaps more fond of good shoes than good food. The idea that women can seek satisfaction in an aggressively sexual way, not as a means to marriage but as a conscious repudiation of it, is itself rather remarkable. Consider "Love and the Modern Spinster" (excerpt):

> Granted, most people think of a "spinster" as someone who doesn't have romantic relationships. Historically, a spinster was a woman whom [sic] love had passed by, who had never "been chosen" for marriage or motherhood. As modern spinsters, however, we do our own choosing. We embrace romance and relationship, but with a consciousness of both the joys and the costs involved. We know that it's nice to wake up next to a warm man, but that the trade-offs are that he'll likely leave the toilet seat up and forget to pick up his underwear. We understand that the ideal and the reality of love must be taken together, and so we feel no impetus to radically change the men we become romantically involved with. And as permanent single people, we also do not invest energy in evaluating whether men are "marriage-material." This orientation gives us a power in relationships that is (sadly) not always accessed by our married (or marriage-minded) sisters.[12]

In a kind of Nietzschean reversal they say that it is the romantic who is cynical since they are on a hopeless quest and find most men lacking, failing to live up to their impossible dreams. In contrast the Bachelor Girl resists the hype and enjoys what she finds. She evades the trap of matrimony, with its impossible expectations and corresponding entrapment. Blogs and other Web sites carry on this tradition. T-shirts and other products express these anti-marriage sentiments, saying, "she's not the marrying kind," or opposing the matrimonial "I do" with a T-shirt saying, "I do not."[13] That "do not" is not a no to sex.

VOLUNTARY SPINSTER

In a recent work titled *Calling It Quits; Late-Life Divorce and Starting Over*, author Deirdre Bair writes of women voluntarily leaving marriages for no other reason than that they are unhappy and unfulfilled.[14] The older woman, a kind of Voluntary Spinster, does not define herself as single or divorced. In spite of the more common narrative of the older man divorcing his wife for a younger woman, research conducted by the AARP found that it is the older women who are leaving the men.[15] These are women whose children are grown and who now want more from life. In spite of the social and economic benefits of staying married, these women opt for a kind of voluntary spinsterhood, for freedom and a second chance.

The Voluntary Older Spinster can often be found in Fay Weldon's intelligent and subversive novels. The novel *Life Force*[16] is told from a number of female characters' points of view. The spinster, Marion, is described by one of her more conventional friends, Nora: "Marion Loos, spinster, art dealer, and gallery owner, is more Rosalie's friend than mine. She and I have of late rather lost touch, . . . I use the word 'spinster' of Marion advisedly: the nature, I suspect, predating the event, or rather lack of it. 'I am a spinster,' Marion will exclaim, 'and I am proud of it.' Don't avoid the word, she suggests: better to concentrate on making the state desirable, and so render the world acceptable. Well, bully for her. She likes her life to be an uphill battle. I don't."[17] Another friend of Marion's, Rosalie, comments on Nora's view: "I know what you're thinking, Nora, . . . You think any woman who doesn't have a husband and children is to be pitied. You're nuts."[18] Nora finds matrimony the easy way. Rosalie and especially Marion need to be persuaded that matrimony is such a great prize.

Leslie, whose aggressive male sexuality is the "life force" of the title, is ultimately rejected by Marion:

> "Leslie," Marion said, "I'm sorry. It was a sweet offer, but I really can't marry you. I don't think it would work. My life is so full as it is, I really can't fit anything more into it. You know how it is with businesswomen. Busy, busy, busy! I would drive you mad."

His response mirrors Nora's view of the unmarried woman's life:

> Leslie said bitterly to Marion, ". . . You'll be sorry. Don't think this offer will come again. You're an old hag and getting older by the day. Men last, women don't," and he went back home to Rothwell Gardens.[19]

Leslie's view of Marion, that she is useless and he is still valuable is mirrored in the Web ephemera. To go back to the online Urban Dictionary, a less popular entry[20] states that a spinster is "a woman who is old and not married. They are usually crazy and are just more proof that women NEED us men. Note: 'When men are old and not married it's stylish': the Trunchbull, from Roald Dahl's *Matilda*."[21] The older woman should be glad for a chance at marriage, not like the modern Marion, who is indifferent to it.

Bachelor v. Spinster

The other matter that contemporary blogs speak of is the centuries-old unfairness of the different ways bachelors and spinsters are viewed.[22] The value of monogamous heterosexuality and reproduction begs comparison between the spinster and the bachelor. As we consider heterosexuality and matrimony normative, one might assume that similar strictures should work against all the unmarried. The spinster and bachelor along with the divorced, homosexual, or lesbian fail equally in their prescribed sexual role, but their cultural standing is not equal. The suspicion surrounding these transgressors elides them with the most stigmatized groups, often the homosexuals. If the spinster and bachelor are equally transgressive, why are the implications of their status so different?

Spinster is still inanalogous to bachelor. Although the latter has the stigma of a possible deviant or homosexual, bachelor more commonly has the connotation of being the bon vivant, the playboy, the envy of the heterosexual male stuck in marriage and convention. The idea that the bachelor is sexually active and presumed to be even more active than the married heterosexual male contrasts with the presumptively asexual spinster. But as we have seen, is and was this really the case, is the single woman not sexual? These formulations go back to basic ideas of male sexuality as active and women's sexuality as passive. If this formulation, which goes back at least to Parmenides, is still in place, then it isn't surprising to find a persistent view of aggressive masculine sexuality and passive feminine receptivity. This then makes monsters of both the sexualized, and therefore predatory, female and the asexual one, who fails to fill her biological function of reproduction. We know these have been reinforced over centuries in writings of sexologists and psychoanalysts, to name but a few.

Bachelor, now used most generally for a young man and, more specifically, for one who is unmarried, was originally used for male and female persons. "The word bachelor, now confined to men in this connotation, was formerly sometimes used of women also."[23] The word is itself derived from a class-based concept. The Oxford dictionaries confirm this origin, *bachelor* always connoting the lowest rank whether in knights or university degrees.[24] "Throughout all its meanings the word has retained the idea of subordination suggested in this origin."[25] So the bachelor is inferior to the married man. But once bachelor is a gendered male, bachelor is less stigmatized than spinster.

The use of *bachelor* and *spinster* as complementary legal terms for those never married is fairly late. Since both of the terms go back to their British usage, it is worth noting that in 2005, in preparation for the December 5 Civil Partnership Act, the terms *bachelor* and *spinster* were removed from the language of registration in favor of the word *single* as a neutral descriptor. The contemporary press mourned the loss of the patriarchic discourse in different ways. The *UK Times Online*:

> The term spinster developed as a way of describing a woman who spins, but developed into the legal definition of an unmarried woman. The occupational description disappeared as the spinning trade died out in the industrial revolution. By the 18th century it had acquired derogatory connotations, synonymous with "old maid." Bachelor has always had more romantic associations. As well as referring to an unmarried man, it could also refer to a man aspiring to be a knight bachelor, or a man (and now woman) who had taken their first degree. Unlike spinster, the term also retained its association with youth, and unmarried men referred to as bachelors were invariably unmarried young men.[26]

William Safire refers to the "Spinster-Bachelor Breakup" in one of his "On Language" columns.[27] He fails to note the common gender-neutral origin for the two words, which were associated with fairly lowly ranks in both cases. *Bachelor*'s origin is obscure, but by this century it had a legal use as "an unmarried man." The European unmarried male as we noted has been subject to similar or analogous coercions meted out to the spinster; he was in turn deemed abnormal (suspected of homosexuality) and subject to taxation for his status and disrespect for convention. *Bachelor* can be used of a young man without negative connotation; it is especially used of an older bachelor whose life choices are questioned. He failed to produce an heir, did not do his duty to the state, and selfishly held on to his money and property.

The term *spinster* came into the printed language in 1362 and is, like many names, a relic of reference to occupation; in this case, a worker who spun wool into yarn. Not all such workers were women, although the occupation itself was occasionally protected to maintain lawful occupation for women.[28] In genealogy the expression *distaff side of the family* is the female line. The distaff around which yarn was wound was sometimes used as a symbol of women weavers, unmarried women, and witches; it is opposed to the spear or male line. Although *spinster* was a legal term appended to the name of a woman or man whose occupation was spinning, by the seventeenth century it came to refer to an as yet unmarried woman. Its meaning was further stigmatized by being related to ideas of women as unnecessary, as a burden when they exist outside their traditional occupation. Unmarried women put a financial strain on the brothers and fathers who must support them if they are not married. By the early twentieth century the European press described thousands of "Surplus Women" after World War I. Women were seen as surplus or unnecessary since there would be no one to marry them and no one with whom they could replenish the stock of Europe. One of the important differences between the modern spinster and her historical cousin is the argument from fulfilling her nature through reproduction.

PRESSURE TO MARRY

It is hard to talk about the spinster without considering normative heterosexual matrimony. It is against these well-known views that the spinster has both her positive and negative characteristics. Although people have occasionally scoffed at the idea of both compulsory heterosexuality and compulsory heterosexual marriage, we continue to find the desire to move women into the unpaid labor of marriage, into sexual availability, and into unpaid domestic service. That some women were very willing to escape this situation, even if its cost was celibacy, is interesting. In eras when women's sexuality was ignored, described out of existence, or out of her control, perhaps this cost was deemed as slight.

Women who questioned the felicity of marriage and have seen other dangers such as dying in childbirth, who viewed wedded bliss as undesirable, and who have voluntarily attempted to avoid the institution of marriage have been subject to various types of social control. Like the bachelor, she has been more heavily taxed than married persons. Attempts to push spinsters into marriage vary. They range from subtle coercion to referring to their unmarried state as unnatural or socially unacceptable, to being seen as unfulfilled without children or the authority of being the matriarch of a family. When speaking of African mores, Leon Clark observes that "[t]he rearing of a family brings with it a rise in social status. The social position of a married man and woman who have children is of greater importance and dignity than that of a bachelor or spinster." [29] The coercion in its extreme form involves a variety of forms of enforcement, sometimes using religious or even civil law to enforce matrimony. This is shown in an extreme form in colonial Ghana in the early twentieth century where "unmarried women, ages 15+, were ordered by chiefs to be married or suffer state detention." These women were imprisoned until they named someone they would marry. That man had to then bail them out of jail. "With the emergence of the cocoa trade, 1921–1935, women's roles in the cash economy began to change significantly, with more financial autonomy suddenly becoming possible. The resulting change in power relations between genders was characterized by officials as a moral crisis. The direct intervention of the state in marriage practices was a drastic attempt to reassert control over women's productive & reproductive labor." [30] Women's economic autonomy was resulting in them choosing not to marry. This was then dealt with by imprisonment.

In a paper on marriage in Malawi, Amy Kahler speaks of marriage as being romanticized and presented as deteriorating from an ideal past. [31] Presenting the institution of marriage as being in jeopardy is one way to socially control the domestic sphere in general and women in particular. Kahler discovers that not only was the institution far from its ideal state in the past, it was described as in danger then too. Thus, ideals of marriage, the married state's unquestioned value, and threats to marriage's stability have worked as a kind of social control in many cultures and at many times. Twenty-first-century America with its approximately 50 percent divorce rate is another case among many instances. Feminists have been active in pointing out the forces pushing us toward the desirability of marriage and a domestic career for women. "Compulsory Heterosexuality" and perhaps more importantly compulsory marriage have served to keep women's labor out of capital economies, political engagement, and have kept women in the dangerous and exhausting business of reproduction. In quoting from such diverse sources I don't mean to suggest that spinsterhood is the same in all parts of Africa, Britain, or in the United States, nor that *bachelor* has the same meaning. After this preliminary exploration it is clear that the situation of the unmarried woman (and man) would benefit by consideration in many contexts.

Old Maids
by Sandra Cisneros[32]

My cousins and I,
we don't marry.
We're too old
by Mexican standards.

And the relatives
have long suspected
we can't anymore
in white.

My cousins and I,
we're all old
maids at thirty.

Who won't dress children,
and never saints—
though we undress them.

The aunts,
they've given up on us.
No longer nudge—You're next.

Instead—
What happened in your childhood?
What left you all mean teens?
Who hurt you, honey?

But we've studied
marriages too long—

Aunt Ariadne,
Tia Vashti,
Comadre Penelope,
querida Malintzin,
Senora Pumpkin Shell—

lessons that served us well.

NOTES

1. The use of blogs to get a sense of contemporary pulse is fraught with problems. They are ephemeral. They are usually unedited; quoting them at length is often pointless. But they do give us a sense of what young women and men are saying about these issues.

2. These are mostly religious.

3. Dana Luciano, "Scouting for Queers," *GLQ: A Journal of Lesbian and Gay Studies* 11.2 (2005): 327–30. Copyright © 2005 Duke University Press.

4. Ibid., Adrienne Rich, "Compulsory Heterosexuality and Lesbian Existence," in *The Signs Reader: Women, Gender, & Scholarship*, eds. Elizabeth Abel and Emily K. Abel (Chicago: University of Chicago Press, 1983).

5. "Spinster War Diaries," http://spinsterwardiaries.blogspot.com/. She reads Sophie Kinsella—happy ending Chick Lit, http://spinsterchronicles.wordpress.com. "This blog (started 18.01.2007) is partly about my life as a thirty something spinster with its ups and downs, toughs and incidents."

6. http://www.hbo.com/city/cast/character/carrie_bradshaw.shtml   (accessed September 12, 2007).

7. Stacey Ballis Has a Blog She Writes for Amazon, http://www.amazon.com/gp/Blog/A2FOKS3JF6DNEF/ref=cm_Blog_dp_artist_Blog.

8. http://www.askaspinster.com/Spinster_Home.html (accessed September 12, 2007), "spin·ster spin: 1. (noun) the rationalization that the freak you're dating is really into you. 2. (verb) asking your girlfriends to help you rationalize the obnoxious, selfish, bizarre, and doltish behavior from the guy you're dating."

"Spin·ster straight: 1. (verb) when spinsters stop being nice and start being real. 2. (noun) the truth, the straight dope, what's up." (N.b., Their descriptions of themselves

"Back in their 20s, life and love seemed so hopeful. Now they're both in their mid [to late, ugh] 30s and still single. The facts are this: Both girls are total babes [and we're not just saying that because we're writing this—the pictures are recent!], extremely intelligent, successful, super fun, and would make any man and mother-in-law happy. So where did these girls go wrong? Sadly, the girls are hopeless romantics that always want to see the good in people—they hope against hope that the next date will be a really nice, cool guy." Sound familiar?)

9. http://celibateinthecity.blogspot.com.

10. Julie Johnsson, "Random Walk: Time for a New Spin on an Outmoded Term," *Crain's Chicago Business* (May 1999), http://findarticles.com/p/articles/mi_hb5253/ is_199905/ "spinster (spin´-ster) n. 1: an unmarried woman 2: an old maid 3: a single woman who owns property in Illinois. Single women face a nasty shock at real estate closings—even apart from the usual mortgage snafus and last-minute charges. As they sign the title to a mortgage or deed, many unmarried women learn that, in the eyes of the law, they are spinsters. "It's not a real flattering term," says Eileen Van Roeyen, regulatory counsel for Chicago Title & Trust Co. "You have the connotation that you have nothing better to do than spin wool, . . ."

11. http://www.urbandictionary.com/define.php?term=spinster (accessed September 12, 2007).

12. http://www.spinsterspin.com, a defunct Web site whose content is still accessible through Wikipedia and other Web-based sites.

13. http://www.cafepress.com/spinsterspin (accessed September 12, 2008).

14. Deirdre Bair, *Calling It Quits; Late-Life Divorce and Starting Over* (New York: Random House, 2007).

15. "The Divorce Experience: A Study of Divorce at Midlife and Beyond," *Research Report*, Xenia Montenegro, AARP Knowledge Management (May 2004), http://www .aarp.org/research/reference/publicopinions/aresearch-import-867.html (accessed September 12, 2007).

16. Fay Weldon's novel *Life Force* (New York: Viking, 1992).

17. Ibid., p. 11.

18. Ibid., p. 12.

19. Ibid., p. 211.

20. http://www.urbandictionary.com/define.php?term=spinster (accessed September 12, 2007), the vote was 69 up, 160 down.

21. Ibid.

22. http://spinsterchronicles.wordpress.com/2007/03/06/why-spinster-and -bachelor/ (accessed September 12, 2007), "Why Spinster and Bachelor?" Posted on March 6, 2007, by Raindreamer. "The English Language is more discriminating than other European languages. In most big European language one talks about either old or young boys and girls, while in English we speak about glam Bachelors and dry Spinsters. Meaning of both of bachelor and spinster have their origins in the practical historical world of Middle English time. Bachelor ment first just a knight-trainee and then trainee of any short of profession. Spinster ment of course a maid spinner, as it was a work of maids young and old as well. Later bachelor became a university term and I think that

short of glamoroush nature of the term relates the freedom of the life in university world. Bachelor is known in French vieux garçon, in German Junggeselle ja in Swedish ungkarl. Several latinic languages also talk about Celibates. Both kind of terms are more neutral than the English one, that is kind of dashing term. That does not necessary mean that the tone is any more sweeter. The stereotypes can be in the language areas as grimm as in English speaking countries. It seems that spinsters are everywhere seen kind of grim and sour, while batchelors are usually sweet and jovial, if not very outgoing and glamorous. Before this century there was great difference in situation. Women needed to strugle to support them selves and felt unfullfilled while not been fulfiling the role of the mother. Men did not have the similar problem. Their place in the society as workers and contributors was never due to maritial status. On the other hand the situation of unmarried mothers was even wortst than one of spinsters."[This excerpt is unedited]

"Old Maid vs Swinging Bachelor," *Notes from Venus*, http://www.notesfromvenus .com/Blog/?p=584 (accessed April 2, 2007), "Here are my pet peeves related to gender equality (or lack thereof):

1. What is the deal with the spinster/bachelor thing? Why is an unmarried woman a spinster while an unmarried man a 'swinging bachelor'?! The very word 'spinster' sounds sad, hopeless and somehow derogatory. Mention the word 'bachelor' and it's so relaxed and free. While we're on the subject, another term that is used to describe an unmarried woman is even worse than spinster and that's old maid.

2. It's just so perfectly ghastly! I have unwittingly played the card game that has the same name and shouted "old maid, old maid!" at the top of my lungs at some hapless victim who happened to have the 'Old Maid' card. Poor Old Maid, no one ever wanted her in the game and so it seems to be in life.

3. I don't know many single, older women who are embraced by society if they flaunt their freedom the way old bachelors do. Society assumes that an old bachelor chooses to remain single while an old spinster is only single because no man wanted to marry her. That is so unfair!"

23. http://www.1911encyclopedia.org/Bachelor.

24. The term *bachelor* is used as a legal status in some places; in the United Kingdom, for instance, until the introduction of the Civil Partnership Act in 2004 any never-married man was listed as a bachelor.

25. http://www.1911encyclopedia.org/Bachelor.

26. Ruth Gledhill, religion correspondent, "New Marriage Rules to Split with Spinster and Bachelor," *Times Online UK*, July 27, 2005, http://www.timesonline.co.uk/tol/news/uk/article548517.ece (accessed September 12, 2007).

27. William Safire, "On Language," *New York Times*, September 4, 2005.

28. ". . . forbade importation of silk and lace by Lombards and other alien strangers, imagining to destroy the craft of the silk spinsters and all such virtuous occupations for women." "Women," in the online 1911 *Encyclopedia Britannica*, http://www.1911 encyclopedia.org/Women (accessed September 12, 2007).

29. Leon Clark, *Through African Eyes* (New York: CITE, 2000), p. 141.

30. Jean Allman, "Rounding Up Spinsters: Gender Chaos and Unmarried Women in Colonial Asante," *Journal of African History* 37, no. 2 (1996): 195–214.

31. Amy Kahler, conference presentation, May 2007. Amy Kahler, "The Moral Lens of Population Control: Condoms and Controversies in Southern Malawi," paper presented at the annual meeting of the African Studies Association, Washington, DC, December 5–8, 2002.

32. Sandra Cisneros, "Old Maids," *Loose Woman* (New York: Knopf, 1994).

9.

MARITAL FAITHFULNESS

Susan Mendus

And so the two swore that at every time of their lives, until death took them, they would assuredly believe, feel and desire exactly as they had believed, felt and desired during the preceding weeks. What was as remarkable as the undertaking itself was the fact that nobody seemed at all surprised at what they swore.[1]

Cynicism about the propriety of the marriage promise has been widespread amongst philosophers and laymen alike for many years. Traditionally, the ground for suspicion has been the belief that the marriage promise is a promise about feelings where these are not directly under the control of the will. G. E. Moore gives expression to this view when he remarks that "to love certain people, or to feel no anger against them, is a thing which it is quite impossible to attain directly by the will" and concludes therefore that the commandment to love your neighbor as yourself cannot possibly be a statement of your duty, "all that can possibly be true is that it would be your duty if you were able."[2] Thus, as Mary Midgley has pointed out, Moore invests the commandment with "about as much interest for us as a keep-fit manual would have for paraplegics."[3] Moore's sentiments would presumably be endorsed by Russell, who tells of how

Philosophy: The Journal of the British Institute of Philosophical Studies 59 (1984): 243–52. By permission of the *Journal* and Dr. Susan Mendus.

his love for his wife "evaporated" during the course of a bicycle ride. He simply "realized," he says, that he no longer loved her and was subsequently unable to show any affection for her.[4] This, anyway, is the most familiar objection to the marriage promise: that it is a promise about feelings, where these are not directly under the control of the will.

A second objection to the marriage promise is that it involves a commitment which extends over too long a period: promising to do something next Wednesday is one thing, promising to do something fifty years hence is quite another, and it is thought to be improper either to give or to extract promises extending over such a long period of time. This second objection has found recent philosophical favor in the writings of Derek Parfit. In "Later Selves and Moral Principles" Parfit refers to those who believe that only short-term promises can carry moral weight and counts it virtue of his theory of personal identity that it "supports" or "helps to explain" that belief.[5]

Here I shall not discuss Parfit's theory of personal identity as such, but only the plausibility of the consequent claim that short-term promises alone carry moral weight: for it is the supposed intuitive plausibility of the latter which Parfit appeals to in defense of his theory of personal identity. If, therefore, the belief that only short-term promises carry moral weight can be undermined, that will serve, indirectly, to undermine any theory of personal identity which supports it.

Claiming that long-term promises do not carry any moral weight seems to be another way of claiming that unconditional promises do not carry any moral weight. Such an unconditional promise is the promise made in marriage, for when I promise to love and to honor I do not mutter under my breath, "So long as you never become a member of the Conservative party," or "Only if your principles do not change radically." Parfit's suggestion seems to be that all promises (all promises which carry any moral weight, that is) are, and can be, made only on condition that there is no substantial change in the character either of promisor or promisee: if my husband's character changes radically, then I may think of the man before me not as my husband, but as some other person, some "later self." Similarly, it would seem that I cannot now promise to love another "till death us do part," since that would be like promising that another person will do something (in circumstances in which my character changes fundamentally over a period of time) and I cannot promise that another person will do something, but only that I will do something. Thus all promises must be conditional; all promises must be short-term. For what it is worth, I am not the least tempted to think that only short-term promises carry any moral weight and it is therefore a positive *disadvantage* for me that Parfit's theory has this consequence. But even if it were intuitively plausible that short-term promises alone carry moral weight, there are better arguments than intuitive ones and I hope I can mention some here.

The force of Parfit's argument is brought out by his "Russian nobleman" example, described in "Later Selves and Moral Principles":

Imagine a Russian nobleman who, in several years, will inherit vast estates. Because he has socialist ideals, he intends now to give the land to the peasants, but he knows that in time his ideals may fade. To guard against this possibility he does two things. He first signs a legal document, which will automatically give away the land and which can only be revoked with his wife's consent. He then says to his wife, "If I ever change my mind and ask you to revoke the document, promise me that you will not consent." He might add, "I regard my ideals as essential to me. If I lose these ideals I want you to think that I cease to exist. I want you to think of your husband then, not as me, but only as his later self. Promise me that you would not do as he asks."[6]

Parfit now comments:

This plea seems understandable and if his wife made this promise and he later asked her to revoke the document she might well regard herself as in no way released from her commitment. It might seem to her as if she had obligations to two different people. She might think that to do what her husband now asks would be to betray the young man whom she loved and married. And she might regard what her husband now says as unable to acquit her of disloyalty to this young man—to her husband's earlier self. [Suppose] the man's ideals fade and he asks his wife to revoke the document. Though she promised him to refuse, he now says that he releases her from this commitment . . . we can suppose she shares our view of commitment. If so, she will only believe that her husband is unable to release her from the commitment if she thinks that it is in some sense not *he* to whom she is committed is. . . . She may regard the young man's loss of ideals as involving replacement by a later self.[7]

Now, strictly speaking, and on Parfit's own account, the wife should not make such a promise: to do so would be like promising that another person will do something, since she has no guarantee that she will not change in character and ideals between now and the time of the inheritance. Further, there is a real question as to why anyone outside of a philosophical example should first draw up a document which can only be revoked with his wife's consent and then insist that his wife not consent whatever may happen. But we can let these points pass. What is important here, and what I wish to concentrate on, is the suggestion that my love for my husband is conditional upon his not changing in any substantial way: for this is what the example amounts to when stripped of its special story about later selves. (In his less extravagant moods Parfit himself allows that talk of later selves is, in any case, a mere "*façon de parler.*")[8]

The claim then is that all promises must be conditional upon there being no change in the character of the promisee: that if my husband's character and ideals change it is proper for me to look upon him as someone other than the person I loved and married. This view gains plausibility from reflection on the fact that people can, and often do, give up their commitments. There is, it will be said, such an institution as divorce, and people do sometimes avail themselves of it. But although I might give up my commitment to my husband, and give as my reason a change in his character and principles, this goes no way towards showing that only short-term promises carry any moral weight, for there is a vital distinction here: the distinction between, on the one hand, the person who promises to love and to honor but who finds that, after a time, she has lost her commitment (perhaps on account of change in her husband's character), and, on the other hand, the person who promises to love and to honor only on condition that there be no such change in character. The former person may properly be said, under certain circumstances, to have given up a commitment; the latter person was never committed in the appropriate way at all. The wife of the Russian nobleman, by allowing in advance that she will love her husband only so long as he doesn't change in any of the aforementioned ways, fails properly to commit herself to him: for now her attitude to him seems to be one of respect or admiration, not commitment at all. Now she *does* mutter under her breath, "So long as you don't become a member of the Conservative party." But the marriage promise contains no such "escape clause." When Mrs. Micawber staunchly declares that she will never desert Mr. Micawber, she means just that. There are no conditions, nor could there be any, for otherwise we would fail to distinguish between respect or admiration *for the principles* of another and the sort of unconditional commitment *to him* which the marriage vow involves. There are many people whose ideals and principles I respect, and that respect would disappear were the ideals and principles to disappear, but my commitment to my husband is distinct from mere respect or admiration in just this sense, that it is not conditional on there being no change in his ideals and principles. I am now prepared to admit that my respect for another person would disappear were he revealed to be a cheat and a liar. I am not now prepared to admit that my love for my husband, my commitment to him, would disappear were he revealed to be a cheat and a liar. Perhaps an analogy will be illuminating here: in his article "Knowledge and Belief," Norman Malcolm distinguishes between a strong and a weak sense of "know" and says:

> In an actual case of my using "know" in a strong sense I cannot envisage a possibility that what I say should turn out to be not true. If I were speaking of another person's assertion about something I *could* think both that he is using "know" in a strong sense and that none the less what he claims he knows to be

so might turn out to be not so. But in my own case I cannot have this conjunction of thoughts, and this is a logical, not a psychological fact. When I say that I know, using "know" in the strong sense, it is unintelligible to me (although perhaps not to others) to suppose that anything could prove that it is not so and therefore that I do not know it.[9]

Such is the case with commitment of the sort involved in the marriage vow. I promise to love and to honor and in so doing I cannot now envisage anything happening such as would make me give up that commitment. But, it might be asked, how can I be clairvoyant? How can I recognize that there is such a thing as divorce and at the same time declare that nothing will result in my giving up my commitment? The explanation lies in the denial that my claim to know (in the strong sense) or commitment (here) has the status of a prediction. My commitment to another should not be construed as a prediction that I will never desert that other. Malcolm again: "The assertion describes my present attitude towards the statement . . . it does not prophesy what my attitude would be if various things happened."[10] But if my statement is not a prediction, then what is it? It is perhaps more like a statement of intention, where my claims about a man's intentions do not relate to his future actions in as simple a way as do my predictions about his future actions.

If I predict that A will do x and A does not do x, then my prediction is simply false. If, on the other hand, if I claim that A intends to do x and he does not, it is not necessarily the case that my statement was false: for he may have had that intention and later withdrawn it. Similarly with commitment: if I claim that A is unconditionally committed to B, that is not a prediction that A will never desert B, it is a claim that there is in A a present intention to do something permanently, where that is distinct from A's having a permanent intention. Thus Mrs. Micawber's claim that she will never desert Mr. Micawber, if construed as a commitment to him, is to that extent different from a prediction that she will never desert him, for her commitment need not be thought never to have existed if she does desert him. Thus an unconditional commitment to another person today, a denial today that anything could happen such as would result in desertion of Mr. Micawber, is not incompatible with that commitment being given up at a later date.

In brief, then, what is wrong in Parfit's example is that the wife *now* allows that her commitment will endure only so long as there is no substantial change in character. She should not behave thus, because her doing so indicates that she has only respect for her husband, or admiration for his principles, not a commitment to him: she need not behave thus, as there can be such a thing as unconditional commitment, analogous to intention and distinct from prediction in the way described.

All this points to the inherent oddity of the "trial marriage." It is bizarre to respond to "wilt thou love her, comfort her, honor her and keep her?" with "Well, I'll try." Again, the response "I will" must be seen as the expression of an intention to do something permanently, not a prediction that the speaker will permanently have that intention.

A further problem with the Russian nobleman example and the claim that only short-term promises carry any moral weight is this: when the wife of the Russian nobleman allows in advance that her commitment to her husband will cease should his principles change in any substantial way, she implies that a list of his present principles and ideals will give an exhaustive explanation of her loving him. But this is not good enough. If I now claim to be committed to my husband I precisely cannot give an exhaustive account of the characteristics he possesses in virtue of which I have that commitment to him: if I could do so, there would be a real question as to why I am not prepared to show the same commitment to another person who shares those characteristics (his twin brother, for example). Does this then mean that nothing fully explains my love for another and that commitment of this sort is irrationally based? I think we need not go so far as to say that: certainly, when asked to justify or explain my love I may point to certain qualities which the other person has, or which I believe him to have, but in the first place such an enumeration of qualities will not provide a complete account of why I love him, rather it will serve to explain, as it were, his "lovableness." It will make more intelligible my loving him, but will not itself amount to a complete and exhaustive explanation of my loving him. Further, it may well be that in giving my list of characteristics I cite some which the other person does not, in fact, have. If this is so, then the explanation may proceed in reverse order: the characteristics I cite will not explain or make intelligible my love, rather my love will explain my ascribing these characteristics. A case in point here is Dorothea's love for Casaubon, which is irrationally based in that Casaubon does not have the characteristics and qualities which Dorothea thinks him to have. Similarly, in the case of infatuation the lover's error lies in wrongly evaluating the qualities of the beloved. In this way Titania "madly dotes" on the unfortunate Bottom, who is trapped in an ass's head, and addresses him thus:

> Come sit thee down upon this flowery bed
> While I thy amiable cheeks do coy
> And stick musk roses in thy sleek, smooth head
> And kiss thy fair, large ears my gentle joy.

And again:

I pray thee, gentle mortal, sing again.
Mine ear is much enamored of thy note;
So is mine eye enthralled to thy shape,
And thy fair virtue's force perforce doth move me
On the first view, to say, to swear, I love thee.[11]

Both cases involve some error on the part of the lover: in one case the error is false belief about the qualities the beloved possesses; in the other it is an error about the evaluation of the qualities the beloved possesses. These two combine to show that there can be such a thing as a "proper object" of love. This will be the case where there is neither false belief nor faulty evaluation. They do not, however, show that in ascribing qualities and characteristics to the beloved the lover exhaustively explains and accounts for his love. The distinction between "proper" love and irrationally based love, or between "proper" love and infatuation, is to be drawn in terms of the correctness of beliefs and belief-based evaluations. By contrast, the distinction between love and respect or admiration is to be drawn in terms of the explanatory power of the beliefs involved. In the case of respect or admiration the explanatory power of belief will be much greater than it is in the case of love. For this reason my respect for John's command of modal logic will disappear, and I am now prepared to admit that it will disappear, should I discover that my belief that he has a command of modal logic is false. Whereas I am not now prepared to admit that my commitment to and love for my husband will disappear if I discover that my beliefs about his qualities and characteristics are, to some extent, false.

W. Newton-Smith makes something like this point in his article "A Conceptual Investigation of Love":

> Concern and commitment cannot be terminated by some change in or revelation about the object of that concern or commitment. We are inclined to accept "I felt affection for her so long as I thought she was pure and innocent" but not "I was really concerned for her welfare as long as I thought she was pure and innocent." Being genuinely concerned or committed seems to involve a willingness on my part to extend that concern or commitment even if I have been mistaken about the person with regard to some feature of her that led to the concern, and even if that person ceases to have those features which led me to be concerned or committed in the first place.[12]

This, though initially plausible, cannot be quite right, for on Newton-Smith's analysis it is difficult to see how I could ever give up a commitment without it being the case that I never was committed in the first place. But we can and do distinguish between those who had a commitment and have now given it up and those who never had a commitment at all. We need not, I think, go so far as to say that "love is not love which alters when it alteration finds," but only that love is not love which allows in advance that it will so alter. The love which shows that it will alter when it alteration finds is at best sentimentality, at worst opportunism. (Of course, the reasons which one cites for giving up a commitment will cast light on whether one was committed at all. Thus "I was committed to her as long as I thought she was an heiress" is highly dubious. "I was committed to her as long as I thought she was pure and innocent" is, I think, not so dubious.) What is at least necessary is that one should not be prepared to say *now* "I will love her as long as she is pure and innocent, but no longer."

I turn now to a somewhat bizarre element in Parfit's talk of ideals. Parfit portrays the Russian nobleman as one who "finds" that his ideals have faded, as one who "loses" his ideals when circumstances and fortune change. What is bizarre in this talk is emphasized by the following extract from Alison Lurie's novel *Love and Friendship*:

> "But, Will, promise me something."
>   "Sure."
>   "Promise me you'll never be unfaithful to me."
>   Silence.
>   Emily raised her head. "You won't promise?" she said incredulously.
>   "I can't, Emily. How can I promise how I'll feel for the next ten years? You want me to lie to you? You could change. I could change. I could meet somebody."
>   Emily pulled away. "Don't you have any principles?" she asked.[13]

The trouble with the inappropriately named Will and the Russian nobleman in Parfit's example is that it is doubtful whether either man has any genuine principles at all. Each is portrayed as almost infinitely malleable, as one whose principles will alter in accordance with changing circumstances. The point about a moral principle however is that it must serve in some sense to rule out certain options as options at all. In his article "Actions and Consequences," John Casey refers us to the example of Addison's Cato who, when offered life, liberty and the friendship of Caesar if he will surrender, and is asked to name his terms, replies:

> Bid him disband his legions,
> Restore the Commonwealth to liberty,
> Submit his actions to the public censure
> And stand the judgment of a Roman Senate.
> Bid him do this and Cato is his friend.[14]

The genuine principles which Cato has determine that certain options will not ultimately be options at all for him. To say this, of course, is not to deny that life and liberty are attractive and desirable to him. Obviously he is, in large part, admirable precisely because they are attractive to him and yet he manages to resist their allure. The point is rather that not *any* sort of life is desirable. The sort of life he would, of necessity, lead after surrender—a life without honor—is not ultimately attractive to him and that it is not attractive is something which springs from his having the principles he does have. What Cato values above all else is honor and his refusal to surrender to Caesar is a refusal to lead a life without honor. By contrast, when the Russian nobleman draws up a legal document giving away his inheritance, we may suspect that he is concerned not with an honorable life or with a life which he now conceives of as honorable, but rather with his present principle. Where Cato values a certain sort of life, the Russian nobleman values a certain principle. It is this which is problematic and which generates, I believe, the bizarre talk of ideals fading. For Cato's adherence to his principles is strengthened, if not guaranteed, by the fact that he treats a certain sort of life as an end in itself and adopts the principles he does adopt because they lead to that end. The Russian nobleman, however, is portrayed more as a man who finds the principle important than as a man who finds the life to which the principle leads important. Obviously, in either case there may be temptation and inner struggle, but the temptation is less likely to be resisted by the Russian nobleman than by Cato, for the nobleman will find his principle undermined and threatened by the prospect of affluence, which is attractive to him. His ideals will fade. For Cato, on the other hand, things are not so simple. He is not faced by a choice between two things, each of which he finds attractive. The fact that he treats a life of honor as an end in itself precludes his finding life attractive under *any* circumstances. For him, life will ultimately be attractive and desirable only where it can be conducted honorably. Nevertheless, he finds life attractive and desirable, but this means only that if he surrenders he will have *sacrificed* his ideals, not that his ideals will have faded. Thus, the nobleman is a victim, waiting for and guarding against attack upon his principles; Cato is an agent who may sacrifice his principles after a struggle, but not one who would find that they had altered.

In conclusion, then, the claim that the marriage vow is either impossible or improper is false. It is possible to commit oneself unconditionally because commitment is analogous to a statement of intention, not to a prediction or a piece of clairvoyance. It is proper, since if we refuse to allow such unconditional commitment, we run the risk of failing to distinguish between, on the one hand, sentimentality and commitment and, on the other hand, respect or admiration and commitment. Further, it is simply not true that I am helpless in circumstances in which I find my commitment wavering: this is because my principles will initially serve to modify my view of the opportunities which present themselves, so that I simply will not see certain things as constituting success because my principles are such as to exclude such things being constitutive of success. In this way, my principles determine what is to count as a benefit and what is to count as an opportunity. As Shakespeare has it:

> Some glory in their birth, some in their skill,
> Some in their wealth, some in their body's force,
> Some in their garments though new fangled ill:
> Some in their hawks and hounds, some in their horse.
> And every humour has his adjunct pleasure,
> Wherein it finds a joy above the rest,
> But these particulars are not my measure,
> All these I better in one general best.
> Thy love is better than high birth to me,
> Richer than wealth, prouder than garments cost,
> Of more delight than hawks and horses be:
> And having these of all men's pride I boast.
> Wretched in this alone, that thou may'st take
> All this away, and me most wretched make.[15,16]

NOTES

1. Thomas Hardy, *Jude the Obscure.*

2. G. E. Moore, "The Nature of Moral Philosophy," in *Philosophical Studies* (London: Routledge and Kegan Paul, 1922), p. 316.

3. Mary Midgley, "The Objection to Systematic Humbug," *Philosophy* 53 (1978): 147.

4. Bertrand Russell, *Autobiography* (London: George Allen and Unwin, 1967–69).

5. Derek Parfit, "Later Selves and Moral Principles," in *Philosophy and Personal Relations*, A. Montefiore, ed. (London: Routledge and Kegan Paul, 1973), p. 144.

6. Ibid., p. 145.

7. Ibid., pp. 145–46.

8. Ibid., pp. 14, 161–62.

9. Norman Malcolm, "Knowledge and Belief," in *Knowledge and Belief*, A. Phillips Griffiths, ed. (Oxford University Press, 1967), p. 81.

10. Ibid., p. 78.

11. W. Shakespeare, *A Midsummer Night's Dream*, Acts III and I.

12. W. Newton-Smith, "A Conceptual Investigation of Love," in *Philosophy and Personal Relations*, pp. 132–33.

13. Alison Lurie, *Love and Friendship* (Harmondsworth: Penguin, 1962), pp. 329–30.

14. As quoted in J. Casey, "Actions and Consequences," from *Morality and Moral Reasoning*, J. Casey, ed. (London: Methuen, 1971), p. 201.

15. W. Shakespeare, Sonnet 91.

16. I wish to thank my colleague, Dr. Roger Woolhouse, for many helpful discussions on the topic of this paper.

10.

IS ADULTERY IMMORAL?

Richard Wasserstrom

Many discussions of the enforcement of morality by the law take as illustrative of the problem under consideration the regulation of various types of sexual behavior by the criminal law. It was, for example, the Wolfenden Report's recommendations concerning homosexuality and prostitution that led Lord Devlin to compose his now famous lecture "The Enforcement of Morals." And that lecture in turn provoked important philosophical responses from H. L. A. Hart, Ronald Dworkin, and others.

Much, if not all, of the recent philosophical literature on the enforcement of morals appears to take for granted the immorality of the sexual behavior in question. The focus of discussion, at least, is on whether such things as homosexuality, prostitution, and adultery ought to be made illegal even if they are immoral, and not on whether they are immoral.

I propose in this paper to consider the latter, more neglected topic, that of sexual morality, and to do so in the following fashion. I shall consider just one kind of behavior that is often taken to be a case of sexual immorality—adultery. I am interested in pursuing at least two questions. First, I want to explore the question of in what respects adulterous behavior falls within the domain of

Reprinted from Richard Wasserstrom, ed., *Today's Moral Problems* (New York: Macmillan Co., 1975), with the permission of the author.

morality at all, for this surely is one of the puzzles one encounters when considering the topic of sexual morality. It is often hard to see on what grounds much of the behavior is deemed to be either moral or immoral, for example, private homosexual behavior between consenting adults. I have purposely selected adultery because it seems a more plausible candidate for moral assessment than many other kinds of sexual behavior.

The second question I want to examine is that of what is to be said about adultery if we are not especially concerned to stay within the area of its morality. I shall endeavor, in other words, to identify and to assess a number of the major arguments that might be advanced against adultery. I believe that they are the chief arguments that would be given in support of the view that adultery is immoral, but I think they are worth considering even if some of them turn out to be nonmoral arguments and considerations.

A number of the issues involved seem to me to be complicated and difficult. In a number of places I have at best indicated where further philosophical exploration is required, without having successfully conducted the exploration myself. This essay may very well be more useful as an illustration of how one might begin to think about the subject of sexual morality than as an elucidation of important truths about the topic.

Before I turn to the arguments themselves, there are two preliminary points that require some clarification. Throughout the paper I shall refer to the immorality of such things as breaking a promise, deceiving someone, and so on. In a very rough way I mean by this that there is something morally wrong in doing the action in question. I mean that the action is, in a strong sense of "prima facie," prima facie wrong or unjustified. I do not mean that it may never be right or justifiable to do the action just that the fact that it is an action of this description always counts against the rightness of the action. I leave entirely open the question of what it is that makes actions of this kind immoral in this sense of "immoral."

The second preliminary point concerns what is meant or implied by the concept of adultery. I mean by "adultery" any case of extramarital sex, and I want to explore the arguments for and against extramarital sex, undertaken in a variety of morally relevant situations. Someone might claim that the concept of adultery is conceptually connected with the concept of immorality and that to characterize behavior as adulterous is already to characterize it as immoral or unjustified in the sense described above. There may be something to this. Hence the importance of making it clear that I want to discuss extramarital sexual relations. If they are always immoral, this is something that must be shown by argument. If the concept of adultery does in some sense entail or imply immorality, I want to ask whether that connection is a rationally based one. If not all cases of extramarital sex are immoral (again, in the sense described above), then the concept of adultery should either be weakened accordingly or restricted to those classes of extramarital sex for which the predication of immorality is warranted.

One argument for the immorality of adultery might go something like this: What makes adultery immoral is that it involves the breaking of a promise, and what makes adultery seriously wrong is that it involves the breaking of an important promise. For, so the argument might continue, one of the things the two parties promise each other when they get married is that they will abstain from sexual relationships with third parties. Because of this promise both spouses quite reasonably entertain the expectation that the other will behave in conformity with it. Hence, when one of them has sexual intercourse with a third party, he or she breaks that promise about sexual relationships that was made when the marriage was entered into and defeats the reasonable expectations of exclusivity entertained by the spouse.

In many cases the immorality involved in breaching the promise relating to extramarital sex may be a good deal more serious than that involved in the breach of other promises. This is so because adherence to this promise may be of much greater importance to them than is adherence to many of the other promises given or received by them in their lifetime. The breaking of this promise may be much more hurtful and painful than is typically the case.

Why is this so? To begin with, it may have been difficult for the nonadulterous spouse to have kept the promise. Hence that spouse may feel the unfairness of having restrained himself or herself in the absence of reciprocal restraint having been exercised by the adulterous spouse. In addition, the spouse may perceive the breaking of the promise as an indication of a kind of indifference on the part of the adulterous spouse. "If you really cared about me and my feelings," the spouse might say, "you would not have done this to me." And third, and related to the above, the spouse may see the act of sexual intercourse with another as a sign of affection for the other person and as an additional rejection of the nonadulterous spouse as the one who is loved by the adulterous spouse. It is not just that the adulterous spouse does not take the feelings of the nonadulterous spouse sufficiently into account; the adulterous spouse also indicates through the act of adultery affection for someone other than the nonadulterous spouse. I will return to these points later. For the present it is sufficient to note that a set of arguments can be developed in support of the proposition that certain kinds of adultery are wrong just because they involve the breach of a serious promise that, among other things, leads to the intentional infliction of substantial pain on one spouse by the other.

Another argument for the immorality of adultery focuses not on the existence of a promise of sexual exclusivity but on the connection between adultery and deception. According to this argument adultery involves deception. And because deception is wrong, so is adultery.

Although it is certainly not obviously so, I shall simply assume in this essay that deception is always immoral. Thus, the crucial issue for my purposes is the asserted connection between extramarital sex and deception. Is it plausible to maintain, as this argument does, that adultery always involves deception and is, on that basis, to be condemned?

The most obvious person upon whom deceptions might be practiced is the nonparticipating spouse; and the most obvious thing about which the nonparticipating spouse can be deceived is the existence of the adulterous act. One clear case of deception is that of lying. Instead of saying that the afternoon was spent in bed with A, the adulterous spouse asserts that it was spent in the library with B or on the golf course with C.

There can also be deception even when no lies are told. Suppose, for instance, that a person has sexual intercourse with someone other than his or her spouse and just does not tell the spouse about it. Is that deception? It may not be a case of lying if, for example, he or she is never asked by the spouse about the situation. Still, we might say, it is surely deceptive because of the promises that were exchanged at marriage. As we saw earlier, these promises provide a foundation for the reasonable belief that neither spouse will engage in sexual relationships with any other person. Hence the failure to bring the fact of extramarital sex to the attention of the other spouse deceives that spouse about the present state of the marital relationship.

Adultery, in other words, can involve both active and passive deception. An adulterous spouse may just keep silent or, as is often the case, the spouse may engage in an increasingly complex way of life devoted to the concealment of the facts from the nonparticipating spouse. Lies, half-truths, clandestine meetings, and the like may become a central feature of the adulterous spouse's existence. These are things that can and do happen, and when they do they make the case against adultery an easy one. Still, neither active nor passive deception is inevitably a feature of an extramarital relationship.

It is possible, though, that a more subtle but pervasive kind of deceptiveness is a feature of adultery. It comes about because of the connection in our culture between sexual intimacy and certain feelings of love and affection. The point can be made indirectly by seeing that one way in which we can in our culture mark off our close friends from our mere acquaintances is through the kinds of intimacies that we are prepared to share with them. I may, for instance, be willing to reveal my very private thoughts and emotions to my closest friends or to my wife but to no one else. My sharing of these intimate facts about myself is, from one perspective, a way of making a gift to those who mean the most to me. Revealing these things and sharing them with those who mean the most to me is one means by which I create, maintain, and confirm those interpersonal relationships that are of most importance to me.

In our culture, it might be claimed, sexual intimacy is one of the chief currencies through which gifts of this sort are exchanged. One way to tell someone—particularly someone of the opposite sex—that you have feelings of affection and love for them is by allowing them, or sharing with them, sexual behaviors that one does not share with others. This way of measuring affection was certainly very much a part of the culture in which I matured. It worked something like this: If you were a girl, you showed how much you liked a boy by the degree of sexual intimacy you would allow. If you liked him only a little you never did more than kiss—and even the kiss was not very passionate. If you liked him a lot and if your feeling was reciprocated, necking and, possibly, petting were permissible. If the attachment was still stronger and you thought it might even become a permanent relationship, the sexual activity was correspondingly more intense and intimate, although whether it led to sexual intercourse depended on whether the parties (particularly the girl) accepted fully the prohibition on non-marital sex. The situation for the boys was related but not exactly the same. The assumption was that males did not naturally link sex with affection in the way in which females did. However, since women did link sex with affection, males had to take that fact into account. That is to say, because a woman would permit sexual intimacies only if she had feelings of affection for the male and only if those feelings were reciprocated, the male had to have and express those feelings too, before sexual intimacies of any sort would occur.

The result was that the importance of a correlation between sexual intimacy and feelings of love and affection was taught by the culture and assimilated by those growing up in the culture. The scale of possible positive feelings toward persons of the other sex ran from casual liking, at one end, to the love that was deemed essential to, and characteristic of, marriage, at the other. The scale of possible sexual behavior ran from brief, passionless kissing or hand-holding, at one end, to sexual intercourse, at the other. And the correlation between the two scales was quite precise. As a result, any act of sexual intimacy carried substantial meaning with it, and no act of sexual intimacy was simply a pleasurable set of bodily sensations. Many such acts were, of course, more pleasurable to the participants because they were a way of saying what their feelings were. And sometimes they were less pleasurable for the same reason. The point is, however, that sexual activity was much more than mere bodily enjoyment. It was not like eating a good meal, listening to good music, lying in the sun, or getting a pleasant back rub. It was behavior that meant a great deal concerning one's feelings for persons of the opposite sex in whom one was most interested and with whom one was most involved. It was among the most authoritative ways in which one could communicate to another the nature and degree of one's affection.

If this sketch is even roughly right, then several things become somewhat clearer. To begin with, a possible rationale for many of the rules of conventional sexual morality can be developed. If, for example, sexual intercourse is associated with the kind of affection and commitment to another that is regarded as characteristic of the marriage relationship, then it is natural that sexual intercourse should be thought properly to take place between persons who are married to each other. And if it is thought that this kind of affection and commitment is only to be found within the marriage relationship, then it is not surprising that sexual intercourse should only be thought to be proper within marriage.

Related to what has just been said is the idea that sexual intercourse ought to be restricted to those who are married to each other, as a means by which to confirm the very special feelings that the spouses have for each other. Because our culture teaches that sexual intercourse means that the strongest of all feelings for each other are shared by the lovers, it is natural that persons who are married to each other should be able to say this to each other in this way. Revealing and confirming verbally that these feelings are present is one thing that helps to sustain the relationship; engaging in sexual intercourse is another.

In addition, this account would help to provide a framework within which to make sense of the notion that some sex is better than other sex. As I indicated earlier, the fact that sexual intimacy can be meaningful in the sense described tends to make it also the case that sexual intercourse can sometimes be more enjoyable than at other times. On this view, sexual intercourse will typically be more enjoyable if strong feelings of affection are present than it will be if it is merely "mechanical." This is so in part because people enjoy being loved, especially by those whom they love. Just as we like to hear words of affection, so we like to receive affectionate behavior. And the meaning enhances the independently pleasurable behavior.

More to the point, an additional rationale for the prohibition on extramarital sex can now be developed. For given this way of viewing the sexual world, extramarital sex will almost always involve deception of a deeper sort. If the adulterous spouse does not in fact have the appropriate feelings of affection for the extramarital partner, then the adulterous spouse is deceiving that person about the presence of such feelings. If, on the other hand, the adulterous spouse does have the corresponding feelings for the extramarital partner but not toward the nonparticipating spouse, the adulterous spouse is very probably deceiving the nonparticipating spouse about the presence of such feelings toward that spouse. Indeed, it might be argued, whenever there is no longer love between the two persons who are married to each other, there is deception just because being married implies both to the participants and to the world that such a bond exists. Deception is inevitable, the argument might conclude, because the feelings of affection that ought to accompany any act of sexual intercourse can only be held toward one other person at any given time in one's life. And if this is so, then the adulterous spouse always deceives either the partner in adultery or the nonparticipating spouse about the existence of such feelings. Thus, extramarital sex involves deception of this sort and is for that reason immoral, even if no deception vis-à-vis the occurrence of the act of adultery takes place.

What might be said in response to the foregoing arguments? The first thing that might be said is that the account of the connection between sexual intimacy and feelings of affection is inaccurate—not in the sense that no one thinks of things that way but in the sense that there is substantially more divergence of opinion than the account suggests. For example, the view I have delineated may describe reasonably accurately the concepts of the sexual world in which I grew up, but it does not capture the sexual *Weltanschauung* of today's youth at all. Thus, whether or not adultery implies deception in respect to feelings depends very much on the persons who are involved and the way they look at the "meaning" of sexual intimacy.

Second, the argument leaves unanswered the question of whether it is desirable for sexual intimacy to carry the sorts of messages described above. For those persons for whom sex does have these implications there are special feelings and sensibilities that must be taken into account. But it is another question entirely whether any valuable end—moral or otherwise—is served by investing sexual behavior with such significance. That is something that must be shown and not just assumed. It might, for instance, be the case that substantially more good than harm would come from a kind of demystification of sexual behavior—one that would encourage the enjoyment of sex more for its own sake and one that would reject the centrality both of the association of sex with love and of love with only one other person.

I regard these as two of the more difficult unresolved issues that our culture faces today in respect of thinking sensibly about the attitudes toward sex and love that we should try to develop in ourselves and in our children.

Much of the contemporary literature that advocates sexual liberation of one sort or another embraces one or the other of two different views about the relationship between sex and love. One view holds that sex should be separated from love and affection. To be sure, sex is probably better when the partners genuinely like and enjoy being with each other. But sex is basically an intensive, exciting, sensuous activity that can be enjoyed in a variety of suitable settings with a variety of suitable partners. The situation in respect to sexual pleasure is no different from that of the person who knows and appreciates fine food and who can have a satisfying meal in any number of good restaurants with any number of congenial companions. One question that must be settled here is whether sex can be thus demystified; another, more important, question is whether it would be desirable to do so. What might we gain and what might we lose if we all lived in a world in which an act of sexual intercourse was no more or less significant or enjoyable than having a delicious meal in a nice setting with a good friend? The answer to this question lies beyond the scope of this essay.

The second view of the relationship between sex and love seeks to drive the wedge in a different place. On this view it is not the link between sex and love that needs to be broken, but rather the connection between love and exclusivity. For a number of the reasons already given it is desirable, so this argument goes, that sexual intimacy continue to be reserved to and shared with only those for whom one has very great affection. The mistake lies in thinking that any "normal" adult will have those feelings toward only one other adult during his or her lifetime—or even at any time in his or her life. It is the concept of adult love, not ideas about sex that needs demystification. What are thought to be both unrealistic and unfortunate are the notions of exclusivity and possessiveness that attach to the dominant conception of love between adults in our culture and others. Parents of four, five, six, or even ten children can certainly claim, and sometimes claim correctly, that they love all of their children, that they love them all equally, and that it is simply untrue to their feelings to insist that the numbers involved diminish either the quantity or the quality of their love. If this is readily understandable in the case of parents and children, there is no necessary reason why it is an impossible or undesirable ideal in the case of adults. To be sure, there is probably a limit to the number of intimate, "primary" relationships that any person can maintain at any given time without affecting the quality of the relationship. But one adult ought surely to be able to love two, three, or even six other adults at any one time without that love being different in kind or degree from that of the traditional, monogamous, lifetime marriage. And between the individuals in these relationships, whether within a marriage or without, sexual intimacy is fitting and good.

The issues raised by a position such as the one described above are also surely worth exploring in detail and with care. Is there something to be called "sexual love" that is different from parental love or the nonsexual love of close friends? Is there something about love in general that links it naturally and appropriately with feelings of exclusivity and possession? Or is there something about sexual love, whatever that may be, that makes these feelings especially fitting? Once again, the issues are conceptual, empirical, and normative all at once: What is love? How could it be different? Would it be a good thing or a bad thing if it were different?

Suppose, though, that having delineated these problems we were now to pass them by. Suppose, moreover, that we were to be persuaded of the possibility and the desirability of weakening substantially either the links between sex and love or the links between sexual love and exclusivity. Would it not then be the case that adultery could be free from all of the morally objectionable features described thus far? To be more specific, let us imagine that a husband and wife have what is today sometimes characterized as an "open marriage." Suppose, that is, that they have agreed in advance that extramarital sex is—under certain circumstances—acceptable behavior for each to engage in. Suppose that as a result there is no impulse to deceive each other about the occurrence or nature of any such relationships and that no deception in fact occurs. Suppose, too, that there is no deception in respect to the feelings involved between the adulterous spouse and the extramarital partner. And suppose, finally, that one or the other or both of the spouses then have sexual intercourse in circumstances consistent with these understandings. Under this description, so the argument might conclude, adultery is simply not immoral. At a minimum adultery cannot very plausibly be condemned either on grounds that it involves deception or on grounds that it requires the breaking of a promise.

At least two responses are worth considering. One calls attention to the connection between marriage and adultery; the other looks to more instrumental arguments for the immorality of adultery. Both deserve further exploration.

One way to deal with the case of the "open marriage" is to question whether the two persons involved are still properly to be described as being married to each other. Part of the meaning of what it is for two persons to be married to each other, so this argument would go, is to have committed oneself to have sexual relationships only with one's spouse. Of course, it would be added, we know that that commitment is not always honored. We know that persons who are married to each other often do commit adultery. But there is a difference between being willing to make a commitment to marital fidelity, even though one may fail to honor that commitment, and not making the commitment at all. Whatever the relationship may be between the two individuals in the case just described, the absence of any commitment to sexual exclusivity requires the conclusion that their relationship is not a marital one. For a commitment to sexual exclusivity is a necessary but not a sufficient condition for the existence of a marriage.

Although there may be something to this suggestion, it is too strong as stated to be acceptable. To begin with it is doubtful that there are many, if any, *necessary* conditions for marriage; but even if there are, a commitment to sexual exclusivity is not such a condition.

To see that this is so, consider what might be taken to be some of the essential characteristics of a marriage. We might be tempted to propose that the concept of marriage requires the following: a formal ceremony of some sort in which mutual obligations are undertaken between two persons of the opposite sex; the capacity on the part of the persons involved to have sexual intercourse with each other; the willingness to have sexual intercourse only with each other; and feelings of love and affection between the two persons. The problem is that we can imagine relationships that are clearly marital and yet lack one or more of these features. For example, in our own society it is possible for two persons to be married without going through a formal ceremony, as in the common-law marriages recognized in some jurisdictions. It is also possible for two persons to get married even though one or both lacks the capacity to engage in sexual intercourse. Thus, two very elderly persons who have neither the desire nor the ability to have intercourse can nonetheless get married, as can persons whose sexual organs have been injured so that intercourse is not possible. And we certainly know of marriages in which love was not present at the time of the marriage, as, for instance, in marriages of state and marriages of convenience.

Counterexamples not satisfying the condition relating to the abstention from extramarital sex are even more easily produced. We certainly know of societies and cultures in which polygamy and polyandry are practiced, and we have no difficulty in recognizing these relationships as cases of marriages. It might be objected, though, that these are not counterexamples because they are plural marriages rather than marriages in which sex is permitted with someone other than one of the persons to whom one is married. But we also know of societies in which it is permissible for married persons to have sexual relationships with persons to whom they are not married, for example, temple prostitutes, concubines, and homosexual lovers. And even if we knew of no such societies, the conceptual claim would still, I submit, not be well taken. For suppose all of the other indicia of marriage were present: suppose the two persons were of the opposite sex; suppose they had the capacity and desire to have intercourse with each other; suppose they participated in a formal ceremony in which they understood themselves voluntarily to be entering into a relationship with each other in which substantial mutual commitments were assumed. If all these conditions were satisfied we would not be in any doubt as to whether or not the two persons were married, even though they had not taken on a commitment of sexual exclusivity and even though they had expressly agreed that extramarital sexual intercourse was a permissible behavior for each to engage in.

A commitment to sexual exclusivity is neither a necessary nor a sufficient condition for the existence of a marriage. It does, nonetheless, have this much to do with the nature of marriage—like the other indicia enumerated above, its presence tends to establish the existence of a marriage. Thus, in the absence of a formal ceremony of any sort an explicit commitment to sexual exclusivity would count in favor of regarding the two persons as married. The conceptual role of the commitment to sexual exclusivity can, perhaps, be brought out through the following example. Suppose we found a tribe that had a practice in which all the other indicia of marriage were present but in which the two parties were *prohibited* even from having sexual intercourse with each other. Moreover, suppose that sexual intercourse with others was clearly permitted. In such a case we would, I think, reject the idea that the two persons were married to each other, and we would describe their relationship in other terms, for example, as some kind of formalized, special friendship relation—a kind of heterosexual "blood-brother" bond.

Compare that case with the following one. Again suppose that the tribe had a practice in which all of the other indicia of marriage were present, but instead of a prohibition on sexual intercourse between the persons in the relationship there was no rule at all. Sexual intercourse was permissible with the person with whom one had this ceremonial relationship, but it was no more or less permissible than with a number of other persons to whom one was not so related (for instance, all consenting adults of the opposite sex). While we might be in doubt as to whether we ought to describe the persons as married to each other, we would probably conclude that they were married and that they simply were members of a tribe whose views about sex were quite different from our own.

What all of this shows is that a *prohibition* on sexual intercourse between the two persons involved in a relationship is conceptually incompatible with the claim that the two of them are married. The *permissibility* of intramarital sex is a necessary part of the idea of marriage. But no such incompatibility follows simply from the added permissibility of extramarital sex.

These arguments do not, of course, exhaust the arguments for the prohibition on extramarital sexual relations. The remaining argument that I wish to consider is—as I indicated earlier—a more instrumental one. It seeks to justify the prohibition by virtue of the role that it plays in the development and maintenance of nuclear families. The argument, or set of arguments, might, I believe, go something like this:

Consider first a far-fetched nonsexual example. Suppose a society were organized so that after some suitable age—say 18, 19, or 20—persons were forbidden to eat anything but bread and water with anyone but their spouse. Persons might still choose in such a society not to get married. Good food just might not be very important to them because they have underdeveloped taste buds. Or good food might be bad for them because there is something wrong with their digestive system. Or good food might be important to them, but they might decide that the enjoyment of good food would get in the way of the attainment of other things that were more important. But most persons would, I think, be led to favor marriage in part because they preferred a richer, more varied diet to one of bread and water. And they might remain married because the family was the only legitimate setting within which good food was obtainable. If it is important to have society organized so that persons will both get married and stay married, such an arrangement would be well suited to the preservation of the family, and the prohibitions relating to food consumption could be understood as fulfilling that function.

It is obvious that one of the more powerful human desires is the desire for sexual gratification. The desire is a natural one, like hunger and thirst, in the sense that it need not be learned in order to be present within us and operative on us. But there is in addition much that we do learn about what the act of sexual intercourse is like. Once we experience sexual intercourse ourselves—and, in particular, once we experience orgasm—we discover that it is among the most intensive, short-term pleasures of the body.

Because this is so it is easy to see how the prohibition on extramarital sex helps to hold marriage together. At least during that period of life when the enjoyment of sexual intercourse is one of the desirable bodily pleasures, persons will wish to enjoy those pleasures. If one consequence of being married is that one is prohibited from having sexual intercourse with anyone but one's spouse, then the spouses in a marriage are in a position to provide an important source of pleasure for each other that is unavailable to them elsewhere in the society.

The point emerges still more clearly if this rule of sexual morality is seen as being of a piece with the other rules of sexual morality. When this prohibition is coupled, for example, with the prohibition on nonmarital sexual intercourse, we are presented with the inducement both to get married and to stay married. For if sexual intercourse is only legitimate within marriage, then persons seeking that gratification that is a feature of sexual intercourse are furnished explicit social directions for its attainment, namely, marriage.

Nor, to continue the argument, is it necessary to focus exclusively on the bodily enjoyment that is involved. Orgasm may be a significant part of what there is to sexual intercourse, but it is not the whole of it. We need only recall the earlier discussion of the meaning that sexual intimacy has in our own culture to begin to see some of the more intricate ways in which sexual exclusivity may be connected with the establishment and maintenance of marriage as the primary heterosexual love relationship. Adultery is wrong, in other words, because a prohibition on extramarital sex is a way to help maintain the institutions of marriage and the nuclear family.

I am frankly not sure what we are to say about an argument such as the preceding one. What I am convinced of is that, like the arguments discussed earlier, this one also reveals something of the difficulty and complexity of the issues that are involved. So what I want now to do in the final portion of this essay is to try to delineate with reasonable precision several of what I take to be the fundamental, unresolved issues.

The first is whether this last argument is an argument for the *immorality* of extramarital sexual intercourse. What does seem clear is that there are differences between this argument and the ones considered earlier. The earlier arguments condemned adulterous behavior because it was behavior that involved breaking a promise, taking unfair advantage of or deceiving another. To the degree to which the prohibition on extramarital sex can be supported by arguments that invoke considerations such as these, there is little question but that violations of the prohibition are properly regarded as immoral. And such a claim could be defended on one or both of two distinct grounds. The first is that actions such as promise-breaking and deception are simply wrong. The second is that adultery involving promise-breaking or deception is wrong because it involves the straightforward infliction of harm on another human being—typically the nonadulterous spouse—who has a strong claim not to have that harm so inflicted.

The argument that connects the prohibition on extramarital sex with the maintenance and preservation of the institution of marriage is an argument for the instrumental value of the prohibition. To some degree this counts, I think, against regarding all violations of the prohibition as obvious cases of immorality. This is so partly because hypothetical imperatives are less clearly within the domain of morality than are categorical ones, and even more because instrumental prohibitions are within the domain of morality only if the end that they serve or the way that they serve it is itself within the domain of morality.

What this should help us see, I think, is the fact that the argument that connects the prohibition on adultery with the preservation of marriage is at best seriously incomplete. Before we ought to be convinced by it, we ought to have reasons for believing that marriage is a morally desirable and just social institution. And such reasons are not quite as easy to find or as obvious as it may seem. For the concept of marriage is, as we have seen, both a loosely structured and a complicated one. There may be all sorts of intimate, interpersonal relationships that will resemble but not be identical with the typical marriage relationship presupposed by the traditional sexual morality. There may be a number of distinguishable sexual and loving arrangements that can all legitimately claim to be called *marriages*. The prohibitions of the traditional sexual morality may be effective ways to maintain some marriages and ineffective ways to promote and preserve others. The prohibitions of the traditional sexual morality may make good psychological sense if certain psychological theories are true, and they may be purveyors of immense psychological mischief if other psychological theories are true. The prohibitions of traditional sexual morality may seem obviously correct if sexual intimacy carries the meaning that the dominant culture has often ascribed to it, and they may seem equally bizarre if sex is viewed through the perspective of the counterculture. Irrespective of whether instrumental arguments of this sort are properly deemed moral arguments, they ought not fully convince anyone until questions such as these are answered.

11.

ADULTERY AND FIDELITY

Mike W. Martin

Adultery has recently entered prominently into evaluations of public figures. Bill Clinton's 1992 presidential campaign was nearly derailed by
allegations about a twelve-year extramarital affair. Shortly thereafter England's
royal family engaged in extensive damage control as public revelations surfaced
about the love trysts of Prince Charles and Lady Diana. Earlier, in 1987, Gary
Hart's "womanizing" forced his withdrawal as the leading democratic presidential candidate. About the same time, charges of adultery contributed to the
downfall of the leading television evangelist Jim Bakker.[1]

It is not clear what most upsets (or intrigues) the public in such cases. Is it
the adultery per se, the deception used to conceal it (from spouses or the public),
the hypocrisy in professing contrary religious beliefs, or the poor judgment in
failing to keep it discrete (including the bravado of Gary Hart in baiting the press
to uncover his affairs)? Nor is it clear how the adultery itself is pertinent to public
service, even if we think the adultery is immoral. Character is not a seamless web,
and integrity can be present in one context (public service) and absent in
another setting (sexual conduct).[2] Many notable leaders had extramarital affairs,

From the *Journal of Social Philosophy* 25, no. 3 (Winter 1994). Reprinted by permission of the *Journal of
Social Philosophy*.

including Franklin D. Roosevelt, Dwight Eisenhower, John F. Kennedy, and Martin Luther King Jr., and public scrutiny of marital intimacy might discourage worthy candidates from seeking public office.

It is clear, however, that adultery is morally complex. Philosophers have devoted little attention to it,[3] largely leaving it as a topic for theology, social science, and literature. Certainly novelists have had much to say: "To judge by literature, adultery would seem to be one of the most remarkable of occupations in both Europe and America. Few are the novels that fail to allude to it."[4] In any case, whether as moral judges assessing the character of adulterers or as moral agents confronted with making our own decisions about adultery, we often find ourselves immersed in confusions and ambiguities that are both personally and philosophically troublesome.

I will seek a middle ground between conventional absolute prohibitions and trendy permissiveness. A humanistic perspective should embrace a pluralistic moral outlook that affirms a variety of forms of sexual relationships, including many traditional marriages. It can justify a strong presumption against adultery for individuals who embrace traditional marital ideals.

The ethics of adultery divides into two parts: making commitments and keeping them. The ethics of making commitments centers primarily on commitments to love, where love is a value-guided relationship, and secondarily on the promise of sexual exclusivity (the promise to have sex only with one's spouse) which some couples make in order to support the commitment to love. The ethics of keeping commitments has to do with balancing initial marital commitments against other moral considerations.

MAKING COMMITMENTS

What is adultery? Inspired by the New Testament, some people employ a wide definition that applies to any significant sexual interest in someone besides one's spouse: "You have heard that it was said, 'Do not commit adultery.' But I tell you that anyone who *looks* at a woman lustfully has already committed adultery with her in his heart."[5] Other people define adultery narrowly to match their particular scruples: for them extramarital genital intercourse may count as adultery, but not oral sex; or falling in love with someone besides one's spouse may count as adultery but not "merely" having sex.[6] Whatever definition we adopt there will always be borderline cases, if only those created by "brinkmanship"—going as far as possible without having intercourse (e.g., lying naked together in bed).[7]

In this paper, "adultery" refers to married persons having sexual intercourse (of any kind) with someone other than their spouses.[8] I am aware that the word "adultery" is not purely descriptive and evokes a range of emotive connotations. Nevertheless, I use the word without implying that adultery is immoral; that is a topic left open for investigation in specific cases. Like "deception," the word "adultery" raises moral questions about possible misconduct but it does not answer them. By contrast, I will use a wider sense of "marriage" that refers to all monogamous (two-spouse) relationships formally established by legal or religious ceremonies *and* closely analogous moral relationships such as committed relationships between homosexual or heterosexual couples who are not legally married.

A moral understanding of adultery turns on an understanding of morality. If we conceive morality as a set of rules, we will object to adultery insofar as it violates those rules. "Do not commit adultery" is not an irreducible moral principle, but many instances of adultery violate other familiar rules. As Richard Wasserstrom insightfully explained, much adultery violates one or more of these rules: Do not break promises (viz., the wedding vows to abjure outside sex, vows which give one's partner "reasonable expectations" of sexual fidelity); do not deceive (whether by lying, withholding information, or pretending about the affair); do not be unfair (by enjoying outside sex forbidden to one's spouse); and do not cause undeserved harm (to one's spouse who suspects or hears of the affair).[9] Wasserstrom points out that all these rules are prima facie: In some situations they are overridden by other moral considerations, thereby justifying some instances of adultery.

Moreover, adultery is not even prima facie wrong when spouses have an "open marriage" in which they give each other permission to have extramarital affairs. In this connection Wasserstrom raises questions about the reasonableness of traditional marital promises of sexual exclusivity. Wouldn't it be wiser to break the conventional ties between sex and love, so that the pleasures of adultery can be enjoyed along with those of marriage? Alternatively, should we maintain the connection between sex and love but break the exclusive tie between sexual love and one's spouse, thus tolerating multiple simultaneous loves for one's spouse and for additional partners? No doubt the linking of love, sex, and exclusivity has an *instrumental* role in promoting marriages, but so would the patently unreasonable practice of allowing people to eat decent meals (beyond bread and water) only with their spouses.

In my view, a rule-oriented approach to morality lacks the resources needed to answer the important questions Wasserstrom raises. We need an expanded conception of morality as encompassing ideals and virtues, in particular the moral ideals of love, which provide the point of marital commitments and the virtues manifested in pursuing those ideals. The ethics of adultery centers on the moral ideals of and commitments to love—which include ideals of constancy (or faithfulness), honesty, trust, and fairness—that make possible special ways of caring for persons. The ideals are morally optional in that no one is obligated to embrace them. Nevertheless, strong obligations to avoid adultery arise for those couples who embrace the ideals as a basis for making traditional marital commitments. The primary commitment is to love each other, while the commitment of sexual exclusivity is secondary and supportive. This can be seen by focusing on three ideas that Wasserstrom devotes little attention to: love, commitments to love, and trust.

1. What is *love*? Let us set aside the purely descriptive (value-neutral) senses in which "love" refers to (a) a strong positive attraction or emotion[10] or (b) a complex attitude involving many emotions—not only strong affection, but also excitement, joy, pride, hope, fear, jealousy, anger, and so on.[11] Let us focus instead on the normative (value-laden) sense in which we speak of "true love" or "the real thing." Cogent disputes arise concerning the values defining true love, though ultimately individuals have a wide area of personal discretion in the ideals they pursue in relationships of erotic love.

In its value-laden senses, "love" refers to special ways of valuing persons.[12] As an attitude, love is valuing the beloved, cherishing her or him as unique. Erotic love includes sexual valuing, but the valuing is focused on the person as a unity, not just a body. As a relationship, love is defined by reciprocal attitudes of mutual valuing. The precise nature of this valuing turns on the ideals one accepts, and hence those ideals are part of the very meaning of "love."

2. According to the traditional ideal (or set of ideals) of interest here, marriage is based on a *commitment to love*: "to have and to hold from this day forward, for better for worse, for richer for poorer, in sickness and in health, to love and to cherish, till death us do part." This is not a commitment to have continuous feelings of strong affection—feelings which are beyond our immediate voluntary control. Instead, it is a commitment to create and sustain a relationship conducive to those feelings, as well as conducive to the happiness and fulfillment of both partners. Spouses assume responsibility for maintaining conditions for mutual caring which in turn foster recurring emotions of deep affection, delight, shared enthusiasm, and joy. The commitment to love is not a promise uttered once during a wedding ceremony; it is an ongoing willingness to assume responsibility for a value-guided relationship.

The commitment to love implies a web of values and virtues. It is a commitment to create a lifelong relationship of deep caring that promises happiness through shared activities (including sexual ones) and through joining interests in mutually supportive ways involving shared decision-making, honesty, trust, emotional intimacy, reciprocity, and (at least in modern versions) fair and equal opportunities for self-expression and personal growth. This traditional ideal shapes how spouses value each other, both symbolically and substantively. Commitments to love throughout a lifetime show that partners value each other as having paramount importance and also value them as a unity, as persons-living-throughout-a-lifetime. Time-limited commitments, such as to remain together only while in college, express at most a limited affirmation of the importance of the other person in one's life.

Valuing each other is manifested in a willingness to make accommodations and sacrifices to support the marriage. For most couples, some of those sacrifices are sexual. The promise of sexual exclusivity is a distinct wedding vow whose supportive status is symbolized by being mentioned in a subordinate clause, "and, forsaking all others, keep thee only unto her/him." Hopefully, couples who make the vow of sexual exclusivity are not under romantic illusions that their present sexual preoccupation with each other will magically abolish sexual interests in other people and temptations to have extramarital affairs. They commit themselves to sexual exclusivity as an expression of their love and with the aim of protecting that love.

How does sexual exclusivity express and protect love? In two ways. First, many spouses place adultery at the top of the list of actions which threaten their marriage. They are concerned, often with full justification, that adultery might lead to another love that would damage or destroy their relationship. They fear that the affection, time, attention, and energy (not to mention money) given to an extramarital partner would lessen the resources they devote to sustaining their marriage. They also fear the potential for jealousy to disrupt the relationship.[13] As long as it does not become excessive, jealousy is a healthy reaction of anger, fear, and hurt in response to a perceived loss of an important good.[14] Indeed, if a spouse feels no jealousy whatsoever, the question is raised (though not answered) about the depth of love.

Second, sexual exclusivity is one way to establish the symbolism that "making love" is a singular affirmation of the partner. The love expressed is not just strong affection, but a deep valuing of each other in the ways defined by the ideals embedded in the marriage. Sex is especially well-suited (far more than eating) to express that love because of its extraordinary physical and emotional intimacy, tenderness, and pleasure. The symbolic meaning involved is not sentimental fluff; it makes possible forms of expression that enter into the substance of love.

In our culture sex has no uniform meaning, but couples are free to give it personal meanings. Janet Z. Giele notes two extremes: "On the one hand, the body may be viewed as the most important thing the person has to give, and sexual intercourse therefore becomes the symbol of the deepest and most far-reaching commitment, which is to be strictly limited to one pair-bond. On the other hand, participants may define sexual activity as merely a physical expression that, since it does not importantly envelop the whole personality nor commit the pair beyond the pleasures of the moment, may be regulated more permissively."[15] Between the two extremes lie many variations in the personal symbolism that couples give to sex, and here we are exploring only those variations found in traditional marital vows.

3. *Trust* is present at the time when couples undertake commitments to love, and in turn those commitments provide a framework for sustaining trust. Trust implies but is not reducible to Wasserstrom's "reasonable expectations" about a partner's conduct. Expectations are epistemic attitudes, whereas trust is a moral attitude of relying on others to act responsibly, with goodwill, and (in marriage) with love and support.[16] We have a reasonable expectation that the earth will continue to orbit the sun throughout our lifetime, but no moral relationship of trust is involved. As a way of giving support to others, underwriting their endeavors, and showing the importance of their lives to us, trust and trustworthiness is a key ingredient in caring.

To be sure, trust is not always good. It is valuable when it contributes to valuable relationships, in particular to worthwhile marriages.[17] Marital trust is confidence in and dependence upon a spouse's morally responsible love. As such, it provides a basis for ongoing intimacy and mutual support. It helps spouses undergo the vulnerabilities and risks (emotional, financial, physical) inherent in intimate relationships.

The trust of marital partners is broad-scoped. Spouses trust each other to actively support the marriage and to avoid doing things that might pull them away from it. They trust each other to maintain the conditions for preserving intimacy and mutual happiness. Violating marital trust does more than upset expectations and cause pain. It violates trust, honesty, fairness, caring, and the other moral ideals defining the relationship. It betrays one's spouse. And it betrays one's integrity as someone committed to these ideals.

To sum up, I have avoided Wasserstrom's narrow preoccupation with the promise of sexual exclusivity. Commitments of sexual exclusivity find their rationale in wider commitments to love each other *if* a couple decides that exclusivity will support their commitments to love *and* where love is understood as a special way to value persons within lasting relationships based on mutual caring, honesty, and trust. Accordingly, marital faithfulness (or constancy) in loving is the primary virtue; sexual fidelity is a supporting virtue. And sexual fidelity must be understood in terms of the particular commitments and understandings that couples establish.

I have also avoided saying that sexual exclusivity is intrinsically valuable or a feature of all genuine love, unlike Bonnie Steinbock: "[sexual] exclusivity seems to be an intrinsic part of 'true love.' Imagine Romeo pouring out his heart to both Juliet *and* Rosaline! In our ideal of romantic love, one chooses to forgo pleasure with other partners in order to have a unique relationship with one's beloved."[18] In my view, the intrinsic good lies in fulfilling love relationships, rather than sexual exclusivity per se, thereby recognizing that some couples sustain genuine love without sexual exclusivity. For some couples sexual exclusivity does contribute to the goods found in traditional relationships, but other couples achieve comparable goods through nontraditional relationships, for example open marriages that tolerate outside sex without love.[19] We can recognize the value of traditional relationships while also recognizing the value of alternative relationships, as chosen autonomously by couples.[20]

KEEPING COMMITMENTS

A complete ethics of keeping commitments of exclusivity would focus on the virtues of responsibility, faithfulness, and self-control. Here, however, I wish to defend Wasserstrom's view that even in traditional relationships the prohibition against adultery is prima facie. However strong the presumption against adultery in traditional relationships, it does not yield an exceptionless, all-things-considered judgment about wrongdoing and blameworthiness in specific cases. I will discuss four of many complicating factors.[21] What if partners wish to change their commitments? What happens when love comes to an end? What if one spouse falls in love with an additional partner? And what about the sometimes extraordinary self-affirmation extramarital affairs may bring?

(i) *Changing Commitments.* Some spouses who begin with traditional commitments later revise them. Buoyed by the exuberance of romance, most couples feel confident they will not engage in adultery (much less be among the 50 percent of couples who divorce). Later they may decide to renegotiate the guidelines for their marriage in light of changing attitudes and circumstances, though still within the framework of their commitments to love each other.[22] One study suggests that 90 percent of couples believe sexual exclusivity to be essential when they marry, but only 60 percent maintain this belief after several years of marriage (with the changes occurring primarily among those who had at least one affair).[23]

Vita Sackville-West and Harold Nicolson provide an illuminating if unusual example. They married with the usual sexual attraction to each other and for several years were sexually compatible. As that changed, they gave each other permission to pursue extramarital affairs, primarily homosexual ones. Yet their original commitment to love each other remained intact. Indeed, for forty-nine years, until Vita died in 1962, their happy marriage was a model of mutual caring, deep affection, and trust: "What mattered most was that each should trust the other absolutely. 'Trust,' in most marriages means [sexual] fidelity. In theirs it meant that they would always tell each other of their infidelities, give warning of approaching emotional crises, and, whatever happened, return to their common center in the end."[24] Throughout much of their marriage they lived apart on weekdays, thereby accommodating both their work and their outside sexual liaisons. On weekends they would reunite as devoted companions, "berthed like sister ships."[25]

Just as we respect the mutual autonomy of couples in forming their initial understanding about their relationship, we should also respect their autonomy in renegotiating that understanding. The account I have offered allows us to distinguish between the primary commitment to love and the secondary commitment of sexual exclusivity. The secondary commitment is made in order to support the primary one, and if a couple agrees that it no longer is needed they are free to revoke it. Renegotiations can also proceed in the reverse directions: Spouses who initially agree on an open marriage may find that allowing extramarital affairs creates unbearable strains on their relationship, leading them to make commitments of exclusivity.

Changing commitments raise two major difficulties. First, couples are sometimes less than explicit about the sexual rules for their relationship. One or both partners may sense that their understandings have changed over the years but fail to engage in discussions that establish explicit new understandings. As a result, one spouse may believe that something is acceptable to the other spouse when in fact it is not. For example, Philip Blumstein and Pepper Schwartz interviewed a couple who, "when it came to a shared understanding about extramarital sex, . . . seemed not to be in the same marriage."[26] The man reported to them, "Sure we have an understanding. It's: 'You do what you want. Never go back to the same one [extramarital partner],'" presumably since that would threaten the relationship. By contrast, the wife reports: "We've never spoken about cheating, but neither of us believe in it. I don't think I'd ever forgive him [if he cheated on me]." Lack of shared understanding generates moral vagueness and ambiguity concerning adultery, whereas periodic forthright communication helps establish clear moral boundaries.[27]

Second, what happens when only one partner wants to renegotiate an original understanding? The mere desire to renegotiate does not constitute a betrayal, nor does it by itself justify adultery if one's spouse refuses to rescind the initial vow of sexual exclusivity. In such cases the original presumption against adultery continues but with an increased risk that the partner wishing to change it may feel adultery is more excusable. Such conflicts may or may not be resolved in a spirit of caring and compromise that enables good relationships to continue. Lacking such resolution, the moral status of adultery may become less clear-cut.

(ii) *Lost Love.* Couples who make traditional commitments sometimes fall out of love, singly or together, or for other reasons find themselves unwilling to continue in a marriage. Sometimes the cause is adultery, and sometimes adultery is a symptom of irresponsibility and poor judgment that erodes the relationship in additional ways.[28] But other times there is little or no fault involved. Lasting love is a creation of responsible conduct *and* luck.[29] No amount of conscientiousness can replace the good fortune of emotional compatibility and conducive circumstances.

In saying that traditional commitments to love are intended to be lifelong, we need not view them as unconditional.[30] Typically they are based on tacit conditions. One condition is embedded in the wedding ceremony in which *mutual* vows are exchanged, namely, that one's spouse will take the marital vows seriously. Others are presupposed as background conditions, for example, that the spouse will not turn into a murderer, rapist, spouse-beater, child-abuser, or psychopathic monster. Usually there are more specific tacit assumptions that evolve before the marriage, for example, that the spouses will support each other's careers. Above all, there is the background hope that with sincere effort the relationship will contribute to the overall happiness of both partners. All these conditions remain largely tacit, as a matter of faith. When that faith proves ill-founded or just unlucky, the ethics of adultery becomes complicated.

As relationships deteriorate, adultery may serve as a transition to new and perhaps better relationships. In an ideal world, marriages would be ended cleanly before new relationships begin. But then, in an ideal world people would be sufficiently prescient not to make traditional commitments that are unlikely to succeed. Contemplating adultery is an occasion for much self-deception, but at least sometimes there may be good reasons for pursuing alternative relationships before officially ending a bad marriage.[31]

(iii) *New Loves.* Some persons claim to (erotically) love both their spouse and an additional lover. They may be mistaken, as they later confess to themselves, but is it impossible to love two (or more) people simultaneously? "Impossible" in what sense?

Perhaps for some people it is a psychological impossibility, but, again, other individuals report a capacity to love more than one person at a time. For many persons it is a practical impossibility, given the demands of time, attention, and affection required in genuine loving. But that would seem to allow that resourceful individuals can finesse (psychologically, logistically, financially, and so forth) multiple simultaneous relationships. I believe that the impossibility is moral and conceptual—*if* one embraces traditional ideals that define marital love as a singular affirmation of one's spouse and *if a* couple establishes sex as a symbolic and substantive way to convey that exclusive love.[32] Obviously people can experience additional romantic attractions after they make traditional vows, but it is morally impossible for them to actively engage in loving relationships with additional partners without violating the love defined by their initial commitments.

Richard Taylor disagrees in *Having Love Affairs*, a book-length defense of adultery. No doubt this book is helpful for couples planning open marriages, but Taylor concentrates on situations where traditional vows have been made and then searches for ways to minimize the harm to spouses that results from extramarital love affairs.[33] In that regard his book is morally subversive in that it systematically presents only one side of the story. Here are five examples of this one-sidedness.

First, with considerable panache Taylor develops a long list of rules for *non*adulterous partners who should be tolerant of their partner's affairs. (a) "Do not spy or pry," since that is self-degrading and shows a lack of trust in one's spouse. (But is a commitment-breaking spouse trustworthy?) (b) "Do not confront or entrap," because that would humiliate the spouse. (But what about being humiliated oneself?) (c) "Stay out of it," since good marriages survive adultery. (No empirical support is offered for that generalization!) (d) "Stop being jealous," since jealousy disrupts marriages. (But what about the case for not provoking jealousy in the first place?)

Taylor also offers rules for the spouse having the affair: Maintain fidelity with one's lover, be honest with one's lover, be discrete rather than boasting about the affair, and do not betray or abandon the lover. In discussing these rules Taylor is oblivious to the infidelity, betrayal of trust, and failure to value one's spouse in the way called for by traditional commitments and the shared understanding between spouses.

Second, Taylor defines infidelity as "a betrayal of the promise to love" and faithfulness as "a state of one's heart and mind," rather than "mere outward conformity to rules." Infidelity can be shown in ways unrelated to adultery, such as in neglecting the spouse's sexual needs, selfishly using shared financial resources, and failing to be caring and supportive.[34] It is true that infidelity takes other forms, but what about the infidelity in violating marital vows and understandings? Moreover, the only place we are reminded that "inner states" of faithfulness are manifested in outward conduct is when Taylor condemns infidelity toward an extramarital lover, not one's spouse.

Third, love affairs are natural and avoiding them is unhealthy. "A man, by nature, desires many sexual partners"; "The suppression of the polygamous impulse in a man is . . . bought at a great price" of frustrated and rueful longing for outside love affairs.[35] Granted, most people (male and female) have desires for multiple sexual partners. Yet many people also have monogamous impulses, as shown in their decisions to enter into traditional marriages. The resulting conflicts make sexual exclusivity notoriously difficult, but they need not result in frustration; often they contribute greatly to overall sexual satisfaction within secure and trusting relationships.

Fourth, "No one can tell another person what is and is not permissible with respect to whom he or she will love. . . . However inadvisable it may be to seek love outside the conventional restraints, the *right* to do so is about as clear as any right can be."[36] Taylor is equivocating of "right," which can mean (1) that others are obligated to leave one alone or (2) that one's conduct is all right. Having a right not to be interfered with by society as one engages in adultery does not imply that one's conduct is "all right" or morally permissible. Indeed, couples who make traditional commitments waive some rights in relation to each other; in particular they waive the right to engage in adultery which violates their marital agreements.

Fifth, and most important, Taylor praises love affairs as inherently good and even the highest good: "the joys of illicit and passionate love, which include but go far beyond the mere joys of sex, are incomparably good."[37] On the same page he says, "This does not mean that love affairs are better than marriage, for they seldom are. Love between married persons can, in the long run, be so vastly more fulfilling" than affairs. I find it difficult to reconcile these claims: Those marriages which are vastly more fulfilling would thereby seem to provide the incomparable goods, not extramarital affairs which violate the commitments defining the marriage. Of course many people find joy in extramarital sex, and for some the joy may be the greatest they find in life. But Taylor provides no basis for saying that happy traditional marriages never produce comparable joys. Nor does he ever explain how extramarital joys are morally permissible for individuals who make traditional marriage vows.

Bonnie Steinbock affirms an opposite view. She suggests that to fall in love with someone other than one's spouse is already a betrayal: "Sexual infidelity has significance as a sign of a deeper betrayal—falling in love with someone else. It may be objected that we cannot control the way we feel, only the way we behave; that we should not be blamed for falling in love, but only for acting on the feeling. While we may not have direct control over our feelings, however, we are responsible for getting ourselves into situations in which certain feelings naturally arise."[38] I agree that spouses who make traditional vows are responsible for avoiding situations that they know (or should know) foster extramarital love.[39] Nevertheless, deeply committed people occasionally do fall in love with third parties without being blameworthy for getting into situations that spark that love. Experiencing a strong romantic attraction is not by itself an infidelity, and questions of betrayal may arise only when a person moves in the direction of acting on the love in ways that violate commitments to one's spouse.

Having said all this, I know of no argument that absolutely condemns all love-inspired adultery as immoral, all things considered and in all respects, even within traditional relationships. Nonetheless, as I have been concerned to emphasize, there is a serious betrayal of one's spouse. But to say that ends the matter would make the commitment to love one's spouse a moral absolute, with no exceptions whatsoever. Tragic dilemmas overthrow such absolutes, and we need to set aside both sweeping condemnations and wholesale defenses of love-inspired adultery.

To mention just one type of case, when marriages are profoundly unfulfilling, and when constricting circumstances prevent other ways of meeting important needs, there is a serious question whether love-inspired adultery is sometimes justifiable or at least excusable—witness *The Scarlet Letter, Anna Karenina, Madame Bovary, Lady Chatterley's Lover,* and *The Awakening.* Moreover, our deep ambivalence about some cases of love-inspired adultery reflect how there is some good and some bad involved in conduct that we cannot fully justify nor fully condemn.

(iv) *Sex and Self-Esteem.* Extramarital affairs are often grounded in attractions less grand than love. Affection, friendship, or simple respect may be mixed with a desire for exciting sex and the enhanced self-esteem from being found sexually desirable. The sense of risk may add to the pleasure that one is so desirable that a lover will take added risks. Are sex and self-esteem enough to justify violating marital vows? It would seem not. The obligations created through marital commitments are moral requirements, whereas sex and self-esteem pertain to one's self-interest. Doesn't morality trump self-interest?

But things are not so simple. Morality includes rights and responsibilities to ourselves to pursue our happiness and self-fulfillment. Some marriages are sexually frustrating or damaging in other ways to self-respect. Even when marriages are basically fulfilling, more than a few individuals report their extramarital affairs were liberating and transforming, whether or not grounded in love. For example, many women make the following report about their extramarital affair: "It's given me a whole new way of looking at myself . . . I felt attractive again. I hadn't felt that way in years, really. It made me very, very confident."[40]

In addition, the sense of personal enhancement may have secondary benefits. Occasionally it strengthens marriages, especially after the extramarital affair ends, and some artists report an increase in creative activity. These considerations do not automatically outweigh the dishonesty and betrayal that may be involved in adultery, and full honesty may never be restored when spouses decide against confessing an affair to their partners.[41] But nor are considerations of enhanced self-esteem and its secondary benefits irrelevant.

I have mentioned some possible justifications or excuses for specific instances of adultery after traditional commitments are made. I conclude with a caveat. Specific instances are one thing; general attitudes about adultery are another. Individuals who make traditional commitments and who are fortunate enough to establish fulfilling relationships based on those commitments ought to maintain a general attitude that for them to engage in adultery would be immoral (as well as stupid). The "ought" is stringent, as stringent as the commitment to sexual exclusivity. Rationalizing envisioned adultery with anecdotes about the joys of extramarital sex or statistics about the sometimes beneficial effects of adultery is a form of moral duplicity. It is also inconsistent with the virtues of both sexual fidelity and faithfulness in sustaining commitments to love.

NOTES

1. Charles E. Shepard, *Forgiven: The Rise and Fall of Jim Bakker and the PTL Ministry* (New York: Atlantic Monthly Press, 1989).

2. Cf. Owen Flanagan, *Varieties of Moral Personality* (Cambridge, MA: Harvard University Press, 1991).

3. R. J. Connelly, "Philosophy and Adultery," in Philip E. Lampe, ed., *Adultery in the United States* (Amherst, NY: Prometheus Books, 1987), pp. 131–64.

4. Denis de Rougemont, *Love in the Western World*, rev. ed., trans. Montgomery Belgion (New York: Harper and Row, 1974), p. 16. Two illuminating literary critics are Tony Tanner, *Adultery in the Novel: Contract and Transgression* (Baltimore: Johns Hopkins University Press, 1979), and Donald J. Greiner, *Adultery in the American Novel: Updike, James, and Hawthorne* (Columbia: University of South Carolina Press, 1985).

5. Matthew 5:27–28, *New International Version*. In targeting males, this scripture presupposes that husbands are the primary adulterers. That presupposition is not surprising given a long history of indulging profligate husbands while severely punishing wayward wives, based in part on the view that wives are their husbands' property, duty-bound to maintain male lines of progeny, and in part on the view that women are chaste creatures who can be held to a higher standard than males. Today, husbands continue to lead in adultery statistics—well over half of them have extramarital affairs—although women are catching up. Annette Lawson cautiously estimates that somewhere between 25 percent and 50 percent of women have at least one extramarital lover during any given marriage, and 50–65 percent of husbands engage in adultery by the age of forty. *Adultery: An Analysis of Love and Betrayal* (New York: Basic Books, 1988), p. 75. A humanistic approach regards male and female adultery as on a par and also proceeds without invoking religious beliefs that condemn all adultery as sinful.

6. Morton Hunt, *The Affair* (New York: World Publishing Company, 1969), p. 9.

7. This is not an imaginary case. See ibid., p. 80.

8. Michael J. Wreen plausibly widens the term "adultery" to apply to nonmarried persons who have sex with married persons, but since my focus is spouses, I will not widen the definition. "What's Really Wrong with Adultery?" *Journal of Applied Philosophy* 3 (1986): 45–49.

9. Richard Wasserstrom, "Is Adultery Immoral?" *Philosophical Forum* 5 (1974): 513–28. Wasserstrom's preoccupation with rules explains why the most interesting part of his essay—the discussion of the connections between sex, love, and sexually exclusive loving relationships—is approached so indirectly, in terms of "deeper deceptions" that violate the rule against deception, rather than directly in terms of violating moral ideals embedded in love.

10. Wasserstrom sometimes uses "love" this way, as on p. 518. But on p. 522 he hints at the value-laden meaning of "love": "the issues are conceptual, empirical, and normative all at once: What is love? How could it be different? Would it be a good thing or a bad thing if it were different?" These questions, which are posed but not pursued, adumbrate my approach.

11. Cf. Annette Baier, "Unsafe Loves," in *The Philosophy of (Erotic) Love*, ed. Robert C. Solomon and Kathleen M. Higgins (Lawrence: University Press of Kansas, 1991), pp. 444 and 449, n. 29.

12. Irving Singer, *The Nature of Love*, 2nd ed. (Chicago: University of Chicago Press, 1984), I, pp. 3ff. In the third volume of this work, Singer sets forth a subjectivist view of the worth of persons. (Chicago: University of Chicago Press, 1987), III, p. 403. I share the more objectivist view of the unique worth of persons defended by Jeffrey Blustein in *Care and Commitment* (New York: Oxford University Press, 1991), pp. 203–16.

13. Roger Scruton, *Sexual Desire* (New York: Free Press, 1986), p. 339.

14. For an illuminating historical study of changing attitudes see Peter N. Stearns, *Jealousy* (New York: New York University Press, 1989).

15. Janet Z. Giele, as quoted by Philip E. Lampe, "The Many Dimensions of Adultery," in *Adultery in the United States*, p. 56.

16. Cf. H. J. N. Horsburgh, "The Ethics of Trust," *Philosophical Quarterly* 10 (1960): 343–54; Annette Baier, "Trust and Antitrust," *Ethics* 96 (1986): 231–60; Lawrence Thomas, "Trust, Affirmation, and Moral Character. A Critique of Kantian Morality," in *Identity, Character, and Morality: Essays in Moral Psychology* (Cambridge, MA: MIT Press, 1990), pp. 235–57; and Mike W. Martin, "Honesty in Love," *Journal of Value Inquiry* (1993).

17. Michael Slote, *Goods and Virtues* (Oxford: Clarendon Press, 1983), pp. 49, 65.

18. Bonnie Steinbock, "Adultery," in *The Philosophy of Sex*, ed. Alan Soble (Savage, MD: Rowman & Littlefield, 1991), p. 191.

19. See Russell Vannoy, *Sex Without Love* (Amherst, NY: Prometheus Books, 1980).

20. I am assuming that the consent involved in agreements between couples is fully voluntary and that a dominant partner does not exert pressures that make consent "intellectual" rather than emotionally wholehearted. Cf. J. F. M. Hunter, *Sex and Love* (Toronto: Macmillan, 1980), p. 42. To be sure, autonomy is not the sole value governing the making of marital commitments. There are reasons which need to be weighed in deciding what kind of commitments to make. Are partners being realistic in choosing between an exclusive relationship (with its element of sexual restriction) or an open relationship (with its risks of jealousy and new loves) as the best way to promote their happiness and love each other? And would permitting extramarital affairs negatively affect third parties (perhaps children)?

21. These are not the only factors—a book would be needed to discuss all relevant factors. For example, what about the effects on third parties, not just children and other

family, but the extramarital lover? Ellen Glasgow describes the joys of her affair with a married man as "miraculous" in *The Woman Within* (New York: Hill and Wang 1980), p. 156. Again, there are factors about how affairs are conducted, including the risk of contracting AIDS and giving it to one's spouse.

22. The mutual renegotiation of relationships is a central aspect of marital equality, as argued by Robert C. Solomon, *About Love* (New York: Simon and Schuster, 1980), pp. 283–300.

23. Lawson, *Adultery*, pp. 72–73.

24. Nigel Nicolson, *Portrait of a Marriage* (New York: Atheneum, 1973), p. 188.

25. Ibid., p. 231.

26. Philip Blumstein and Pepper Schwartz, *American Couples* (New York: William Morrow, 1983), pp. 286–87.

27. Cf. J. E. and Mary Ann Barnhart, "Marital Faithfulness and Unfaithfulness," *Journal of Social Philosophy* 4 (April 1973): 10–15.

28. E.g., Herbert S. Strean, *The Extramarital Affair* (New York: Free Press, 1980); and Frank Pittman, *Private Lies: Infidelity and the Betrayal of Intimacy* (New York: W. W. Norton, 1989).

29. Cf. Martha C. Nussbaum, *The Fragility of Goodness* (New York: Cambridge University Press, 1980), pp. 259–362.

30. Contrary to Susan Mendus, "Marital Faithfulness," *Philosophy* 59 (1984): 246. For criticisms of Mendus, see Alan Soble, *The Structure of Love* (New Haven, CT: Yale University Press, 1990), p. 166; and Mike W. Martin, "Love's Constancy," *Philosophy* 68 (1993): 63–77.

31. An interesting example of deciding against adultery is the subject of Lotte Hamburger and Joseph Hamburger, *Contemplating Adultery* (New York: Fawcett Columbine, 1991).

32. Robert Nozick develops a slightly different argument based on the intimate mutual identification involved in forming a couple or a "we." See *The Examined Life* (New York: Simon and Schuster, 1989), pp. 82, 84.

33. Richard Taylor, *Having Love Affairs* (Amherst, NY: Prometheus Books, 1982), pp. 67-68.

34. Ibid., pp. 59–60.

35. Ibid., pp. 70, 72–73. The possible frustrations of monogamy are discussed by Edmund Leites in his illuminating book, *The Puritan Conscience and Modern Sexuality* (New Haven, CT: Yale University Press, 1986).

36. Ibid., p. 48. For these and other ambiguities of "rights" see Ronald Dworkin, *Taking Rights Seriously* (Cambridge, MA: Harvard University Press, 1977), pp. 188–89.

37. Ibid., p. 12.

38. Bonnie Steinbock, "Adultery," in Alan Soble, ed., *The Philosophy of Sex*, p. 192.

39. For an interesting example, see Janice Rosenberg, "Fidelity," in Laurie Abraham et al., *Reinventing Love* (New York: Plume, 1993), pp. 101–106.

40. Lynn Atwater, *The Extramarital Connection* (New York: Irvington Publishers, 1982), p. 143. The same theme is developed in Dalma Heyn, *The Erotic Silence of the American Wife* (New York: Signet, 1993).

41. Dalma Heyn (ibid.) urges that not confessing adultery to one's spouse is especially justified for women whose adultery is likely to provoke physical abuse or a divorce that would leave them and their children impoverished. Others argue that even when the adultery is immoral that confession wreaks more harm than the benefits of restoring full honesty in the relationship. (E.g., Laura Green, "Never Confess," in *Reinventing Love*, pp. 192–97.) The case for promoting honesty by confessing to one's spouse an infidelity is made by Frank Pittman in *Private Lies*.

12.

APARTHEID AND HOMOPHOBIA
Both Crimes against Humanity
Archbishop Desmond Tutu

A student once asked me if I could have one wish granted to reverse an injustice, what would it be? I had to ask for two. One is for world leaders to forgive the debts of developing nations which hold them in such thrall. The other is for the world to end the persecution of people because of their sexual orientation, which is every bit as unjust as that crime against humanity, apartheid.

This is a matter of ordinary justice. We struggled against apartheid in South Africa, supported by people the world over, because black people were being blamed and made to suffer for something we could do nothing about—our very skins. It is the same with sexual orientation. It is a given. I could not have fought against the discrimination of apartheid and not also fight against the discrimination which homosexuals endure, even in our churches and faith groups. And I am proud that in South Africa, when we won the chance to build our own new constitution, the human rights of all have been explicitly enshrined in our laws. My hope is that, one day, this will be the case all over the world and that all will have equal rights.

For me, this struggle is a seamless rope. Opposing apartheid was a matter of

This edited version of the Foreword by Archbishop Desmond Tutu to "Sex, Love & Homophobia," published today by Amnesty International UK, was first printed in The *Times* newspaper, 1 July 04.

justice. Opposing discrimination against women is a matter of justice. Opposing discrimination on the basis of sexual orientation is a matter of justice.

It is also a matter of love. Every human being is precious. We are all, all of us, part of God's family. We all must be allowed to love each other with honour.

Yet, all over the world, lesbian, gay, bisexual, and transgender people are persecuted. We treat them as pariahs and push them outside our communities. We make them doubt that they too are children of God—and this must be nearly the ultimate blasphemy. We blame them for what they are. Churches say that the expression of love in a heterosexual monogamous relationship includes the physical, the touching, embracing, kissing, the genital act—the totality of our love makes each of us grow to become increasingly godlike and compassionate. If this is so for the heterosexual, what earthly reason have we to say that it is not the case with the homosexual?

In a new book, Amnesty International has reported on the stories of people around the world who simply wish to love one another as an expression of their everyday lives, just like anyone, anywhere. These include Poliyana Mangwiro who was a leading member of Gays and Lesbians of Zimbabwe despite Robert Mugabe's protestations that homosexuality is "against African traditions." And Simon Nkoli, the ANC activist who after spending four years in prison under apartheid went on to be the face of the struggle for gay rights in the new South Africa. These are the voices of the struggle for justice.

But the voices of hate, fear, and persecution are also strong and lamentably often supported by faith leaders. From Egypt to Iran, Nigeria to India, Burma to Jamaica, gay men, lesbians, and transgender people are harassed, imprisoned, beaten, and forced from their communities. Some states even make homosexuality punishable by death. The Churches are not vocal enough in opposing these vicious injustices, while some Christians even encourage such persecution.

Hatred and prejudice are such destructive forces. They destroy human beings, communities, and whole societies—and they destroy the hater, too, from the inside. Reading the words of homophobia that are quoted in the Amnesty book is frightening, it is terrifying. It shows we all have within us a seed, a potential, that can grow into prejudice, hatred, and destruction. But prejudice is a bleak wasteland. A loving, understanding humanity is sustained by justice.

A parent who brings up a child to be a racist damages that child, damages the community in which they live, damages our hopes for a better world. A parent who teaches a child that there is only one sexual orientation and that anything else is evil denies our humanity and their own too. We cannot answer hate with hate. We can only answer it with love, understanding, and a belief in and commitment to justice. This is how we will build a world of human understanding, compassion, and equality: a true rainbow world.

FURTHER INFORMATION:

Amnesty International UK: LGBT books

13.

SAME-SEX MARRIAGE IN SOUTH AFRICA

The Constitutional Court's Judgment

Beth Goldblatt

The 1st of December 2005 was a proud day for South Africa as it joined the ranks of a handful of countries that provide full legal recognition to same-sex partnerships. The Constitutional Court was asked by a lesbian couple (Fourie & Bonthuys) to address their exclusion from the common law definition of marriage, which says that marriage is "a union of one man with one woman, to the exclusion, while it lasts, of all others." The court was asked, in a separate case brought by the Lesbian and Gay Equality Project[1] (together with a number of same sex couples), to remedy the problematic marriage formula in the Marriage Act 25 of 1961 that refers to a person taking another person as his or her "lawful wife (or husband)." The state opposed both cases. The two cases were heard and decided together. Sachs J. gave a judgment on behalf of the majority finding that the common law and the formula in the Marriage Act were inconsistent with the Constitution and invalid to the extent that they prevent same-sex couples from enjoying the status and benefits coupled with responsibilities accorded to heterosexual couples.[2] The decision was based primarily on the right to equality in South Africa's Bill of Rights that affords "equal protection and benefit of the law" and includes a prohibition against unfair discrimination on the basis of a set of

With kind permission from Springer Science + Business Media. *Feminist Legal Studies* 14 (2006): 261–70; Copyright Springer, 2006.

listed grounds including sexual orientation. The Constitution requires that the common law and legislation be developed in accordance with the spirit, purport, and objects of the Bill of Rights.[3] The only real debate within the Court concerned the appropriate remedy to be ordered. The majority decided to suspend the declaration of invalidity for one year from the date of judgment to allow the legislature to correct the defects in the common law and Marriage Act. In the event that this was not done in time the offending words in the marriage formula would be read as including the words "or spouse" after the words "or husband." The common law would become invalid to the extent that it did "not permit same-sex couples to enjoy the status and benefits coupled with responsibilities it accords to heterosexual couples."[4] O'Regan J., dissenting only on the issue of remedy, found that the Court should have developed the common law to include same-sex partners in the definition of marriage and should have read in wording to address the invalidity of the marriage formula in the legislation. This would provide gay and lesbian couples with immediate protection of their rights.

Despite the delay in remedy, the decision is warmly welcomed and many in South Africa are now eagerly awaiting the day, later this year, on which full rights will be extended to same sex couples.

This note briefly discusses the following: the history of the litigation and the reasoning set out in the Constitutional Court's decision; the series of cases on the rights of gays and lesbians that built up towards the marriage decision; the difference in approach taken by the Court towards same-sex marriage and domestic partnership; and lastly, the debate within the Court over remedy.

THE HISTORY OF THE LITIGATION AND THE COURT'S REASONING

Fourie and Bonthuys approached the High Court in 2002 to compel the state to register their marriage without framing a challenge to the constitutionality of the Marriage Act. The Court refused to grant the order.[5] The couple decided to apply to the Constitutional Court for direct access to appeal the decision, thereby bypassing the Supreme Court of Appeal (S.C.A.). The Constitutional Court refused the application stating that the matter dealt with the development of the common law and should therefore properly be heard by the S.C.A.[6] The S.C.A. only considered the common law definition of marriage as the challenge to the Marriage Act had not been included in the appellant's case. Cameron J. A., on behalf of the majority, in a thorough and progressive judgment, developed the common law definition of marriage, in line with the Constitution, to include same-sex partners.[7] The result of the decision was that the common law changed but the marriage formula did not, and so gay and lesbian couples were still unable to marry. The one loophole pointed out by the S.C.A. was the provision in the Marriage Act that allowed the Minister of Home Affairs to approve different marriage formulae for ministers of religion who were entitled to officiate over marriages. This meant that, at least in theory, certain same-sex marriages could occur following the S.C.A. judgment. The state appealed against the decision to the Constitutional Court "on the basis that it went too far" and the couple cross-appealed "on the grounds that it did not go far enough."[8] The Lesbian and Gay Equality Project had brought a separate application to challenge the offending legislation to the High Court and were granted direct access to the Constitutional Court to be heard together with the *Fourie* case.

The judgment held that gay and lesbian couples must be given appropriate provision to celebrate their unions in the same way that heterosexual couples are able to do. Sachs J. stressed the need for tolerance and "respect across difference." He said (at 60):

> ... [W]hat is at stake is not simply a question of removing an injustice experienced by a particular section of the community. At issue is a need to affirm the very character of our society as one based on tolerance and mutual respect. The test of tolerance is not how one finds space for people with whom, and practices with which, one feels comfortable, but how one accommodates the expression of what is discomfiting.

The judgment discussed the many benefits and consequences of marriage as illustration of the importance of the institution and the need to extend such benefits to all couples. Their exclusion was a violation of their equality rights. The court also dealt with four arguments advanced in favour of leaving traditional (heterosexual) marriage intact. First, the court countered the argument that marriage is defined by its procreative potential (and thus excludes same-sex unions) by stating that many heterosexual couples cannot or do not wish to have children. Second, in response to the argument that opening up marriage would violate the religious freedom of many, Sachs J. said that "(i)t is one thing for the Court to acknowledge the important role that religion plays in our public life. It is quite another to use religious doctrine as a source for interpreting the Constitution."[9] The constitutional claims of same sex couples need not prejudice the religious rights of anyone else. The judge pointed to a provision of the Marriage Act that allows (religious) marriage officers to refuse to solemnise marriages that do not accord with their beliefs. He said that "the two sets of interests involved do not collide, they co-exist in a constitutional realm based on accommodation of diversity."[10] Third, the argument that international law protected heterosexual marriage was answered by the Court in saying that these laws do not necessarily preclude same-sex marriage. And fourth, it was argued that s.15(3) of the Constitution (part of the freedom of religion, belief, and opinion right) that refers to the sanctioning of legislation recognising alternative systems of family law was an indication that same-sex partnerships should be given legislative protection separate from marriage. Sachs J. said that the existence of the section did not constitute a bar to the claims of the applicants.[11]

THE CULMINATION OF A SERIES OF SEXUAL ORIENTATION CASES

During the constitutional negotiating and drafting process in the early 1990s in South Africa, gay and lesbian activists lobbied successfully for the inclusion of sexual orientation as a ground of unfair discrimination in the Bill of Rights (Stychin 1996; Croucher 2002). A group of gay and lesbian organisations formed a coalition (the National Coalition for Gay and Lesbian Equality [N.C.G.L.E.])[12] in 1994 to campaign and litigate, using the constitutional right, for the removal of discrimination against gays and lesbians (Louw 2004). The litigation strategy envisaged a step-by-step approach that would start with a challenge to the criminalisation of sodomy and proceed to various aspects of same-sex family relationships culminating in a marriage case. Despite the N.C.G.L.E.'s plans, unaffiliated litigants brought some of their own cases in a different order. None of these turned out to be overly problematic and in general, the plan ran its course and proved to be highly successful, both in changing the law, and in shifting (sections of) public opinion towards the rights of gays and lesbians.

One of the first cases, brought by a policewoman (assisted by the N.C.G.L.E.), asked the court to set aside the rules of a medical scheme that prevented her female partner from being registered as a dependant. The court agreed on the basis that the couple had a legal duty to support each other.[13] The N.C.G.L.E. then successfully challenged the sodomy laws in the Constitutional Court.[14] The judgment "created a jurisprudential foundation on which to build far-reaching gay and lesbian rights to equality" (Louw 2004, p. 71). This was followed by another important N.C.G.L.E. case concerning the right of a person to make a permanent residence application where a same-sex partnership existed with a South African.[15] In an important equality judgment, the Court crafted an order that read into the legislation after the word "spouse," "or partner in a permanent same-sex life partnership." Further significant victories followed in two cases brought by High Court judges in same-sex partnerships: one concerned the entitlement of the judge's partner to benefit from her pension in terms of benefits reserved for spouses;[16] the other concerned the rights of both partners to be registered as adoptive parents of their adopted children although the law concerned only allowed married people this right.[17]

These cases paved the way for the Constitutional Court's affirmation of the rights of gays and lesbians to the same benefits as married heterosexuals in the *Fourie* case. This means that South African family law, which still locates marriage at its centre, will now be inclusive of same-sex partners for all purposes. An interesting question is whether the earlier judgments that extended rights and benefits to 'permanent same-sex life partners' will still apply now if gays and lesbians can choose to marry. If same-sex couples choose not to marry but are still entitled to benefit from such judgments, the implication is that they will now have greater rights in these areas than do heterosexual life partners. However, many same-sex couples do not wish to marry and other than in the specific cases that have been addressed through litigation, they will lack rights in many important areas (such as intestate succession). The challenge facing the development of South African family law is to expand our conception of family not only to a plurality of marital forms but to a more pluralistic conception of family itself. The Constitutional Court's unwillingness to lead this expansion is now discussed in relation to a recent judgment on domestic partnerships.

COMPARING THE COURT'S APPROACH TO SAME-SEX MARRIAGE AND DOMESTIC PARTNERSHIPS

In South Africa there is no legal recognition or protection of domestic partnerships within family law (although piecemeal statutory recognition has been extended for a range of benefits). There is a high incidence of domestic partnerships, particularly in the black community where historical factors such as migrancy and family dislocation remain legacies of Apartheid policies. Women tend to suffer when domestic partnerships end either through death or separation since, as the poorer members of the partnership, they are left with nothing. Until recently, this position had not been challenged in the courts. Where same-sex partnerships were given recognition by courts, this was always limited to gay and lesbian couples. Thus, in *N.C.G.L.E. v. Home Affairs*,[18] the Constitutional Court was careful to say that "other conjugal relationships not presently recognised as valid by law" were not covered by the decision which gave rights to same-sex life partners.[19]

Recently however, a woman who had been in a domestic partnership that ended with the death of her partner challenged a statute entitled the Maintenance of Surviving Spouses Act 27 of 1990 as violating her right to equality (on the ground of marital status) for failing to include permanent life partners in its ambit. Having succeeded in the High Court, she lost in the Constitutional Court.[20] The Court in *Volks* reasoned that since there was no duty to maintain a domestic partner in law during the lifetime of the parties, such an obligation could not be imposed after the death of one of the parties. The majority said that the "fundamental difference" between marriage and domestic partnership in law did not result in unfair discrimination as marriage had a special place in our law and society.[21]

The Court's assumption was that domestic partners choose this form of family arrangement over marriage knowing that theirs does not attract the same legal benefits as marriage. Yet, socio-legal research conducted in South Africa highlights the lack of choice faced by (usually) women partners who though wishing to marry, put up with their partners' refusal for want of a better alternative (Goldblatt 2003). Many women depend for their economic survival on men for whom they cook, clean, and look after children. Their 'choice' is highly constrained if it exists at all.

The Court expressed sympathy for this type of partnership saying that there was a "strong argument that partners ought to be obliged to maintain each other during their lifetime in certain circumstances,"[22] but failed to address this in the case before it. Judge Skweyiya said that the solution to vulnerability and economic dependence was law reform that regulated domestic partnerships.[23]

Steinberg points to the contradictions between the *Fourie* and *Volks* judgments:

> The spirit of *Fourie* is strikingly antiteleological: its hallmark is its insistence that life unions need not and ought not conform to any received doctrine. Yet *Volks* is all about sexual doctrine. The court's majority judgments are clearly grounded on the doctrine that the unions of those who publicly vow to a life-long, monogamous commitment must be privileged over those who do not. (Steinberg 2006, p. 6.)

The same-sex marriage judgment uses a formal equality framework that easily allows gays and lesbians the full benefits of an existing institution. The domestic partnership case requires the use of a more substantive equality framework since it involves recognising a new form of legal regulation of family. The Court's deferral of the problem to the legislature points to a discomfort in dealing with the complexities of such families. Another possible reason to distinguish between the judgments is the history of involvement of an organised and vocal gay and lesbian movement in South Africa while women in domestic partnerships remain an underrepresented, vulnerable group.[24]

DIFFERENT FINDINGS ON REMEDY

The only troubling feature of the majority's judgment in *Fourie* is its decision on the remedy. Sachs J. said that the legislature should be given a period of one year within which to address the constitutional invalidities highlighted by the Court. He justified this as best serving the principle of separation of powers and the need to legitimize the changes to the law by allowing these to go through Parliament. He said that legislation would provide greater security to people around the sensitive issue of the status of their relationships. He noted the work of the South African Law Reform Commission that had been investigating the recognition of same-sex marriage. The Commission had come up with a proposal to enact a Reformed Marriage Act that allowed same-sex marriage while renaming the current Marriage Act the "Conventional Marriage Act" and reserving it for use by opposite-sex couples. Sachs J. took this as evidence of the possibility of a number of ways in which the law could be changed to accomplish full benefits for same-sex partnerships. He said that equal treatment might not "invariably require identical treatment" if human dignity and the achievement of equality were "promoted . . . by the measure concerned."[25] The Court said that wording would be read in to the Marriage Act to allow same-sex marriage should Parliament fail to meet its deadline of 30 November 2006.

O'Regan J. disagreed with the majority judgment on the matter of remedy. She said that immediate relief should have been given to the applicants. Allowing gays and lesbians to marry would in no way undermine the institution of marriage. Changes to the Marriage Act and development of the common law would not prevent Parliament from making appropriate legislative changes in the future. In any event, the possible legislative choices were narrow. While separation of powers was important, this could not "be used to avoid the obligation of a court to provide appropriate relief that is just and equitable to litigants who successfully raise a constitutional complaint."[26] An order of the court has legitimacy since it flows from the Constitution itself.

O'Regan J. ultimately chose the more courageous path (Rickard 2005). It seems that the fear of a lack of credibility in the changes to marriage by the Court motivated the majority to require legislative reform. However, the nuances of judge-made or Parliament-made law are often unclear to the public. Some moral outcry was voiced when the judgment came out but this quickly dissipated. It remains to be seen whether the government will meet the court's deadline and introduce new laws in time. It is also unclear whether such new laws will adequately address the concern of gays and lesbians for full legal recognition and whether opposition groups will accept such laws.

A kinder interpretation of the majority's referral of the matter to the legislature is that the Court was trying to send a message to Parliament to take greater responsibility for contentious issues of law and 'morality.' The Justice Ministry has for many years neglected to address the questions of same-sex marriage and the regulation of domestic partnerships. Sachs J.'s decision sets up a positive rights framework within which to draft new legislation. Should Parliament fail to meet its obligation to introduce new laws, this will reflect poorly on our young democracy.

ACKNOWLEDGMENTS

Thanks to Cathi Albertyn, Jonathan Berger, and Paul Jammy for their helpful comments on this note. I would like to acknowledge the enormous contribution of the late Professor Ronald Louw to the struggle for the rights of gays and lesbians in South Africa.

REFERENCES

Croucher, S. "South Africa's Democratisation and the Politics of Gay Liberation," *Journal of Southern African Studies* 28, no. 2 (2002): 315–30.
Goldblatt, B. "Regulating Domestic Partnerships—A Necessary Step in the Development of South African Family Law," *South African Law Journal* 120, no. 3 (2003): 610–29.
Louw, R. "A Decade of Gay and Lesbian Equality Litigation." In *Constitutional Democracy in South Africa 1994–2004*, edited by M. du Plessis & S. Pete. LexisNexis Butterworths: Durban, 2004, pp. 65–79.
Rickard, C. "At Heart, Ruling Lacks Courage," *Sunday Times*, December 4, 2005.
Steinberg, J. "Two Judgments That Show a New Light, an Old Shadow," *Business Day*, January 17, 2006.
Stychin, C. F. "Constituting Sexuality: The Struggle for Sexual Orientation in the South African Bill of Rights," *Journal of Law and Society* 23, no. 4 (1996): 455–83.

NOTES

1. An organisation established to litigate and promote the rights of gays and lesbians in South Africa.

2. *Minister of Home Affairs and Another v. Fourie and Others; Lesbian and Gay Equality Project and Others v. Minister of Home Affairs and Others* (2006) (3) B.C.L.R. 355 (C.C.) The case is hereinafter referred to as *Fourie*.

3. Section 39(2) of the Constitution of the Republic of South Africa Act 108 of 1996.

4. Para. 1(c)(i) of the Order.

5. *Fourie and Another v. Minister of Home Affairs and Another (The Lesbian and Gay Equality Project intervening as amicus curiae)* Case no. 17280/02, unreported.

6. *Fourie and Another v. Minister of Home Affairs and Another* (2003) (5) S.A. 301 (C.C.).

7. *Fourie and Another v. Minister of Home Affairs and Others* (2005) (3) S.A. 429 (S.C.A.). The minority decision of Farlam J.A. also developed the common law to allow same-sex marriage but read in wording to the Marriage Act that allowed such marriages to occur. He said that the changes should be suspended for two years to allow Parliament to enact appropriate legislative remedies.

8. *Fourie, supra* n. 2, para. 33.

9. *Fourie,* ibid., para. 92.

10. *Fourie,* ibid., para. 98.

11. *Fourie,* ibid., para. 109.

12. The Gay and Lesbian Equality Project who brought the case discussed in this note is a successor of the now disbanded N.C.G.L.E.

13. *Langemaat v. Minister of Safety and Security and Others* (1998) (3) S.A. 312 (T).

14. *National Coalition for Gay and Lesbian Equality and Another v. Minister of Justice and Others* (1999) (1) S.A. 6 (C.C.).

15. *National Coalition for Gay and Lesbian Equality v. Minister of Home Affairs* (2000) (2) S.A. 1 (C.C.).

16. *Satchrvell v. President of the Republic of South Africa* (2002) (6) S.A. 1 (C.C.).

17. *Du Toit v. Minister of Population and Welfare Development* (2003) (2) S.A. 198 (C.C.).

18. *Supra* n. 12, at p. 293 C–D.

19. This is because the cases were argued narrowly around the rights of same-sex partners only and because the decision was based on the inability of gays and lesbians to marry.

20. *Volks N. O. v. Robinson and Others* (2005) (5) B.C.L.R. 446 (C.C.).

21. *Volks,* ibid., paras. 52, 55–56.

22. *Volks,* ibid., para. 60.

23. *Volks,* ibid., paras. 63–68.

24. The movement for gay and lesbian rights has weakened significantly in the last decade, however its existence during this period was crucial to the legal improvements witnessed in South Africa. The women's movement has lacked the same coherence in developing its own litigation strategy.

25. *Fourie, supra* n. 2, para. 152.

26. *Fourie,* ibid., para. 170.

14.

MORAL REASONING IN JUDICIAL DECISIONS ON SAME-SEX MARRIAGE

Alicia Ouellette

The relevance of the morality of homosexuality is a point of sharp disagreement for judges confronted with legal challenges to laws that limit marriage to heterosexual couples. Judges ruling in favor of same-sex marriage eschew moral opprobrium as a legitimate basis for legal decision-making in favor of a traditional liberal vision of the neutral state. By contrast, judges who support the exclusion of same sex couples from marriage unapologetically endorse the majority's preference for heterosexual procreative sex to legitimate legal barriers to marriage for same-sex couples. Thus, the threshold question in a study of the role of morality in the same-sex marriage decisions is whether the judges view moral preference as a legitimate state interest in the first place. The next step in the analysis—that which yields more surprising results—is a study of the effort of pro-marriage judges to "bracket"[1] morality. That analysis reveals that even judges who claim to base decisions on traditional liberal values of equality, tolerance, and privacy do not remain morally neutral toward homosexual relationships when they justify the grant of marriage rights. Instead, they make the case that same-sex relationships are normatively valuable for the very reasons that heterosexual marriages are normatively valuable. It is only the judges who take the middle ground—condemning discriminatory laws without granting the affirmative right to marriage itself—who come close to achieving moral neutrality toward homosexuality and same-sex relationships in their opinions.

This paper explores the role of morality and morality-based reasoning in a sampling of judicial decisions for and against same-sex marriage. It starts with an explanation of the legal context in which the marriage cases came before state courts. Next, it demonstrates the disagreement over the legitimacy of moral judgments as basis for marriage laws. Then, focusing exclusively on the courts' treatment of the justifications proffered in defense of same-sex marriage bans,[2] it examines the reasoning employed by judges who reject same sex-marriage claims and the reasoning employed by the Massachusetts judges and others who have voted to grant access to marriage to people of the same gender. Finally, it contrasts the decisions that grant same-sex couples equality in the form of civil unions without granting full acceptance through marriage. What becomes strikingly apparent in this study are the sharp disagreements as to whether moral justifications for law are appropriate at all, and the difficulty all judges face in refraining from morality-based decision-making in same-sex marriage cases.

A. CHANGING MORES, RADICAL TIMES: THE SUPREME COURT'S TURNAROUND ON SODOMY LAWS

At the same time that the historic Massachusetts same-sex marriage case was winding its way though the state courts, the US Supreme Court was deciding a series of cases that radically changed the legal parameters for state regulation of sexual relationships between consenting adults. Over just two decades, the Court moved from express approval of morality-based sexual regulations, to condemnation of laws that disadvantage people because of moral disapproval of their sexual conduct. An understanding of the cases that led to the Supreme Court's about-face on sex laws is helpful to understanding the relevance of morality to the same-sex marriage cases.

Early cases defined a constitutional right to personal privacy, but gave no consideration of its application to homosexuality or access to marriage. The first privacy case, decided in 1891,[3] concerned searches of employees in civil cases. In rejecting compulsory searches, the Supreme Court explained: "No right is held more sacred, or is more carefully guarded, by the common law, than the right of every individual to the possession and control of his own person, free from all restraint or interference of others. . . ." In 1965, the Court expanded the right of personal privacy to reproductive choices when it held in favor of a right of married persons to use contraceptives.[4] Then, in 1972, the Court clarified that the right to reproductive privacy is not bound by marriage when it struck down a statute that prohibited the use of contraception by unmarried adults.[5] In the decision, the Court said, "If the right of privacy means anything, it is the right of the individual, married or single, to be free from unwarranted governmental intrusion into matters so fundamentally affecting a person as the decision whether to bear or beget a child."[6] The court extended the right of privacy to include decisions to terminate a pregnancy in its January 22, 1973, decision in *Roe v. Wade,*[7] a decision reaffirmed in on June 29, 1992, in *Planned Parenthood v. Casey.*[8]

As a result of these decisions, it was clear by the mid 1980s that the right to privacy applied to matters concerning reproduction. Not so for matters concerning sex. In 1986, the United States Supreme Court upheld as constitutional a Georgia law that criminalized sodomy between consenting adults.[9] The defendant in *Bowers v. Hardwick* was a gay man who had been convicted under the Georgia statute. He argued that he had a constitutional right to privacy that extended to private, consensual sexual conduct. Reframing the legal question as whether the constitution created "a fundamental right to engage in homosexual sodomy," the Court rejected the defendant's arguments and answered that the constitution provided no such right. The judges writing in favor of the majority rejected the plaintiff's claims about the importance of sexual intimacy between members of the same sex, and emphasized historical negative judgments about homosexual sex. Said Justice Byron White in the majority, "the presumed belief of a majority of the electorate in Georgia that homosexual sodomy is immoral and unacceptable" is an adequate rationale to support the criminalization of sodomy because "[t]he law . . . is constantly based on notions of morality."[10] Justice Warren Burger's concurrence was even more direct. He quoted William Blackstone's characterization of sodomy as a "crime not fit to be named," and concluded that "[t]o hold that the act of homosexual sodomy is somehow protected as a fundamental right would be to cast aside millennia of moral teaching."[11]

With moral teaching clearly approved as a legitimate basis for legislation, states passed laws that went beyond the direct regulation of homosexual sex to legislation directed at gays and lesbians themselves. For example, the voters of Colorado changed the state's constitution to prohibit all legislative, executive, or judicial action that would protect gays and lesbians from discrimination based on their sexual orientation. The amendment (known as Amendment 2) was designed to protect the association rights of citizens who morally disapproved of homosexuality from having to associate with gays and lesbians. Amendment 2 was challenged on federal constitutional basis in a case that made its way to the Supreme Court.[12] In its decision, the Supreme Court backed away from its previous stance about moral opprobrium as basis for law. In striking down the Colorado law, the Supreme Court held that Amendment 2 classified "homosexuals not to further a proper legislative end but to make them unequal to everyone else. This Colorado cannot do. A State cannot so deem a class of persons a stranger to its laws" even when a majority of citizens morally disapprove of the class.[13] Importantly, the decision was based on equal protection, not the right to privacy. Nonetheless, the notion that the majority's moral disapproval of the sexual conduct of a minority was an illegitimate basis for law making began to take root. Indeed, the dissent in the case lamented, "Amendment 2 is a modest attempt by seemingly tolerant Coloradans to preserve traditional sexual mores against the efforts of a politically powerful minority to revise those mores through use of the laws. That objective, and the means chosen to achieve it, is [. . .] unimpeachable under any constitutional doctrine hitherto pronounced."[14]

Then came the revolution. Seventeen years after the Court upheld sodomy laws as legitimate morality-based legislation in *Bowers*, the Supreme Court reversed course and held that the US Constitution precludes government intrusion into deeply personal decisions about consensual sexual relationships between adults.[15] In *Lawrence v. Texas*, two men convicted of "deviate sexual intercourse" under a Texas statute that criminalized oral and anal sex by consenting same-sex couples argued that the Texas law was unconstitutional for the very reasons rejected by the court in *Bowers*. In its decision, the *Lawrence* Court took the unusual step of overruling itself and striking down the Texas statute. Writing for the majority, Justice Anthony M. Kennedy declared *Bowers* wrongly decided and held that the defendants were free as adults to engage in private sexual conduct in the exercise of their liberty rights guaranteed by the Due Process Clause of the Fourteenth Amendment.

Critical to the holding in *Lawrence* was the rejection of morality judgments as legitimate bases for legislation that interferes with private, consensual sexual relationships. Justice O'Connor's concurrence was most direct on this point. In scrutinizing the Texas statute and the rationale proffered in its defense by the State of Texas, she found no basis for the statute other than moral disapproval of sodomy. Echoing the sentiments of the majority in its due process analysis, O'Connor rejected moral disapproval as a legitimate basis for a law that discriminates among groups of persons. The Texas law discriminates, she said, because "the law serves more as a statement of dislike and disapproval against homosexuals than as a tool to stop criminal behavior." A law "branding one class of persons as criminals solely based on the State's moral disapproval of that class and conduct associated with that class"[16] cannot stand.

Not surprisingly, the dissent in *Lawrence* objected forcefully to the dismissal of morality as basis for law. In the dissent's view, "[A] governing majority's belief that certain sexual behavior is 'immoral and unacceptable' constitutes a rational basis for regulation."[17] The majority's decision, it claimed, called into question laws against bigamy, same-sex marriage, adult incest, prostitution, masturbation, adultery, fornication, bestiality, and obscenity. Indeed, the dissent claimed that the majority opinions are hypocritical. Rather than removing morality from the equation, the majority departed from its role as neutral observer by imposing its own view of morality on the "many Americans who do not want persons who openly engage in homosexual conduct as partners in their business, as scoutmasters for their children, as teachers in their children's schools, or as boarders in their home."[18]

With these decisions as backdrop, the top courts in several states were confronted with challenges to laws that prohibited same-sex couples from marrying. The application in the marriage cases of the rule that morality judgments are not a legitimate basis for laws that regulate sexual conduct is a source of major disagreement among judges.

B. Bracketing and Embracing Morality

The most obvious divide between judges who have voted to uphold laws that prohibit marriage by people of the same gender, and those who vote to abolish the barriers is in their view of the role of majoritarian moral judgments as legitimate bases for marriage laws. Judges who reject claims to same-sex marriage, "traditional marriage judges," accept moral judgments about homosexuality as legitimate basis for barriers to marriage. Those judges who favor marriage rights for same-sex couples, "pro-marriage judges," view the Supreme Court's admonishment that moral disapproval of homosexuality is not a legitimate basis for law as the starting point for analysis in marriage cases.

1. Moral Judgments Uphold the Status Quo

Traditional marriage judges do not purport to bracket moral judgment in their decisions on marriage laws. To be sure, they do not couch their decisions in quotes from Thomas Aquinas or others who condemn homosexuality. Instead, they uphold as legitimate majoritarian decision-making based on "tradition," "history,"[19] and a preference for natural procreation that adopts "the notion that marriage, often linked to procreation, is a union forged between one man and one woman."[20] For example, one judge wrote "the historical conception of marriage as a union between a man and a woman is reflected in the civil institution of marriage."[21] Another said, "New York's marriage laws are part of a long-standing tradition."[22] And the dissent in the Massachusetts case asserted, "In this Commonwealth and in this Country, the roots of the institution are deeply set in history as a civil union between a single man and single woman."[23] These calls on tradition and history implicitly incorporate moral value judgments about intimate relationships between members of the same sex.

The historical roots of marriage are unabashedly value laden in their preference for heterosexual relationships. Said a Massachusetts court in 1810, the purpose of marriage "is to regulate, chasten, and define the intercourse between the sexes; and to multiply, preserve, and improve the species."[24] That this purpose chooses a particular moral vision was confirmed by the Supreme Court in 1885:

> [N]o legislation can be supposed more wholesome and necessary in the founding of a free, self-governing commonwealth . . . than that which seeks to establish it on the basis of the idea of the family, as consisting in and springing from the union for life of one man and one woman . . . the sure foundation of all that is stable and noble in our civilization; the best guaranty of that reverent morality which is the source of all beneficent progress in social and political improvement."[25]

And the Court later explained that marriage creates "the most important relation in life . . . having more to do with the morals and civilization of a people than any other institution."[26] Thus, "civil marriage is the institutional mechanism by which societies have sanctioned and recognized particular family structures."[27]

The moral vision supporting traditional marriage has its roots in natural law theory.[28] Simply put, the natural law view of homosexuality is that sex acts between people of the same sex are abhorrent because they are not generative.[29] Nonreproductive sex acts are "part of our animal nature rather than our divine nature: part, that is, of the declension. It is only a small step to view that sex is, at best, a necessary evil (necessary to the survival of the human race . . .) to the correlative view that nonprocreative sex, like gluttony, is an unqualified evil."[30] Thus viewed, homosexuality is immoral, "akin to 'copulation of humans with animals' in that both are destructive of human character and relationships."[31] Under the natural law framework, "[a] political community is therefore entitled to protect its institutions (such as marriage and the family) from the influence and effect of homosexuals and their relationships."[32] Communities may accomplish that protection be penalizing immoral sex acts, and by providing the special status that is marriage to those who engage in moral sex acts.[33]

The majoritarian positions endorsed by traditional marriage judges track natural law arguments. They equate marriage with procreation. "Marriage," they claim, "was instituted to address the fact that sexual contact between a man and a woman can naturally result in pregnancy and childbirth."[34] Defining the institution thus, judges explain why heterosexual relationships may be afforded special treatment by the state. "Heterosexual intercourse has a natural tendency to lead to the birth of children; homosexual intercourse does not . . . [A]n important function of marriage is to create more stability and permanence in the relationships that cause children to be born."[35] Thus, traditional-marriage judges argue, state legislatures can give special status—marriage—to those heterosexual relationships as "an inducement" to opposite sex couples promote procreation.[36]

The marriage as procreation view is repeated time and again in decisions denying access to marriage by same-sex couples. Said another judge, "The binary nature of marriage—its inclusion of one woman and one man—reflects the biological fact that human procreation cannot be accomplished without the genetic contribution of both a male and a female. Marriage creates a supportive environment for procreation to occur and the resulting offspring to be nurtured."[37] Another added, "Paramount among its many important functions, the institution of marriage has systematically provided for the regulation of heterosexual behavior, brought order to the resulting procreation, and ensured a stable family structure in which children will be reared, educated, and socialized. . . . The institution of marriage provides the important legal and normative link between heterosexual intercourse and procreation on the one hand and family responsibilities on the other."[38]

Like the traditional values argument, the marriage as procreation argument incorporates and accepts as legitimate a moral preference for heterosexuality and moral disapproval of homosexuality as basis for law. As pointed out by a pro-marriage Massachusetts judge, "The 'marriage is procreation' argument singles out the one unbridgeable difference between same-sex and opposite-sex couples, and transforms that difference into the essence of legal marriage. . . . the marriage restriction impermissibly 'identifies persons by a single trait and then denies them protection across the board . . . In so doing, the State's action confers an official stamp of approval on the destructive stereotype that same-sex relationships are inherently unstable and inferior to opposite-sex relationships and are not worthy of respect."[39]

In response to the argument that barring from marriage even same-sex couples who are raising children is rational, traditional-marriage judges rely most directly on majoritarian moral judgment. They claim that opposite sex couples make the best parents for children. For example, one judge argued that "continuing to limit the institution of civil marriage to members of the opposite sex [despite technological advances and changes in adoption laws that allow gays and lesbians to become parents] furthers the legitimate purpose of ensuring, promoting, and supporting an optimal social structure for the bearing and raising of children."[40] The view that married heterosexuals are "optimal" parents is said to be rational given "studies that document negative consequences that too often follow children either born outside of marriage or raised in households lacking either a father or a mother figure, and scholarly commentary contending that children and families develop best when mothers and fathers are partners in their parenting."[41] Some judges go further and endorse outright disapproval of same-sex relationships and how they affect children. For example, Judge Robert Smith of the New York Court of Appeals argued, "The Legislature could rationally believe that it is better, other things being equal, for children to grow up with both a mother and a father."[42] Judge Smith did not invoke studies to support the position. Instead he based his argument on "intuition and experience." A "person's preference for the sort of sexual activity that cannot lead to the birth of children is relevant to the state's interest in fostering relationships that will serve the children best."[43]

Thus, the traditional-marriage judges accept the majoritarian view that champions heterosexual relations because of their natural tendency to lead to procreation, and denounces the value of same-sex relationships. This reasoning affirms the right of the voting majority to confer the benefits of marriage based on its collective moral judgment that homosexuality and homosexual relationships are unworthy of respect.

2. Bracketing Morality to Grant Access to Marriage

Unlike traditional-marriage judges, pro-marriage judges reject moral opprobrium as legitimate basis for marriage laws. The most important decision in this respect, the (Massachusetts) November 2003 ruling in *Goodridge v. Department of Public Health*, is also the most important decision in favor of marriage rights for same-sex couples. Decided just five months after the Supreme Court called for moral bracketing in public reasoning in *Lawrence*, the Massachusetts Supreme Judicial Court held that the Massachusetts law that kept same-sex couples from marrying violated their constitutional rights and denied "the dignity and equality of all individuals."

The *Goodridge* decision is paradigmatic of the decisions by other judges who have written in favor of striking marriage bans in that it starts with the assertion that the job of judges is protecting the liberty of all citizens, "not to mandate our own moral code."[44] In *Goodridge*, the court acknowledged that "many people hold deep-seated religious, moral, and ethical convictions that marriage should be limited to the union of one man and one woman, and that homosexual conduct is immoral. Many hold equally strong religious, moral, and ethical convictions that same-sex couples are entitled to be married, and that homosexual persons should be treated no differently than their heterosexual neighbors. Neither view answers the question before us."[45] The court further explained that "matters of belief and conviction are properly outside the reach of judicial review or government interference. But neither may the government, under the guise of protecting "traditional" values, even if they be the traditional values of the majority, enshrine in law an invidious discrimination."[46]

Similarly, Judge Judith Kaye, writing for the dissent in the New York marriage cases repeatedly rejected moral disapproval of homosexuals as a legitimate basis for law.[47] Quoting the Supreme Court, she rejected the argument that moral judgments, even long held moral judgments, are legitimate basis for law. "The fact that the governing majority state has traditionally viewed a particular practice as immoral is not a sufficient reason for upholding a law prohibiting the practice."[48]

Thus, pro-marriage judges reject moral disapproval of gays and lesbians as legitimate basis for law. Their opinions thus appear to be consistent with Rawlsian liberalism in its preference for equality and neutrality. The question remains whether they incorporate some other form of moral reasoning in the place of moral disapprobation.

C. Does One Moral Judgment Replace Another?

While pro-marriage judges claim to bracket moral judgment from judicial decision-making, a close look at their opinions reveals that the decisions are far from morally neutral. Pro-marriage judges engage in moral reasoning of a different sort than their traditional-marriage colleagues. These judges decouple marriage from sex to distill a value in marriage, a public good, which can be realized by gay and lesbian relationships in the same way that it can be realized by heterosexual relationships.[49] Having made the normative case those honoring same-sex relationships in marriage promotes the public good, pro-marriage judges conclude that excluding them from the institution is irrational.

Pro-marriage judges take issue with majority view that marriage is about procreation. Instead, they see marriage itself as a public good and same-sex relationships as fully capable of promoting that good. Marriage, said Judge Kaye of the New York Court of Appeals, is about "emotional support and public commitment;"[50] it promotes a "stable society."[51] Justice Marshall of the Supreme Judicial Court of Massachusetts agrees: "marriage is a vital social institution. The commitment of two individuals to each other nurtures love and mutual support; it brings stability to our society."[52] "Civil marriage anchors an ordered society by encouraging stable relationships over transient ones. It is central to the way the Commonwealth identifies individuals, provides for the orderly distribution of property, ensures that children and adults are cared for and supported whenever possible from private rather than public funds, and tracks important epidemiological and demographic data."[53]

The marriage as procreation argument is illogical, point out the pro-marriage judges: "Our laws of civil marriage do not privilege procreative heterosexual intercourse between married people able to procreate over every other form of adult intimacy and every other means of creating a family. [The laws] contain no requirement that the applicants for a marriage license attest to their ability or intention to conceive children by coitus."[54] "Marriage is about much more than producing children . . . Indeed, the protections that the State gives to couples who do marry—such as the right to own property as a unit or to make medical decisions for each other—are focused largely on the adult relationship, rather than on the couple's possible role as parents . . . The breadth of protections that the marriage laws make unavailable to gays and lesbians is 'so far removed' from . . . the goal of promoting procreation that the justification is . . . 'impossible to credit.'"[55]

Focused then on the broader good of social stability created by marriage, pro-marriage judges argue that same-sex couples can realize the same social stability through marriage that heterosexual couples can achieve. "The State's interest in a stable society is rationally advanced when families are established and remain intact irrespective of the gender of the spouses."[56] To buttress the argument, the judges make the normative case in favor of same-sex unions. For example, one judge described the plaintiffs in the case as follows:

> a doctor, a police officer, a public school teacher, a nurse, an artist and a state legislator . . . They come from upstate and down, from rural, urban and suburban settings. Many have been together in committed relationships for decades, and many are raising children—from toddlers to teenagers. Many are active in their communities, serving on their local school board, for example, or their cooperative apartment building board. *In short, plaintiffs represent a cross-section of New Yorkers who want only to live full lives, raise their children, better their communities and be good neighbors.*[57]

Giving these plaintiffs access to marriage will "anchor [. . .] an ordered society," the very public good achieved by marriage in the first place. Because we ought to behave as a society by doing what will best advance the public good, and because same-sex couples can contribute to the good through marriage, the only rational tact, say the pro-marriage judges, is to give same-sex couples access to the institution. Barriers to marriage fall as irrational and illegitimate.

Through this argument, pro-marriage judges engage in moral reasoning of a different sort than that employed by traditional-marriage judges. Viewing marriage itself as a social good, pro-marriage judges make the normative judgment that same-sex couples are just as capable as opposite-sex couples in promoting social good through marriage. Excluding these capable couples from the institution is unfair and irrational because it defeats the good advanced by the institution. While free of reliance on the moral opprobrium as basis for law, this line of argument is hardly morally neutral.

To be sure, pro-marriage judges also engage additional arguments that are more neutral toward homosexuality. These arguments, steeped in equality, focus on the denial of the benefits of marriage to same-sex couples. "Civil marriage provides tangible legal protections and economic benefits to married couples and their children, and tens of thousands of children are currently being raised by same-sex couples in New York. Depriving these children of the benefits and protections available to the children of opposite-sex couples is antithetical to their welfare."[58] The only justifications offered to support such discrimination," said the Massachusetts Court, are those "rooted in persistent prejudices against persons who are (or who are believed to be) homosexual. 'The Constitution cannot control such prejudices but neither can it tolerate them. Private biases may be outside the reach of the law, but the law cannot, directly or indirectly, give them effect.'"[59]

This fairness argument is morally neutral in its position on the virtue of homosexuality toward same-sex relationships. Fairness alone is not enough, however, to require the grant of full access to marriage. That result is achieved by coupling the fairness argument with the normative argument that posits that same-sex couples are worthy of the privilege of marriage because of their ability to contribute to the public good. As the Massachusetts Court acknowledges in construing "civil marriage to mean the voluntary union of two persons as spouses, to the exclusion of all others:" "This reformulation redresses the plaintiffs' constitutional injury *and furthers the aim of marriage to promote stable, exclusive relationships.*"[60] Redressing inequities could be achieved without stamping the marriage label on same-sex relationships. Civil unions, domestic partnerships, or other mechanisms are available to allow same-sex couples to access the same rights and privileges available to heterosexual couples through marriage.[61] It is the normative judgment that giving same-sex couples the right to marriage will advance the public goods of marriage that supports the result reached by the pro-marriage judges.

D. IS THERE A PATH TO MORAL NEUTRALITY?

When confronted with demands for legal recognition of same-sex relationships, the top courts in Vermont and New Jersey refused to grant the plaintiff couples the full legal acceptance they sought. Recognizing that the denial of access to the rights that accompany legal recognition of a monogamous relationship disadvantaged gays and lesbians, the courts required the states to eliminate barriers to equality.

The courts did not, however, grant gays and lesbians full access to marriage. Instead, the Courts demanded only that the state legislators devise a scheme to provide equal access to the rights and privileges attendant to marriage. In this way, the decisions of the New Jersey and Vermont Courts are the most morally neutral toward homosexuality and homosexual relationships of those handed down in same-sex marriage cases.[62] Consistent with Rawlsian liberalism, they embrace the notion of justice as fairness while recognizing that "there are many conflicting reasonable comprehensive doctrines with their [own] conceptions of the good."[63]

The New Jersey and Vermont Courts start their analysis with application of the constitutional principles of liberty and equality enunciated by the Supreme Court in *Romer* and *Lawrence* to prohibit the states from denying gays and lesbians access to the benefits and privileges available to married opposite-sex couples, but analyze separately the question of "whether committed same-sex partners have a constitutional right to define their relationship by the name marriage, the word that historically has characterized the union of a man and a woman."[64] In this second part of the analysis, the New Jersey and Vermont Courts neither affirm nor deny the morality of homosexuality or homosexual relationships. They merely tolerate difference without mandating acceptance.[65] The Vermont Court held, for example, that "the State is constitutionally required to extend to same-sex couples the common benefits and protections that flow from marriage under Vermont law. That the State could do so through a marriage license is obvious. But it is not required to do so."[66]

The New Jersey Court explained that the neutral principle of equal treatment requires that "committed same-sex couples must be afforded on equal terms the same rights and benefits enjoyed by married opposite couples,"[67] but that granting access to marriage requires "social acceptance" of their relationships.[68] The court was unwilling to take that step. "To be clear, it is not our role to suggest whether the Legislature should either amend the marriage statutes to include same sex couples or enact a civil union scheme. Our role here is limited to constitutional adjudication, and therefore we must steer clear of the swift and treacherous currents of social policy."

The Vermont Court quoted Sunstein in explaining its position: "When a democracy is in moral flux, courts may not have the best or final answers. Judicial answers may be wrong. They may be counterproductive even if they are right. Courts do best by proceeding in a way that is catalytic rather than preclusive, and that is closely attuned to the fact that courts are participants in the system of democratic deliberation."[69]

Thus, the courts concluded that notions of equality and tolerance require that states provide parity in the benefits associated with marriage, but liberalism's "central organizing idea . . . the neutrality of the state toward moral

ideals, or, to use the more current phrase, conceptions of the good life"[70] prevented the courts from approving of gays and lesbians in the normative sense
necessary to move from tolerance to full acceptance through marriage rights.[71]

E. Conclusion

Judicial decisions on the constitutionality of legal barriers to marriage by same-sex
couples are complex on many levels. Judges disagree as to the scope of rights
involved, the degree of scrutiny the laws should receive, and what if anything constitutes legitimate state purposes in the regulation of marriage. This paper does not
begin to discuss many of the issues raised in the cases. Rather, the paper focuses on
the judges' treatment of the rationales proffered in support of traditional marriage
laws to determine whether and to what extent moral reasoning and moral judgments affect the analyses. This focus reveals a deep divide between the views of
pro-marriage and traditional-marriage judges. Traditional-marriage judges not
only accept moral condemnation of homosexual sex as a legitimate basis for traditional marriage laws, they embrace as legitimate the majority's view that that procreative sex is deserving of special status and protection unavailable to homosexual
sex. Pro-marriage judges reject moral condemnation of gays and lesbians as a legitimate basis for laws affecting sexual relationships, but engage in a different type of
moral reasoning to conclude that states must bestow full marriage rights on same-
sex couples because such couples are equally capable of contributing to the
public good advanced by marriage. It is only judges that stop short of granting
full marriage rights, but deem illegal the deprivation of equal access to the legal
benefits that accompany marriage, who approximate moral neutrality toward
gays and lesbians. Moral neutrality in judicial decision-making is not necessarily
a desirable goal. To the extent that judges seek to achieve it, however, the decisions of the New Jersey and Vermont courts appear to be the best models.

Notes

1. Carlos A. Ball, "Moral Foundations for a Discourse on Same-Sex Marriage:
Looking beyond Political Liberalism," *Georgetown Law Journal* 85 (1997): 1871.
2. This focus is deliberately narrow. The opinions themselves address a multitude
of legal issues including standard of review, due process, equal protection, privacy, and
state constitutional rights, which are not addressed in this paper.
3. *Union Pacific Railway Co. v. Botsford,* 141 U.S. 250, 251 (1891).
4. *Griswold v. Connecticut,* 381 U.S. 479 (1965).
5. *Eisentadt v. Baird,* 405 U.S. 438 (1972).

6. Ibid., at 453.

7. 410 U.S. 113 (1973).

8. 505 U.S. 833 (1992).

9. *Bowers v. Hardwick*, 478 U.S. 186 (1986).

10. Ibid., at 196.

11. Ibid., at 197.

12. *Romer v. Evans*, 517 U.S. 620 (1995).

13. Ibid., at 868.

14. Ibid., at 868 (Scalia, J. dissenting).

15. *Lawrence v. Texas*, 539 U.S. 558 (2003).

16. Ibid., at 585.

17. Ibid., at 589.

18. Ibid., at 602.

19. *Goodridge*, at 990 (Cordy, J. dissenting).

20. *Standhart v. Superior Court of the State of Arizona*, 77 P.3d 451, 459 (2003).

21. *Hernandez*, at 367 (Graffeo, J. concurring).

22. *Hernandez*, at 374 (Graffeo, J. concurring).

23. *Goodridge*, at 977 (Spina, J. dissenting).

24. *Goodridge*, at 985 (Cordy, J. dissenting) (quoting *Milford v. Worcester*, 7 Mass. 48, 52 (1810)).

25. *Murphy v. Ransey*, 114 U.S. 15, 45 (1885).

26. *Maynard v. Hill*, 125 U.S. 190, 205 (1888).

27. *Goodridge*, at 995 (Cordy, J. dissenting).

28. For a more expansive view of this argument, see John Finnis, "Law, Morality, and Sexual Orientation," *Notre Dame Law Review* 69 (1994): 1049–76; Ball, at 1909.

29. John Finnis, "Law, Morality, and Sexual Orientation," *Notre Dame Law Review* 69 (1994): 1049–76; Robert P. George, *In Defense of Natural Law* (New York: Oxford University Press, 1999).

30. Summa Theolagia, in *Homosexuality and Ethics* 42–44 (Edward Batchellor Jr., ed., 1980); see also, Pim Pronk, *Against Nature? Types of Moral Argumentation Regarding Homosexuality* 26–36 (1993).

31. Ball, at 1911.

32. Ibid.

33. For more on this theory, see John Finnis, "Sexual Morality and the Possibility of 'Same-Sex Marriage': The Good of Marriage and the Morality of Sexual Relations: Some Philosophical and Historical Observations," *American Journal of Jurisprudence* 42 (1997): 97.

34. *Hernandez*, at 378–79 (Graffeo, J. concurring).

35. Ibid.

36. Those courts that confront the fact that technology allows same-sex couples to reproduce, offer the following tortured rationale to explain why the law need not respond to the reality that same-sex couples are procreating: "The legislature could find that unstable relationships between people of the opposite sex present a greater danger that children will be born into or grow up in unstable homes than is the case with same-sex couples, and thus that promoting the stability in opposite-sex relationships will help chil-

dren more." *Hernandez*, at 359. See also *Morrison v. Sadler*, 821 N.E.2d 15 (Ind. 2005) (adopting a "natural procreation" argument).

37. *Hernandez*, at 370 (Graffeo, J. concurring).

38. *Goodridge*, at 995 (Spina, J. dissenting); see also *Conaway v. Deane*, 932 A.2d 571 (Maryland 2007).

39. *Goodridge*, at 962 (quoting *Romer v. Evans*, 517 U.S. 620, 233 (1996)).

40. *Goodridge*, at 998 (Cordy, J. dissenting). See also *Citizens for Equal Protection v. Bruning*, 455 F.3d 859, 867 (8th Cir. 2006) (describing as legitimate the view that "two committed heterosexuals are the optimal partnership for raising children").

41. *Goodridge*, at 998–99 (Cordy, J. dissenting). The existence of studies that conclude that children raised be same-sex couples are arguments that undermine the validity of these studies are deemed irrelevant by traditional-marriage judges. Said Judge Robert Smith, "Plaintiffs seem to assume that they have demonstrated the irrationality of the view that opposite-sex marriages offer advantages to children by showing there is no scientific evidence to support it. Even assuming no such evidence exists, this reasoning is flawed. In the absence of conclusive scientific evidence, the Legislature could rationally proceed on the commonsense premise that children will do best with a mother and father in the home." *Hernandez*, at 360.

42. *Hernandez*, at 360; see also *Goodridge*, 440 Mass. at 358–59 (Sosman, J. dissenting) (referring to the commonsense premise that children will do best with a mother and father in the home.)

43. *Hernandez*, at 365.

44. *Goodridge v. Dep't of Health*, 798 N.E.2d 941(Mass. 2003), quoting *Lawrence v. Texas*, 539 U.S. 558 (2003).

45. Ibid., at 312.

46. *Opinions of the Justices*, 802 N.E.2d 565 (2004).

47. *Hernandez v. Robles*, 7 NY.3d at 394.

48. *Hernandez*, at 387 (Kaye, J. dissenting).

49. This framework is essentially consistent with perfectionist liberalism as explained by Joseph Raz (*The Morality of Freedom*, 1986), and was described as Aristotelian approach by Michael Sandel, in "Moral Argument and Liberal Toleration, Abortion and Homosexuality," in *New Communitarian Thinking: Persons, Virtues, Institutions, and Communities*, Amitai Etzioni, ed., University of Virginia Press, 1995.

50. *Hernandez v. Robles*, 7 N.Y.3d 338,392 (2006).

51. *Hernandez*, at 393.

52. *Goodridge*, at 948.

53. *Goodridge*, at 954.

54. *Hernandez*, at 380.

55. *Hernandez*, at 392.

56. *Hernandez*, at 393.

57. *Hernandez*, at 380.

58. *Hernandez*, at 393.

59. *Goodridge*, at 968 (quoting *Palmore v. Sidoti*, 466 U.S. 429, 433 (1984)).

60. *Goodridge*, at 343.

61. Ball, "Moral Foundations."

62. True moral neutrality is impossible of course. The conception of justice as fairness has a normative content. "For Rawls, the choice is not between a conception of justice that eschews values and one that does not; instead the choice is between a conception of justice 'whose content is given by certain ideals, principles and standards . . . articulating political values' and conceptions of justice, such as those formulated by Plato, Aristotle, the Christian tradition, and utilitarianism, all of which incorporate values based on broader philosophical religious, and moral comprehensive doctrines." Carlos A. Ball, "Moral Foundations for a Discourse on Same-sex marriage: Looking beyond Political Liberalism," *Georgetown Law Journal* 85 (1997): 1871, 1889 (quoting John Rawls, *Political Liberalism*, at 134–35 (1997).

63. For a complete articulation of this view, see Bruce Ackerman, *Social Justice in the Liberal State*, pp. 349–78 (1980); Ronald Dworkin, *Taking Rights Seriously*, pp. 90–100 (1977); John Rawls, *The Theory of Justice* 31 (1971).

64. *Lewis v. Harris*, 188 N.J. 415 (N.J. 2006).

65. This assertion should not be construed as one celebrating the civil union-type solution. It is instead an observation that the judges reaching the middle ground solution have most fully achieved moral neutrality.

66. *Baker v. Vermont*, 744 A.2d, 864, 887 (1999).

67. *Lewis*, at 457.

68. *Lewis*, at 458.

69. *Baker v. Vermont*, 744 A.2d at 888, quoting C. Sunstein, "Forward, Leaving Things Undecided," *Harvard Law Review* 110, no. 4 (1996): 1010.

70. Stephen A. Garbaum, "Why the Liberal State Can Promote Moral Ideals after All," *Harvard Law Review* 104, no. 1350 (1991): 1251.

71. "'Tolerance' and 'acceptance' are not synonyms; one may tolerate another without accepting them because the latter (but not the former) requires a normative judgment." Ball, at 1875.

15.

IS IT WRONG TO DISCRIMINATE ON THE BASIS OF HOMOSEXUALITY?

Jeff Jordan

Much like the issue of abortion in the early 1970s, the issue of homosexuality has exploded to the forefront of social discussion. Is homosexual sex on a moral par with heterosexual sex? Or is homosexuality in some way morally inferior? Is it wrong to discriminate against homosexuals—to treat homosexuals in less favorable ways than one does heterosexuals? Or is some discrimination against homosexuals morally justified? These questions are the focus of this essay.

In what follows, I argue that there are situations in which it is morally permissible to discriminate against homosexuals because of their homosexuality. That is, there are some morally relevant differences between heterosexuality and homosexuality which, in some instances, permit a difference in treatment. The issue of marriage provides a good example. While it is clear that heterosexual unions merit the state recognition known as marriage, along with the attendant advantage—spousal insurance coverage, inheritance rights, ready eligibility of adoption—it is far from clear that homosexual couples ought to be accorded that state recognition.

From the *Journal of Social Philosophy* 25, no. 1 (Spring 1995). Reprinted by permission of the *Journal of Social Philosophy*.

The argument of this essay makes no claim about the moral status of homosexuality per se. Briefly put, it is the argument of this essay that the moral impasse generated by conflicting views concerning homosexuality, and the public policy ramifications of those conflicting views justify the claim that it is morally permissible, in certain circumstances, to discriminate against homosexuals.[1]

THE ISSUE

The relevant issue is this: does homosexuality have the same moral status as heterosexuality? Put differently, since there are no occasions in which it is morally permissible to treat heterosexuals unfavorably, whether because they are heterosexual or because of heterosexual acts, are there occasions in which it is morally permissible to treat homosexuals unfavorably, whether because they are homosexuals or because of homosexual acts?

A negative answer to the above can be termed the "parity thesis." The parity thesis contends that *homosexuality has the same moral status as heterosexuality*. If the parity thesis is correct, then it would be immoral to discriminate against homosexuals because of their homosexuality. An affirmative answer can be termed the "difference thesis" and contends that there are morally relevant differences between heterosexuality and homosexuality which justify a difference in moral status and treatment between homosexuals and heterosexuals. The difference thesis entails that *there are situations in which it is morally permissible to discriminate against homosexuals*.

It is perhaps needless to point out that the difference thesis follows as long as there is at least one occasion in which it is morally permissible to discriminate against homosexuals. If the parity thesis were true, then on no occasion would a difference in treatment between heterosexuals and homosexuals ever be justified. The difference thesis does not, even if true, justify discriminatory actions on every occasion. Nonetheless, even though the scope of the difference thesis is relatively modest, it is, if true, a significant principle which has not only theoretical import but important practical consequences as well.[2]

A word should be said about the notion of discrimination. To discriminate against X means treating X in an unfavorable way. The word "discrimination" is not a synonym for "morally unjustifiable treatment." Some discrimination is morally unjustifiable; some is not. For example, we discriminate against convicted felons in that they are disenfranchised. This legal discrimination is morally permissible even though it involves treating one person unfavorably different from how other persons are treated. The difference thesis entails that there are circumstances in which it is morally permissible to discriminate against homosexuals.

AN ARGUMENT FOR THE PARITY THESIS

One might suppose that an appeal to a moral right, the right to privacy, perhaps, or the right to liberty, would provide the strongest grounds for the parity thesis. Rights talk, though sometimes helpful, is not very helpful here. If there is reason to think that the right to privacy or the right to liberty encompasses sexuality (which seems plausible enough), it would do so only with regard to private acts and not public acts. Sexual acts performed in public (whether heterosexual or homosexual) are properly suppressible. It does not take too much imagination to see that the right to be free from offense would soon be offered as a counter consideration by those who find homosexuality morally problematic. Furthermore, how one adjudicates between the competing rights claims is far from clear. Hence, the bald appeal to a right will not, in this case anyway, take one very far.

Perhaps the strongest reason to hold that the parity thesis is true is something like the following:

1. Homosexual acts between consenting adults harm no one. And,
2. respecting persons' privacy and choices in harmless sexual matters maximizes individual freedom. And,
3. individual freedom should be maximized. But,
4. discrimination against homosexuals, because of their homosexuality, diminishes individual freedom since it ignores personal choice and privacy. So,
5. the toleration of homosexuality rather than discriminating against homosexuals is the preferable option since it would maximize individual freedom. Therefore,
6. the parity thesis is more plausible than the difference thesis.

Premise (2) is unimpeachable: if an act is harmless and if there are persons who want to do it and who choose to do it, then it seems clear that respecting the choices of those people would tend to maximize their freedom.[3] Step (3) is also beyond reproach: since freedom is arguably a great good and since there does not appear to be any ceiling on the amount of individual freedom—no "too much of a good thing"—(3) appears to be true.

At first glance, premise (1) seems true enough as long as we recognize that if there is any harm involved in the homosexual acts of consenting adults, it would be harm absorbed by the freely consenting participants. This is true, however, only if the acts in question are done in private. Public acts may involve more than just the willing participants. Persons who have no desire to participate, even if only as spectators, may have no choice if the acts are done in public. A real probability of there being unwilling participants is indicative of the public realm and not the private. However, since where one draws the line between private acts and public acts is not always easy to discern, it is clear that different moral standards apply to public acts than to private acts.[4]

If premise (1) is understood to apply only to acts done in private, then it would appear to be true. The same goes for (4): discrimination against homosexuals for acts done in private would result in a diminishing of freedom: since (1)–(4) would lend support to (5) only if we understand (1)–(4) to refer to acts done in private. Hence, (5) must be understood as referring to private acts; and, as a consequence, (6) also must be read as referring only to acts done in private.

With regard to acts which involve only willing adult participants, there may be no morally relevant difference between homosexuality and heterosexuality. In other words, acts done in private. However, acts done in public add a new ingredient to the mix; an ingredient which has moral consequence. Consequently, the argument (1)–(6) fails in supporting the parity thesis. The argument (1)–(6) may show that there are some circumstances in which the moral status of homosexuality and heterosexuality are the same, but it gives us no reason for thinking that this result holds for all circumstances.[5]

Suppose one person believes that X is morally wrong, while another believes that X is morally permissible. The two people, let's stipulate, are not involved in a semantical quibble; they hold genuinely conflicting beliefs regarding the moral status of X. If the first person is correct, then the second person is wrong; and, of course, if the second person is right, then the first must be wrong. This situation of conflicting claims is what we will call an "impasse." Impasses arise out of moral disputes. Since the conflicting parties in an impasse take contrary views, the conflicting views cannot all be true, nor can they all be false.[6] Moral impasses may concern matters only of a personal nature, but moral impasses can involve public policy. An impasse is likely to have public policy ramifications if large numbers of people hold the conflicting views, and the conflict involves matters which are fundamental to a person's moral identity (and, hence, from a practical point of view, are probably irresolvable) and it involves acts done in public. Since not every impasse has public policy ramifications, one can mark off "public dilemma" as a special case of moral impasses: those moral impasses that have public policy consequences. Public dilemmas, then, are impasses located in the public square. Since they have public policy ramifications and since they arise from impasses, one side or another of the dispute will have its views implemented as pubic policy. Because of the public policy ramifications, and also because social order is sometimes threatened by the volatile parties involved in the impasse, the state has a role to play in resolving a public dilemma.[7]

A public dilemma can be actively resolved in two ways: The first is when the government allies itself with one side of the impasse and, by state coercion and sanction, declares that side of the impasse the correct side. The American Civil War was an example of this: the federal government forcibly ended slavery by aligning itself with the Abolitionist side of the impasse.[8] Prohibition is another example. The Eighteenth Amendment and the Volstead Act allied the state with the Temperance side of the impasse. State-mandated affirmative action programs provide a modern example of this. This kind of resolution of a public dilemma we can call a "resolution by declaration." The first of the examples cited above indicates that declarations can be morally proper, the right thing to do. The second example, however, indicates that declarations are not always morally proper. The state does not always take the side of the morally correct; nor is it always clear which side is the correct one.

The second way of actively resolving a public dilemma is that of accommodation. An accommodation in this context means resolving the public dilemma in a way that gives as much as possible to all sides of the impasse. A resolution by accommodation involves staking out some middle ground in a dispute and placing public policy in that location. The middle ground location of a resolution via accommodation is a virtue since it entails that there are no absolute victors and no absolute losers. The middle ground is reached in order to resolve the public dilemma in a way which respects the relevant views of the conflicting parties and which maintains social order. The Federal Fair Housing Act and, perhaps, the current status of abortion (legal but with restrictions) provide examples of actual resolutions via accommodation.[9]

In general, governments should be, at least as far as possible, neutral with regard to the disputing parties in a public dilemma. Unless there is some overriding reason why the state should take sides in a public dilemma—the protection of innocent life, or abolishing slavery, for instance—the state should be neutral, because no matter which side of the public dilemma the state takes, the other side will be the recipient of unequal treatment by the state. A state which is partial and takes sides in moral disputes via declaration, when there is no overriding reason why it should, is tyrannical. Overriding reasons involve, typically, the protection of generally recognized rights.[10] In the case of slavery, the right to liberty; in the case of protecting innocent life, the right involved is the negative right to life. If a public dilemma must be actively resolved, the state should do so (in the absence of an overriding reason) via accommodation and not declaration since the latter entails that a sizable number of people would be forced to live under a government which "legitimizes" and does not just tolerate activities which they find immoral. Resolution via declaration is appropriate only if there is an overriding reason for the state to throw its weight behind one side in a public dilemma.

Is moral rightness an overriding reason for a resolution via declaration? What better reason might there be for a resolution by declaration than that it is the right thing to do? Unless one is prepared to endorse a view that is called "legal moralism"—that immorality alone is a sufficient reason for the state to curtail individual liberty—then one had best hold that moral rightness alone is not an overriding reason. Since some immoral acts neither harm nor offend nor violate another's rights, it seems clear enough that too much liberty would be lost if legal moralism were adopted as public policy.[11]

Though we do not have a definite rule for determining a priori which moral impasses genuinely constitute public dilemmas, we can proceed via a case-by-case method. For example, many people hold that cigarette smoking is harmful and, on that basis, is properly suppressible. Others disagree. Is this a public dilemma? Probably not. Whether someone engages in an imprudent action is, as long as it involves no unwilling participants, a private matter and does not, on that account, constitute a public dilemma. What about abortion? Is abortion a public dilemma? Unlike cigarette smoking, abortion is a public dilemma. This is clear from the adamant and even violent contrary positions involved in the impasse. Abortion is an issue which forces itself into the public square. So, it is clear that, even though we lack a rule which filters through moral impasses designating some as public dilemmas, not every impasse constitutes a public dilemma.

The theistic tradition, Judaism and Christianity and Islam, has a clear and deeply entrenched position on homosexual acts: they are prohibited. Now it seems clear enough that if one is going to take seriously the authoritative texts of the respective religions, then one will have to adopt the views of those texts, unless one wishes to engage in a demythologizing of them with the result that one ends up being only a nominal adherent of that tradition.[12] As a consequence, many contemporary theistic adherents of the theistic tradition, in no small part because they can read, hold that homosexual behavior is sinful. Though God loves the homosexual, these folk say, God hates the sinful behavior. To say that act X is a sin entails that X is morally wrong, not necessarily because it is harmful or offensive, but because X violates God's will. So, the claim that homosexuality is sinful entails the claim that it is also morally wrong. And, it is clear, many people adopt the difference thesis just because of their religious views: because the Bible or the Koran holds that homosexuality is wrong, they too hold that view.

Well, what should we make of these observations? We do not, for one thing, have to base our moral conclusions on those views, if for no other reason than not every one is a theist. If one does not adopt the religion-based moral view, one must still respect those who do; they cannot just be dismissed out of hand.[13] And, significantly, this situation yields a reason for thinking that the difference thesis is probably true. Because many religious people sincerely believe homosexual acts to be morally wrong and many others believe that homosexual acts are not morally wrong, there results a public dilemma.[14]

The existence of this public dilemma gives us reason for thinking that the difference thesis is true. It is only via the difference thesis and not the parity thesis, that an accommodation can be reached. Here again, the private/public distinction will come into play.

To see this, take as an example the issue of homosexual marriages. A same-sex marriage would be a public matter. For the government to sanction same-sex marriage—to grant the recognition and reciprocal benefits which attach to marriage—would ally the government with one side of the public dilemma and against the adherents of religion-based moralities. This is especially true given that, historically, no government has sanctioned same-sex marriages. The status quo has been no same-sex marriages. If the state were to change its practice now, it would be clear that the state has taken sides in the impasse. Given the history, for a state to sanction a same-sex marriage now would not be a neutral act.

Of course, some would respond here that by not sanctioning same-sex marriages the state is, and historically has been, taking sides to the detriment of homosexuals. There is some truth in this claim. But one must be careful here. The respective resolutions of this issue—whether the state should recognize and sanction same-sex marriage—do not have symmetrical implications. The asymmetry of this issue is a function of the private/public distinction and the fact that marriage is a public matter. If the state sanctions same-sex marriages, then there is no accommodation available. In that event, the religion-based morality proponents are faced with a public, state-sanctioned matter which they find seriously immoral. This would be an example of a resolution via declaration. On the other hand, if the state does not sanction same-sex marriages, there is an accommodation available: in the public realm the state sides with the religion-based moral view, but the state can tolerate private homosexual acts. That is, since homosexual acts are not essentially public acts, they can be, and historically have been, performed in private. The state, by not sanctioning same-sex marriages, is acting in the public realm, but it can leave the private realm to personal choice.[15]

THE ARGUMENT FROM CONFLICTING CLAIMS

It was suggested in the previous section that the public dilemma concerning homosexuality, and in particular whether states should sanction same-sex marriages, generates an argument in support of the difference thesis. The argument, again using same-sex marriages as the particular case, is as follows:

7. There are conflicting claims regarding whether the state should sanction same-sex marriages. And,
8. this controversy constitutes a public dilemma. And,
9. there is an accommodation possible if the state does not recognize same-sex marriages. And,
10. there is no accommodation possible if the state does sanction same-sex marriages. And,
11. there is no overriding reason for a resolution via declaration. Hence,
12. the state ought not sanction same-sex marriages. And,
13. the state ought to sanction heterosexual marriages. So,
14. there is at least one morally relevant case in which discrimination against homosexuals, because of their homosexuality, is morally permissible. Therefore,
15. the difference thesis is true.

Since proposition (14) is logically equivalent to the difference thesis, then, if (7)–(14) are sound, proposition (15) certainly follows.

Premises (7) and (8) are uncontroversial. Premises (9) and (10) are based on the asymmetry that results from the public nature of marriage. Proposition (11) is based on our earlier analysis of the argument (1)–(6). Since the strongest argument in support of the parity thesis fails, we have reason to think that there is no overriding reason why the state ought to resolve the public dilemma via declaration in favor of same-sex marriages. We have reason, in other words, to think that (11) is true.

Proposition (12) is based on the conjunction of (7)–(11) and the principle that, in the absence of an overriding reason for state intervention via declaration, resolution by accommodation is the preferable route. Proposition (13) is just trivially true. So, given the moral difference mentioned in (12) and (13), proposition (14) logically follows.

The first objection to the argument from conflicting claims would contend that it is unsound because a similar sort of argument would permit discrimination against some practice which, though perhaps controversial at some earlier time, is now widely thought to be morally permissible. Take mixed-race marriages, for example. The opponent of the argument from conflicting claims could argue that a similar argument would warrant prohibition against mixed-race marriages. If it does, we would have good reason to reject (7)–(14) as unsound.

There are three responses to this objection. The first response denies that the issue of mixed-race marriages is in fact a public dilemma. It may have been so at one time, but it does not seem to generate much, if any, controversy today. Hence, the objection is based upon a faulty analogy.

The second response grants for the sake of the argument that the issue of mixed-race marriages generates a public dilemma. But the second response points out that there is a relevant difference between mixed-race marriages and same-sex marriages that allows for a resolution by declaration in the one case but not in the other. As evident from the earlier analysis of the argument in support of (1)–(6), there is reason to think that there is no overriding reason for a resolution by declaration in support of the parity thesis. On the other hand, it is a settled matter that state protection from racial discrimination is a reason sufficient for a resolution via declaration. Hence, the two cases are only apparently similar, and, in reality, they are crucially different. They are quite different because, clearly enough, if mixed-race marriages do generate a public dilemma, the state should use resolution by declaration in support of such marriages. The same cannot be said for same-sex marriages.

One should note that the second response to the objection does not beg the question against the proponent of the parity thesis. Though the second response denies that race and sexuality are strict analogues, it does so for a defensible and independent reason: it is a settled matter that race is not a sufficient reason for disparate treatment; but, as we have seen from the analysis of (1)–(6), there is no overriding reason to think the same about sexuality.[16]

The third response to the first objection is that the grounds of objection differ in the respective cases: one concerns racial identity; the other concerns behavior thought to be morally problematic. A same-sex marriage would involve behavior which many people find morally objectionable; a mixed-race marriage is objectionable to some, not because of the participants' behavior, but because of the racial identity of the participants. It is the race of the marriage partners which some find of primary complaint concerning mixed-race marriages. With same-sex marriage, however, it is the behavior which is primarily objectionable. To see this latter point, one should note that, though promiscuously Puritan in tone, the kind of sexual acts that are likely involved in a same-sex marriage are objectionable to some, regardless of whether done by homosexuals or heterosexuals.[17] So again, there is reason to reject the analogy between same-sex marriages and mixed-race marriages. Racial identity is an immutable trait and a complaint about mixed-race marriages necessarily involves, then, a complaint about an immutable trait. Sexual behavior is not an immutable trait and it is possible to object to same-sex marriages based on the behavior which would be involved in such marriages. Put succinctly, the third response can be formulated as follows: objections to mixed-race marriages necessarily involve objections over status, while objections to same-sex marriages could involve objections over behavior. Therefore, the two cases are not analogous since there is a significant modal difference in the grounds of the objections.

The second objection to the argument from conflicting claims can be stated so: if homosexuality is biologically based—if it is inborn[18]—then how can discrimination ever be justified? If it is not a matter of choice, homosexuality is an immutable trait which is, as a consequence, morally permissible. Just as it would be absurd to hold someone morally culpable for being of a certain race, likewise it would be absurd to hold someone morally culpable for being a homosexual. Consequently, according to this objection, the argument from conflicting claims "legitimizes" unjustifiable discrimination.

But this second objection is not cogent, primarily because it ignores an important distinction. No one could plausibly hold that homosexuals act by some sort of biological compulsion. If there is a biological component involved in sexual identity, it would incline but it would not compel. Just because one naturally (without any choice) has certain dispositions, it is not in itself a morally cogent reason for acting upon that disposition. Most people are naturally selfish, but it clearly does not follow that selfishness is in any way permissible on that account. Even if it is true that one has a predisposition to do X as a matter of biology, and not as a matter of choice, it does not follow that doing X is morally permissible. For example, suppose that pyromania is an inborn predisposition. Just because one has an inborn and, in that sense, natural desire to set fires, one still has to decide whether or not to act on that desire.[19] The reason that the appeal to biology is specious is that it ignores the important distinction between being a homosexual and homosexual acts. One is status; the other is behavior. Even if one has the status naturally, it does not follow that the behavior is morally permissible, nor that others have a duty to tolerate the behavior.

But, while moral permissibility does not necessarily follow if homosexuality should turn out to be biologically based, what does follow is this: in the absence of a good reason to discriminate between homosexuals and heterosexuals, then, assuming that homosexuality is inborn, one ought not discriminate between them. If a certain phenomenon X is natural in the sense of being involuntary and nonpathological, and if there is no good reason to hold that X is morally problematic, then that is reason enough to think that X is morally permissible. In the absence of a good reason to repress X, one should tolerate it since, as per supposition, it is largely nonvoluntary. The argument from conflicting claims, however, provides a good reason which overrides this presumption.

A second argument for the difference thesis, similar to the argument from conflicting claims, is what might be called the "no-exit argument." This argument is based on the principle that:

A. No just government can coerce a citizen into violating a deeply held moral belief or religious belief.

Is (A) plausible? It seems to be since the prospect of a citizen being coerced by the state into a practice which she finds profoundly immoral appears to be a clear example of an injustice. Principle (A), conjoined with there being a public dilemma arising over the issue of same-sex marriages, leads to the observation that if the state were to sanction same-sex marriages, then persons who have profound religious or moral objections to such unions would be legally mandated to violate their beliefs since there does not appear to be any feasible "exit right" possible with regard to state-sanctioned marriage. An exit right is an exemption from some legally mandated practice, granted to a person or group, the purpose of which is to protect the religious or moral integrity of that person or group. Prominent examples of exit rights include conscientious objection and military service, homeschooling of the young because of some religious concern, and property used for religious purposes being free from taxation.

It is important to note that marriage is a public matter in the sense that, for instance; if one is an employer who provides health care benefits to the spouses of employees, one must provide those benefits to any employee who is married. Since there is no exit right possible in this case, one would be coerced, by force of law, into subsidizing a practice one finds morally or religiously objectionable.[20]

In the absence of an exit right, and if (A) is plausible, then the state cannot morally force persons to violate deeply held beliefs that are moral or religious in nature. In particular, the state morally could not sanction same-sex marriages since this would result in coercing some into violating a deeply held religious conviction.

A CONCLUSION

It is important to note that neither the argument from conflicting claims nor the no-exit argument licenses wholesale discrimination against homosexuals. What they do show is that some discrimination against homosexuals, in this case refusal to sanction same-sex marriages, is not only legally permissible but also morally permissible. The discrimination is a way of resolving a public policy dilemma that accommodates, to an extent, each side of the impasse and further, protects the religious and moral integrity of a good number of people. In short, the arguments show us that there are occasions in which it is morally permissible to discriminate on the basis of homosexuality.[21]

NOTES

1. The terms "homosexuality" and "heterosexuality" are defined as follows. The former is defined as sexual feelings or behavior directed toward individuals of the same sex. The latter, naturally enough, is defined as sexual feelings or behavior directed toward individuals of the opposite sex.

2. Sometimes the term "gay" is offered as an alternative to "homosexual." Ordinary use of "gay" has it as a synonym of a male homosexual (hence, the common expression, "gays and lesbians"). Given this ordinary usage, the substitution would lead to a confusing equivocation. Since there are female homosexuals, it is best to use "homosexual" to refer to both male and female homosexuals, and reserve "gay" to signify male homosexuals, and "lesbian" for female homosexuals in order to avoid the equivocation.

3. Perhaps we should distinguish the weak difference thesis (permissible discrimination on *some* occasions) from the strong difference thesis (given the relevant moral differences, discrimination on *any* occasion is permissible).

4. This would be true even if the act in question was immoral.

5. The standard answer is, of course, that the line between public and private is based on the notion of harm. Acts which carry a real probability of harming third parties are public acts.

6. For other arguments supporting the moral parity of homosexuality and heterosexuality, see Richard Mohr, *Gays/Justice: A Study of Ethics, Society and Law* (New York: Columbia University Press, 1988); and see Michael Ruse, "The Morality of Homosexuality" in *Philosophy and Sex*, eds. R. Baker and F. Elliston, 2d ed. (Amherst, NY: Prometheus Books, 1984), pp. 370–90.

7. Perhaps it would be better to term the disputing positions "contradictory" views rather than "contrary" views.

8. Resolutions can also be passive in the sense of the state doing nothing. If the state does nothing to resolve the public dilemma, it stands pat with the status quo, and the public dilemma is resolved gradually by sociological changes (changes in mores and in beliefs).

9. Assuming, plausibly enough, that the disputes over the sovereignty of the Union and concerning states' rights were at bottom disputes about slavery.

10. The Federal Fair Housing Act prohibits discrimination in housing on the basis of race, religion, and sex. But it does not apply to the rental of rooms in single-family houses, or to a building of five units or less if the owner lives in one of the units. See 42 U.S.C. Section 3603.

11. Note that overriding reasons involve generally recognized rights. If a right is not widely recognized and the state nonetheless uses coercion to enforce it, there is a considerable risk that the state will be seen by many or even most people as tyrannical.

This claim is, perhaps, controversial. For a contrary view see Richard George, *Making Men Moral* (Oxford: Clarendon Press, 1993).

12. See, for example, Leviticus 18:22, 21:3; and Romans 1:22–32; and Koran IV:13.

13. For an argument that religiously based moral views should not be dismissed out

of hand, see Stephen Carter, *The Culture of Disbelief: How American Law and Politics Trivialize Religious Devotion* (New York: Basic Books, 1993).

14. "Two assumptions are these: that the prohibitions against homosexual activity are part of the religious doctrine and not just an extraneous addition; second, that if X is part of one's religious belief or religious doctrine, then it is morally permissible to hold X. Though this latter principle is vague, it is, I think, clear enough for our purposes here (I ignore here any points concerning the rationality of religious belief in general, or in particular cases).

15. This point has implications for the moral legitimacy of sodomy laws. One implication would be this: the private acts of consenting adults should not be criminalized.

16. An *ad hominem point*: if this response begs the question against the proponent of the parity thesis, it does not beg the question any more than the original objection does by presupposing that sexuality is analogous with race.

17. Think of the sodomy laws found in some states which criminalize certain sexual acts, whether performed by heterosexuals or homosexuals.

18. There is some interesting recent research which, though still tentative, strongly suggests that homosexuality is, at least in part, biologically based. See Simon LeVay, *The Sexual Brain* (Cambridge, MA: MIT Press, 1993), pp. 120–22; and J. M. Bailey and R. C. Pillard, "A Genetic Study of Male Sexual Orientation," *Archives of General Psychiatry* 48 (1991): 1089–96; and C. Burr, "Homosexuality and Biology," *Atlantic* 271/273 (March 1993): 64; and D. Hamer, S. Hu, V. Magnuson, N. Hu, A. Pattatucci, "A Linkage between DNA Markers on the X Chromosome and Male Sexual Orientation," *Science* 261 (July 16, 1993): 321–27; and see the summary of this article by Robert Pool, "Evidence for Homosexuality Gene," *Science* 261 (July 16, 1993): 291–92.

19. I do not mean to suggest that homosexuality is morally equivalent or even comparable to pyromania.

20. Is the use of subsidy here inappropriate? It does not seem so since providing health care to spouses, in a society where this is not legally mandatory, seems to be more than part of a salary and is a case of providing supporting funds for a certain end.

21. I thank David Haslett, Kate Rogers, Louis Pojman, and Jim Fieser for helpful and critical comments.

16.

RAWLS'S PRINCIPLE OF JUSTICE AS FAIRNESS AND ITS APPLICATION TO THE ISSUE OF SAME-SEX MARRIAGE

John Scott Gray

This essay attempts to offer an alternative in the ongoing debate surrounding the permissibility of same-sex marriage. The discussion surrounding same-sex marriage has generally centered on the questions of what the definition of marriage is and to what degree same-sex partners can be included within that definition. The two positions, both for and against same-sex marriage rights, fundamentally differ in their conclusions regarding same-sex marriage, while constructing their arguments concerning what constitutes marriage on similar grounds. Those grounds involve assumptions concerning a fixed naturalistic status of marriage. I will use the term naturalistic as a representational tool to describe the arguments in question. By this term, I am including positions grounded in the natural law tradition, ethical naturalism, and ethical essentialism. Put in the most simplistic terms, these arguments define marriage, then decide whether or not same-sex marriage fits their pre-conceived definition. These arguments begin from a conception that the issue at hand, marriage, has a fixed and finished essence, and by doing so end the discussion of what marriage should be before it has even occurred. These naturalistic arguments usually appeal to assertions regarding the facts of the matter as they "naturally appear" in the world, either because of G/god, physical laws, or because various cultural or

Taken from *South African Journal of Philosophy* 23, no. 2 (2004): 158–70. Reprinted by permission.

historical movements have shaped marriage into this current form.[1] We will consider another type of argument, one that preempts the natural/unnatural question and focuses instead on the grounds in which a state has the right to limit an action regardless of a natural or unnatural designation. To accomplish this endeavor, I will turn to the principle of justice as fairness as articulated by John Rawls. Rawls states in *Political Liberalism* that "Justice as fairness works from the fundamental ideas of society as a fair system of cooperation together with the conception of the person as free and equal. These ideas are taken as central to the democratic ideal" (Rawls, 1993: 167). Rawls calls for social institutions that do not confer arbitrary and discriminatory advantages on one class of persons at the expense of others. There are limited exceptions when specific inequalities may be acceptable, as dictated by the difference principle, but I choose to assert that that principle does not apply to our consideration of same-sex marriage.

This essay will be broken into two sections. In the first section, I will examine the concept of the original position as a starting point for considering which political philosophy is most conducive for achieving a just state, as well as the system of justice as fairness that Rawls asserts would be chosen. I will also consider the way those principles guide the creation of the basic structure of society, including societies' institutions, particularly the family. The second section applies justice as fairness to the problem at hand. We will take a closer look at Rawls's idea of the family as a basic institution that is in accord with the principles of justice as they are understood in the original position. Rawls's theory will serve as a springboard for my argument that a just society should in fact recognize same-sex marriage. We will also consider whether gay and lesbian issues (and conversely, heterosexual issues) have a place in the original position.

Finding that the veil of ignorance limits one's knowledge of their sexuality, we consider the ways in which the original position and the principles of justice as fairness foster the family and marriage as political and social institutions within the basic structure. Finding that the emphasis in the formulation of the family is not necessarily on the gender or sexuality of the participants in that family, but on the role that they carry out with regards to the reproduction of the social structure, we will conclude that justice as fairness does in fact allow for same-sex marriage. We will then consider an important objection to this conclusion, addressing the degree to which allowing same-sex marriage would violate the basic liberties of others by forcing them to accept such unions. In the end, by carrying out our project, we will prove that John Rawls was very perceptive when he stated that his theory "will prove a worthwhile theory . . . if it singles out with greater sharpness the graver wrongs a society should avoid" (Rawls, 1971: 201).

SECTION I: CLARIFYING JUSTICE AS FAIRNESS: THE ORIGINAL POSITION AS STARTING POINT AND RAWLS'S TWO PRINCIPLES OF JUSTICE

In the original position, Rawls attempts to capture the thinking of "rationally autonomous representatives of citizens in society. As such representatives, the parties are to do the best they can for those they represent subject to the restrictions of the original position" (Rawls, 1993: 305). The limitations of the original position include the veil of ignorance. Because Rawls is seeking a fair system of cooperation, the original position is an attempt to ensure that agreements reached by the founders of a society are fair. The veil helps achieve this by placing fairness as the central point of political consideration, in that the veil dictates that those parties consider the grounding principles of their political philosophy and basic social structures in an atmosphere that is not colored by their particular socio-economic background or prejudices. According to Rawls:

> . . . the fact that we occupy a particular social position is not a good reason for us to propose, or to expect others to accept, a conception of justice that favors those in this position. . . . To model this conviction in the original position, the parties are not allowed to know the social position of those they represent, or the particular comprehensive doctrine of the person each represents (Rawls, 1993: 24).

This enforced ignorance on the individuals burdened with deciding the terms of social cooperation includes not having information regarding race, religion, sex, as well as individual traits (Rawls calls them endowments) that include the degree of intelligence a person possesses as well as physical strength. While Rawls does not specifically include sexual orientation as a piece of information that those in the original position should not possess, this critic believes that excluding that information is consistent with the intent of the original position, a point we will consider later.

From the original position, Rawls believes his two principles would be chosen. Those two principles of justice were continually re-worked throughout Rawls's career, but the version that appeared in section 46 of *A Theory of Justice*, states:

First Principle

Each person is to have an equal right to the most extensive total system of equal basic liberties compatible with a similar system of liberty for all.

Second Principle

Social and economic inequalities are to be arranged so that they are both:

(a) to the greatest benefit of the least advantaged, consistent with the just savings principle, and
(b) attached to offices and positions open to all under conditions of fair equality of opportunity. (Rawls, 1971: 302)[2]

These two principles are the foundation in which the basic structures of society are constructed. In particular, the first principle is intended to apply "not only to the basic structure . . . but more specifically to what we think of as the constitution, whether written or unwritten" (Rawls, 2001: 46). There are three stages of political development that follow the adoption of the two principles of justice behind the veil of ignorance. First, at the constitutional convention the actual basic structure of the political body is laid out. These structures are the governing bodies that assign rights and duties to its citizens, including basic liberties such as:

> . . . political liberty (the right to vote and be eligible for public office) together with freedom of speech and assembly; liberty of conscious and freedom of thought; freedom of the person along with the right to hold (personal) property; and freedom from arbitrary arrest and seizure as defined by the concept of the rule of law. These liberties are all required to be equal by the first principle. . . . (Rawls, 1971: 61)

Major political and social institutions should be constructed with regards to these basic liberties in accordance with the first principle of justice's assertion that people must have a right to the most extensive total system of equal basic liberties. In the second stage of political development, the legislature, which Rawls assumes would necessarily be created in the constitutional development of a political structure in accordance with justice as fairness, makes laws in accordance with the jurisdiction that is laid down in the constitutional stage as well as in continued accordance with the two principles of justice. The third stage was originally referred to by Rawls as the judiciary stage, but he later broadened its scope to include the ways "in which the rules are applied by administrators and followed by citizens generally . . ." (Rawls, 2001: 48).[3] The key aspect in the application of justice as fairness in these various stages is that the social/political institutions that are created and enforced must not institute arbitrary advantages. Those major institutions distribute the rights and duties to the citizens of the state and they include:

. . . the political constitution and the principal economic and social arrangements. Thus the legal protection of freedom of thought and liberty of conscience, competitive markets, private property in the means of production, and the monogamous family are examples of major social institutions. (Rawls, 1971: 7)

The fact that Rawls includes the family as one of the basic social institutions that justice as fairness is applicable to will be of particular importance in our attempt in section two to apply Rawls's theory to same-sex marriage. For now, it will suffice to recognize that all of these institutions are constructed in the developing state, within the system, laid down in the basic structure. As Rawls emphasizes, the basic structures of the political and social institutions that comprise the state are the primary subject of justice as fairness because these structures "define men's rights and duties and influence their life-prospects, what they can expect to be and how well they can hope to do . . . its effects are so profound and present from the start" (Rawls, 1971: 7). These political and social institutions, because they are constructed to follow the principles of justice as fairness, help achieve what Rawls calls the shared common good.

The shared common good arises because our political and social institutions work toward a well-ordered society. This order does not imply that the people seek the same conception of good in terms of a comprehensive doctrine that drives them, for, according to Rawls, it is possible to take different roads to the same destination:

. . . in the well-ordered society of justice as fairness citizens do have final ends in common. While it is true that they do not affirm the same comprehensive doctrine, they do affirm the same political conception of justice; and this means that they share one very basic political end, and one that has high priority: namely, the end of supporting just institutions and of giving one another justice accordingly. . . . (Rawls, 1993: 202)

By a particular comprehensive doctrine, Rawls is referring to a person's individual religious, philosophical, or moral doctrine that dictates their specific positions regarding the good and the value of particular goods in the world. Individuals may still hold onto their own comprehensive doctrines in a society based on justice as fairness because the political structure that we are constructing is focused on "political values that characterize the domain of the political; it is not proposed as an account of moral values generally" (Rawls, 1993: 125). Doctrines based on naturalism or natural law theory are included here as a comprehensive moral doctrine that people may choose to adopt. According to Rawls, it is perfectly fine for people to have moral standards that are dictated by a divine or natural process, and they can even view the political structures that arise out of justice as fairness as derived out of natural law. Because the focus is on political institutions, Rawls asserts that "Political constructivism does not criticize, then, religious, philosophical, or metaphysical accounts of the truth of moral judgments and of their validity" (Rawls, 1993: 127). The only requirement that Rawls places on these various comprehensive doctrines is that they be reasonable. Reasonable persons "are sufficiently intelligent and conscientious in exercising their powers of practical reason, and whose reasoning exhibits none of the familiar defects of reasoning . . ." (Rawls, 1993: 119). They must be reasonable because they participate in the overlapping consensus of views that operate underneath the political system constructed under the two principles of justice.

The role of the overlapping consensus in a well-ordered society is one of the central concepts that guides Rawls's theory of justice, particularly in his re-working of the principle in writings after *A Theory of Justice*. According to Rawls, the idea of a well-ordered society involves three points:

> First . . . it is a society in which everyone accepts, and knows that everyone else accepts, the very same principles of justice; and second . . . its basic structure—that is, its main political and social institutions and how they fit together as one system of cooperation—is publicly known, or with good reason believed, to satisfy these principles. And third, its citizens have a normally effective sense of justice and so they generally comply with society's basic institutions, which they regard as just. (Rawls, 1993: 35)

The way to achieve this well-ordered society is not through political force, but through achieving an overlapping consensus. It is in just this way that Rawls in part avoids grounding his theory in naturalistic assumptions, because in and after the original position those deciding the political structure do not turn to the various comprehensive doctrines that exist in the world, be they religious, philosophical, or moral. As Rawls puts it, justice as fairness "elaborates a political conception as a freestanding view . . . We leave aside comprehensive doctrines that now exist, or that have existed, or that might exist" (Rawls, 1993: 40).

Rawls believes that the two principles of justice as fairness are acceptable to an overlapping consensus, asserting that a majority of people from conflicting backgrounds will affirm these principles, while doing so for various different reasons.[4] In fact, this is one of the primary strengths that political liberalism has over other political systems. In the original position and behind the veil of ignorance, the fundamental ideas that are chosen are ones that find a favorable ear in holders of various comprehensive doctrines (Rawls, 2001: §11).

As to the issue of the kinds of practices to which Rawls's theory is meant to apply, a few words may be added. Rawls has been criticized for the theoretical nature of his work by some commentators, including Robert Paul Wolff. Wolff complains that the answer to the question of whether or not Rawls is right is "extraordinarily difficult to get a grip on . . . despite the care with which Rawls develops subsidiary themes in his theory. The problem, in part, stems from the fact that Rawls says little or nothing about the concrete facts of social, economic, and political reality" (Wolff, 1977: 195). Of course, Rawls admits that this was his intention, in that he is actively trying to achieve a higher level of abstraction, declaring that it is an ideal theory with which he begins. This abstraction is part of the basic limitation that Rawls places on his own theory with regard to the scope of the project itself. Rawls admits that the project is not intended to lay out a complete political system down to the particular individual laws, but is trying to lay out just principles that he believes will be agreeable and applicable to the creation of an overriding ideal structure. It is for this reason that Rawls begins behind the veil of ignorance in the original position, so that an individual's comprehensive moral doctrine or an egoistic desire to receive more than what reason would call their fair share can be limited. In fact, Rawls asserts that reasonable persons are moved by a desire for "a social world in which they, as free and equal, can cooperate with others on terms all can accept. They insist that reciprocity should hold within that world so that each benefits along with others" (Rawls, 1993: 50).[5] Persons also possess the capacity for a sense of justice and a conception of the good. I must emphasize the fact that Rawls does not require that citizens have a conception of the good, only that, as part of the overlapping consensus, their comprehensive moral doctrine has a conception of the good that they are trying to achieve in their lives. Even in these statements regarding the nature of persons, the emphasis is on the way that those persons interact within the larger system of political and social institutions.

Furthermore, the principles of justice for institutions must be distinguished from those for individuals, because the different subject matter would call for a different type of principle. While institutions are made up of and fundamentally affect the lives of individuals, they do not do so on an individual basis. However, if Rawls's theory does not apply to the problems of particular individuals, one could question its applicability to the issue of same-sex marriage. The family, however, is one of the major institutions that are the primary subject of Rawls's work. If we consider the question of same-sex marriage in terms of the ways in which the institution of marriage and the family would be constructed in a just system such as the one that Rawls lays out and we determine that our current system fundamentally differs from that construction, then that will serve as a basis for a further re-evaluation of our current structure. We will not be directly looking at the particular arguments that could be offered for or against the permissibility of a particular same-sex marriage today, but will instead consider marriage as a basic political/social institution as Rawls defines it and examine how that vision differs from our current practice. It is on this level of the abstract that we can apply Rawls to marriage and then apply those considerations to same-sex marriage as part of the broader institution.

Having attained an idea of the underlying principles that guide Rawls's political theory and also determining that Rawls's theory of justice can in fact apply to our question at hand, we are prepared to begin our detailed consideration of justice as fairness and its relation to same-sex marriage.

SECTION II: THE JUSTICE OF ALLOWING SAME-SEX MARRIAGE

A. Gays and Lesbians in the Original Position

First, we must return to the veil of ignorance and the original position. Since gays and lesbians do count as equal citizens because they possess the minimum requirements, including the capacities for a sense of justice, a conception of the good, and the ability to be cooperating members of society, it is clear that they would be represented in the original position. As we said before, the original position is the tool that Rawls asserts can help us to come to a political conception that nullifies "the effects of specific contingencies which put men at odds and tempt them to exploit social and natural circumstances to their own advantage" (Rawls, 1971: 136). The choosers behind the veil are aware only of general facts, but are unaware of their own individual characteristics and the place that they would hold in society.[6] With regard to their society, they do not even know the history of their own culture and this lack of knowledge would seem to include whether or not it has historically been anti-homosexual or against same-sex marriage (although they would know of the existence of homophobia, along with racism and sexism as general traits that exist in the world). They also do not know the characteristics they will have as individuals once the veil is lifted, such as, their age, class, intelligence, physical capabilities, or their natural endowments. Rawls would later add racial/ethnic information as well as sex. Because sexual orientation is an individual characteristic, it would also be knowledge that is denied to a chooser in the original position, although Rawls does not specifically affirm this. Knowledge of one's sexual orientation is as much an individual characteristic as other traits of which the choosers are deprived because it might prejudice them. We would certainly not want someone who is lesbian or gay to use that knowledge to create political institutions that favor their position any more than we would want someone to know of their economic status and abuse that information in their conception of what is just.

A second point is that while those in the original position know that those for whom they are selecting principles have a conception of the good, behind the veil they do not "know the content of these conceptions . . . they do not know the particular final ends and aims these persons pursue; nor the objects of their attachments and loyalties . . ." (Rawls, 1993: 310).[7] Because those in the original position do not know the identity of their attachments after the veil is lifted, they would be unaware of the sex, for example, of those to whom they have romantic attachments.

As we said before, avoiding the choosing of principles more beneficial to one group over another is the principal reason that the veil of ignorance was created in the first place. As Rawls says, the veil "removes differences in bargaining advantages, so that in this and other respects the parties are symmetrically situated" (Rawls, 2001:87). While the person in the original position does possess general psychological knowledge of human beings, including the kinds of goals that persons tend to seek, those goals include a wide range of possibilities. Most people seek out romantic partners, sometimes for short-term relationships and sometimes for relationships that last a lifetime. Most people choose to make the relationship with that lifetime partner public by getting married, yet some do not. Many people desire to have children and raise a family, while some do not. And within all of these relationships are variations in the kind of partner that is sought, including same-sex partners, opposite-sex partners, multiple partners, and sometimes no partner at all. All of these possibilities are options for the person behind the veil of ignorance. Because people in the original position do not know where they are or who they are as individuals, they are more likely to construct a system of the greatest equality to try and guarantee that they are included as an equal citizen. Depriving the choosers' knowledge of their sexual orientation allows the choosers to truly consider what the fair terms of social cooperation within the state should be. These fair terms of cooperation will find their expression in both the principles of justice themselves and in the basic structure of political and social institutions.

B. The Family as an Institution

Before we commence our consideration of the family as a political and social institution, I must first address how marriage relates to the family. Rawls does not specifically refer to marriage as part of the family. While he may have several reasons for not doing this, a central concern may have been the implication that marriage was the only method for achieving a family. As we shall see, Rawls places few requirements on what constitutes a family, including the members involved or the ways in which they choose to symbolize that involvement. To talk directly about marriage as the genesis of the family could lead some to conclude that only through marriage can a family be said to exist. While marriage may be one way to create a family, it is not the only way, although that does not preclude us from considering marriage as one possible instantiation of the family. Furthermore, although he did write of the importance of the monogamous family structure in *A Theory of Justice*, Rawls would abandon that formulation in his later works, perhaps because the requirement of monogamy itself was too restrictive a requirement to place on the family.

Because the family is one of the major social institutions that we are attempting to include in a scheme of fair cooperation, and marriage is one of the central ways in which people generally begin the process of creating a family, the question of same-sex marriage is an important one. Rawls is clear about the importance of the family as an institution within the basic structure in *Justice as Fairness*, because the family plays an important role in establishing:

> . . . the orderly production and reproduction of society and of its culture from one generation to the next . . . Accepting this, essential to the role of the family is the arrangement in a reasonable and effective way of the raising and caring for children, ensuring their moral development and education into the wider culture. (Rawls, 2001: 162–63)

Unlike other arguments regarding marriage that use procreation as the basis for their conception of marriage, Rawls does not draw conclusions about what procreation means for the family. In fact, Rawls would state in a 1997 article that while the family is important because it is the most common method of having and raising children, that does not in itself dictate what the family is. The idea of procreation does not determine what should be the internal structure of the family, but is only one reason why Rawls thinks the family is a fundamental political and social institution. Procreation is simply one of the things that Rawls would like to see occur within the institution of the family in general, but it is not a requirement for any particular group of people to be considered a family. In an often overlooked footnote in "The Idea of Public Reason Revisited," Rawls states that "no particular form of the family (monogamous, heterosexual, or otherwise) is required by a political conception of justice so long as the family is arranged to fulfill these tasks effectively . . ." (Rawls, 1999: 596).[8] Those tasks not only include raising children, but also educating them on the importance of justice, thereby raising cooperative citizens for the future of the state. The family stands as one of the principal methods of teaching and mentoring future generations and in that role it maintains a central part in the transmission of political ideals. Because of this, Rawls does favor situations in which children "grow up in a small intimate group in which elders (normally our parents) have a certain moral and social authority" (Rawls, 2001: 163). This parental authority is not absolute, for the two principles of justice apply in the formation of the basic institution of the family and it indirectly applies within the family. The basic liberties provided for by the first principle of justice still hold within the family, even though they may not be viewed as strictly political principles. For Rawls, political justice is central to the basic structure and secondary to the actions within that structure. By creating a just basic structure, justice as fairness also creates background justice which reinforces and adjusts the public's conception of what justice is, also serving as a constant public reminder of the original two principles. While background justice does not dictate the particular way in which a parent must address a specific situation with their children, it does dictate that the concepts of equality and due process do not disappear inside the institution itself. Background justice also fosters "social attitudes of encouragement and support" that create an underlying feeling amongst the populace that anything is possible given hard work and determination, that their chosen political structure is just, and every citizen is equal (Rawls, 2001: 57).

The importance that the basic structure has in the formulation of background justice is just one of the reasons why it is one of the primary aspects of justice as fairness. According to Rawls, the basic structure has a "profound and pervasive influence on the persons who live under its institutions" (Rawls, 2001: 55). This influence must be carefully scrutinized because the basic structure can fundamentally alter the life-prospects of citizens, either for good or for ill. Rawls says that life-prospects are influenced by three kinds of contingencies, including: the social class that we are born into, our native endowments, and luck; which he calls respectively, social, natural, and fortuitous contingencies. While our good or bad luck may be outside of the control of political and social institutions, to a great extent the basic structure can manipulate the ways in which the other two contingencies operate within the state. This adjustment of our social viewpoint takes many forms and is primarily carried out by the operation of the difference principle, but another method of manipulation is through education and training. This education does, in part, include the difference principle, in that those who are more blessed by natural endowment in a certain field train those who are less endowed, but it also includes educating people "to recognize one another as free and equal . . ." (Rawls, 2001: 56). Such an education does not simply take place in K–12 and in college, but is also undertaken in all of our interactions with the social and political structures in a just society. Living in a society whose institutions are founded on and implement the two principles of justice, thereby treating its citizens as free and equal persons, creates an atmosphere of background justice.

According to Rawls, one further consideration regarding the family addresses the various social conceptions that currently exist regarding the family. These conceptions concern certain beliefs regarding gender roles within the family, a belief in the importance of monogamy, as well as concerns regarding the sexual orientation of the members of a family. According to Rawls, these beliefs are not political positions that necessarily arise from the state's interest in and construction of the family as an institution, but instead "reflect religious or comprehensive moral doctrines" (Rawls, 1999: 587). Rawls denies that any of these aspects are inherent in the family and a state-sanctioned inclusion of these beliefs in our construction of the family as an institution would have to be arrived at through a consideration of the political values that would call for such a requirement along with its adherence to the principles of justice.

We have seen that, while it is true that Rawls does lay upon the institution of the family the burden of sustaining and reproducing our society and culture from one generation to the next, this is only one aspect of the family. Rawls does not even go so far as to directly tie the notion of marriage to the family, but instead seems content to leave marriage as one possible manifestation of a family. He does not tie himself to any conception of what the family should be except for his requirement that, as a whole, it serve the reproduction and transmission of our political and social mindset. Because of this openness, it seems clear that a same-sex couple, particularly one that incorporated the raising of children, could count as a family. By my reckoning, that conclusion would also entitle those couples to the institution of marriage.

C. Inequality in the Structure of Marriage?

If the formulation of the family as a social and political institution does not rely on sex or gender as a basic requirement, it seems that same-sex couples could qualify. The next question to address is whether or not those couples do in fact qualify as a family within a just political structure grounded in the two principles of justice as fairness.

As we have already stated, the first principle of justice is also considered in the formation of marriage and the family as social institutions. The first principle guarantees that persons have "the same indefeasible claim to a fully adequate scheme of equal basic liberties, which scheme is compatible with the same scheme of liberties for all . . ." (Rawls, 2001: 42). This principle includes the political idea that citizens under this system of justice are free and equal persons. This freedom includes a conception of the good, which for many gay and lesbian couples includes a desire to find a partner, get married, and create a family.

The fact that one has a conception of the good does not entail that they have a right to that good. Rawls outlines two reasons to reject a conception of the good that is not in line with the political conception of justice as fairness and the overlapping consensus, although he says there may be more. These two reasons to reject a conception of the good include:

... those doctrines and their associated ways of life [that] may be in direct conflict with the principles of justice; or else they may be admissible but fail to gain
adherents under the political and social conditions of a just constitutional regime.
The first case is illustrated by a conception of the good requiring the repression
or degradation of certain persons on, say, racial, or ethnic, or perfectionist
grounds, for example, slavery in ancient Athens or in the antebellum South.
Examples of the second case may be certain forms of religion. (Rawls, 2001: 154)[9]

A homosexual conception of the good that chooses to seek marriage as a principal end and aim for the achievement of a worthwhile life would not seem to
violate either of these two exceptions. Furthermore, because the family is a goal
that is not only chosen within particular comprehensive doctrines, but is also a
central part of the basic structure, the request on the part of same-sex partners
for inclusion within a state-sanctioned institution is valid. The basic structure is
constructed to be in unison with the principles of justice in such a way as to "set
out a framework of thought within which [questions of justice] can be approached" (Rawls, 2001: 12). The question of same-sex marriage, when
approached in a Rawlsian framework, is not one of the various questions of justice as it is applied on domestic and global levels, but is, instead, a fundamental
question on the level of institutions themselves.

As I said earlier, I am choosing not to address the ways in which the difference principle could be applied to the questions of same-sex marriage. One
reason for this is the simple fact that it cannot be applied, for the second principle of justice cannot be used to relegate homosexual marriage to a lesser status.
Doing so would not seem to readily improve the situation of the worst off and
also would violate equal opportunity; creating an unjust arrangement. One
could, however, argue that the difference principle would dictate that the central
problem involved in our consideration of same-sex marriage is that a primary
good is not being distributed equally, and that those in the worse position are not
gaining from that inequality. It could be said that the primary good that is
involved here is "The social bases of self-respect . . . essential if citizens are to
have a lively sense of their worth as persons and to be able to advance their ends
with self-confidence" (Rawls, 2001:59). The reason why I am not defending this
perhaps fruitful line of argument has to do with where I am placing my focus. I
choose instead to consider the larger (and prior) questions regarding the formation of the basic structure itself and the institutions that comprise that structure.
While it is these institutions that distribute the primary goods, I am not looking
at the ways in which our current institution can be adjusted, but at the way in
which the original position would choose to construct them in the first place.

Considering the question of same-sex marriage on the level of the family
institution, I assert that those in the original position would include same-sex

marriage as one possible instance of a family. The first principle of justice promises equal basic liberties and these liberties are to be taken into consideration in the construction of the political and social institutions, both in the original position and at the constitutional convention. Those liberties include political liberties (vote and participation in politics), freedom of thought, and they also include "rights and liberties specified by the liberty and integrity (physical and psychological) of the person . . ." (Rawls, 2001: 44). The integrity of persons includes their status as free and equal. These various liberties are important for Rawls because they "provide the political and social conditions essential for the adequate development and full exercise of the two moral powers of free and equal persons" (Rawls, 2001:45). The capacity for a conception of the good may appear to delve into the area of primary goods covered by the difference principle, however, the special status of the family as an institution that must be constructed in accordance with both principles entails that, in particular, access to the family should be free and equal. Allowing for inequality on this fundamental level undermines the principles of justice as well as background justice. Because justice as fairness expresses some of what Rawls calls our greatest values including "the values of equal political and civil liberty . . . [and] the bases of mutual respect between citizens," limitations to liberty (in particular, limitations that are fundamental and occur on the level of political and social institutions), can only be made under extreme circumstances. As Rawls himself said, doctrines that deny freedom, while they may seem to be a fact of life, must be contained "like war and disease—so that they do not overturn political justice" (Rawls, 1993: 64).

D. Would Allowing Same-Sex Marriage Violate Values?

There are many people who would object to my application of Rawls on this point and I would be remiss if I did not address one central concern. This concern is the assertion that some would make regarding the degree to which having to accept a same-sex couple as a family, with a right to marriage, would violate their personal liberties. This is a question that Rawls himself is sensitive to, for he understood that the fact that there were so many comprehensive moral doctrines in the world might on the surface seem to contradict the possibility of a single statement of justice. Rawls asserts, however, that the principles of justice as fairness arrived at behind the veil and the social and political institutions that followed from those principles would be agreeable to an overlapping consensus of reasonable persons within the state. This consensus does not entail that the values of the various comprehensive moral doctrines would always agree with the positions of the state. When that disagreement exists, it is not meant to devalue those comprehensive moral doctrines, because according to Rawls:

. . . political liberalism does not say that the values articulated by a political conception of justice, though of basic significance, outweigh the transcendent values (as people may interpret them)—religious, philosophical, or moral— with
which the political conception may possibly conflict. To say that would go beyond the political (Rawls, 2001: 37).

Rawls would not require, for example, that Southern Baptist ministers conduct
ceremonies for same-sex marriages, for they would be free within their comprehensive doctrine to protest and be contemptuous of such relationships. Such a
position on the part of those ministers would not violate the principles of justice, since they would not interfere with the ability of same-sex couples to be
married, for they could turn to another congregation or even to a justice of the
peace to be married. Those against same-sex marriage would still be free to
express their freedom of speech by speaking to their congregations about the
dangers that they believe are tied to homosexual activity. When we decide that
our political conception of justice as fairness allows for same-sex marriage, this
is only a political statement about rights with regard to political and social institutions, which still leaves "the concept of a true moral judgment to comprehensive doctrines" (Rawls, 1993: 116).

BIBLIOGRAPHY

Rawls, J. *A Theory of Justice.* Cambridge: Harvard University Press, 1971.
———. *Political Liberalism.* New York: Columbia University Press, 1993.
———. "The Idea of Public Reason Revisited." *University of Chicago Law Review* 64
    (Summer 1997): 765–807.
———. *Collected Papers.* Cambridge: Harvard University Press, 1999.
———. *Justice as Fairness: A Restatement.* London: Belknap Press of Harvard University
    Press, 2001.
Wolff, R. P. *Understanding Rawls.* Princeton, NJ: Princeton University Press, 1977.

NOTES

1. It is important to note that I am not asserting that these arguments are valid or
invalid because of their reliance on naturalistic assumptions, only that the application of
a naturalistic foundation for a particular conception of marriage is problematic because
both sides use it to come to opposing conclusions. As I have already said, both sides
attempt to demarcate aspects of marriage that are an inherent part of the institution, and
then argue that same-sex marriage does or does not fulfill those requirements.

2. In his later work, Rawls will rearrange the two aspects of the second principle in such

a way that equality of opportunity is lexically prior to (must be satisfied before) the assertion that any inequalities must work toward the greatest benefit of the least advantaged.

3. It should be noted that in some cases, Rawls speaks of these three stages as three stages that are separate from the original position behind the veil of ignorance (see Rawls, 1993: 180). Yet, in others, he includes the original position as the first stage and counts the constitutional, legislative, and judicial/administrative stages as two through four (see Rawls, 1993: 397 and Rawls, 2001: 48).

4. These various comprehensive doctrines that combine to form the overlapping consensus must, however, satisfy the requirement of reasonable pluralism. The idea here is that overlapping consensus may not always be possible according to Rawls, particularly in many historical conditions, because the consensus may be "overwhelmed by unreasonable and even irrational (and sometimes mad) comprehensive doctrines" (Rawls, 1993: 126). Political liberalism does not, however, judge the position of another as irrational simply because they choose to disagree with it. Only when a disagreement arises because of an unreasonable position (what Rawls calls "a lack of reasonableness, or rationality, or conscientiousness of one or more of the persons involved") can one disregard someone from the overlapping consensus, if the unreasonableness can be identified by independent grounds that are agreed upon by both sides. The unreasonable person's rights as they exist under the two principles of justice as fairness still hold in either case.

5. Rawls contrasts this conception of reasonable persons with his assertion that unreasonable persons "plan to engage in cooperative schemes but are unwilling to honor, or even to propose, except as a necessary public pretense, any general principles or standards for specifying fair terms of cooperation. They are ready to violate such terms as suits their interests when circumstances allow" (Rawls, 1993: 50).

6. While knowledge of their individual situation or the specific situation of the society to which they belong is forbidden, they are, however, allowed general information about "the basis of social organization and the laws of human psychology . . . whatever general filters affect the choice of the principles of justice. There are no limitations on general information . . ." (Rawls, 1971: 137–38).

7. Again, while Rawls forbids particular information, he does allow general knowledge of the broad plans of life.

8. This citation refers to the article's appearance in Rawls's *Collected Papers*, although it was originally published in *University of Chicago Law Review* 64 (Summer 1997): 765–807.

9. Rawls offers the example of a religion that bases its views on a belief that it must control the "machinery of state" in order to prosper.

Part 2.

GENDER, SEXUALITY, AND PERVERSION

17.

"PRICKS" AND "CHICKS"
A Plea for "Persons"

Robert B. Baker

There is a school of philosophers who believe that one starts philosophizing not by examining whatever it is one is philosophizing about but by examining the words we use to designate the subject to be examined. I must confess my allegiance to this school. The import of my confession is that this is an essay on women's liberation.

There seems to be a curious malady that affects those philosophers who in order to analyze anything must examine the way we talk about it; they seem incapable of talking about anything without talking about their talk about it and, once again, I must confess to being typical. Thus I shall argue, first, that the way in which we identify something reflects our conception of it; second, that the conception of women embedded in our language is male chauvinistic; third, that the conceptual revisions proposed by the feminist movement are confused; and finally, that at the roots of the problem are both our conception of sex and the very structure of sexual identification.

"Pricks" and "Chicks": A Plea for "Persons," by Robert Baker. First published in *Philosophy and Sex*, first edition (Amherst, NY: Prometheus Books, 1980). Copyright © Robert Baker. Reprinted by permission of author.

IDENTIFICATION AND CONCEPTION

I am not going to defend the position that the terms we utilize to identify something reflect our conception of it; I shall simply explain and illustrate a simplified version of this thesis. Let us assume that any term that can be (meaningfully) substituted for x in the following statements is a term used to identify something: "Where is the x?" "Who is the x?" Some of the terms that can be substituted for x in the above expressions are metaphors; I shall refer to such metaphors as metaphorical identifications. For example, southerners frequently say such things as "Where did that girl get to?" and "Who is the new boy that Lou hired to help out at the filling station?" If the persons the terms apply to are adult Afro-Americans, then "girl" and "boy" are metaphorical identifications. The fact that the metaphorical identifications in question are standard in the language reflects the fact that certain characteristics of the objects properly classified as boys and girls (for example, immaturity, inability to take care of themselves, need for guidance) are generally held by those who use identifications to be properly attributable to Afro-Americans. One might say that the whole theory of southern white paternalism is implicit in the metaphorical identification "boy" (just as the rejection of paternalism is implicit in the standardized Afro-American forms of address, "man" and "woman," as in, for example, "Hey, man, how are you?").

Most of what I am going to say in this essay is significant only if the way we metaphorically identify something is not a superficial bit of conceptually irrelevant happenstance but rather a reflection of our conceptual structure. Thus if one is to accept my analysis he must understand the significance of metaphorical identifications. He must see that, even though the southerner who identifies adult Afro-American males as "boys" feels that this identification is "just the way people talk"; but for a group to talk that way it must think that way. In the next few paragraphs I shall adduce what I hope is a persuasive example of how, in one clear case, the change in the way we identified something reflected a change in the way we thought about it.

Until the 1960s, Afro-Americans were identified by such terms as "Negro" and "colored" (the respectable terms) and by the more disreputable "nigger," "spook," "kink," and so on. Recently there has been an unsuccessful attempt to replace the respectable identifications with such terms as "African," and "Afro-American," and a more successful attempt to replace them with "black." The most outspoken champions of this linguistic reform were those who argued that nonviolence must be abandoned for Black Power (Stokely Carmichael, H. Rap Brown), that integration must be abandoned in favor of separation (the Black Muslims: Malcolm X, Muhammad Ali), and that Afro-Americans were an internal colony in the alien world of Babylon who must arm themselves against the possibility of extermination (the Black Panthers: Eldridge Cleaver, Huey Newton). All of these movements and their partisans wished to stress that Afro-Americans were different from other Americans and could not be merged with them because the difference between the two was as great as that between black and white. Linguistically, of course, "black" and "white" are antonyms; and it is precisely this sense of oppositeness that those who see the Afro-American as alienated, separated, and nonintegratable wish to capture with the term "black." Moreover, as any good dictionary makes clear, in some contexts "black" is synonymous with "deadly," "sinister," "wicked," "evil," and so forth. The new militants were trying to create just this picture of the black man—civil rights and Uncle Tomism are dead, the ghost of Nat Turner is to be resurrected, Freedom Now or pay the price, the ballot or the bullet, "Violence is as American as cherry pie." The new strategy was that the white man would either give the black man his due or pay the price in violence. Since conceptually a "black man" was an object to be feared ("black" can be synonymous with "deadly," and so on), while a "colored man" or a "Negro" was not, the new strategy required that the "Negro" be supplanted by the "black man." White America resisted the proposed linguistic reform quite vehemently, until hundreds of riots forced the admission that the Afro-American was indeed black.

Now to the point: I have suggested that the word "black" replaced the word "Negro" because there was a change in our conceptual structure. One is likely to reply that while all that I have said above is well and good, one had, after all, no choice about the matter. White people are identified in terms of their skin color as whites; clearly, if we are to recognize what is in reality nothing but the truth, that in this society people are conscious of skin color, to treat blacks as equals is merely to identify them by their skin color, which is black. That is, one might argue that while there was a change in words, we have no reason to think that there was a parallel conceptual change. If the term "black" has all the associations mentioned above, that is unfortunate; but in the context the use of the term "black" to identify the people formerly identified as "Negroes" is natural, inevitable, and, in and of itself, neutral; black is, after all, the skin color of the people in question. (Notice that this defense of the natural-inevitable-and-neutral conception of identification quite nicely circumvents the possible use of such seemingly innocuous terms as "Afro-American" and "African" by suggesting that in this society it is *skin color* that is the relevant variable.)

The great flaw in this analysis is that the actual skin color of virtually all of the people whom we call "black" is not black at all. The color tones range from light yellow to a deep umber that occasionally is literally black. The skin color of most Afro-Americans is best designated by the word "brown." Yet "brown" is not a term that is standard for identifying Afro-Americans. For example, if someone asked, "Who was the brown who was the architect for Washington, DC?" we would not know how to construe the question. We might attempt to read "brown" as a proper name ("Do you mean Arthur Brown, the designer?"). We would have no trouble understanding the sentence "Who was the black (Negro, colored guy, and so forth) who designed Washington, DC?" ("Oh, you mean Benjamin Banneker"). Clearly, "brown" is not a standard form of identification for Afro-Americans. I hope that it is equally clear that "black" has become the standard way of identifying Afro-Americans not because the term was natural, inevitable, and, in the context, neutral, but because of its occasional synonymy with "sinister" and because as an antonym to "white" it best fitted the conceptual needs of those who saw race relations in terms of intensifying and insurmountable antonymies. If one accepts this point, then one must admit that there is a close connection between the way in which we identify things and the way in which we conceive them—and thus it should be also clear why I wish to talk about the way in which women are identified in English.[1] (Thus, for example, one would expect Black Muslims, who continually use the term "black *man*"— as in "the black *man's* rights"—to be more male chauvinistic than Afro-Americans who use the terms "black *people*" or "black *folk*.")

WAYS OF IDENTIFYING WOMEN

It may at first seem trivial to note that women (and men) are identified sexually; but conceptually this is extremely significant. To appreciate the significance of this fact it is helpful to imagine a language in which proper names and personal pronouns do not reflect the sex of the person designated by them (as they do in our language). I have been told that in some Oriental languages pronouns and proper names reflect social status rather than sex, but whether or not there actually exists such a language is irrelevant, for it is easy enough to imagine what one would be like. Let us then imagine a language where the proper names are sexually neutral (for example, "Xanthe"), so that one cannot tell from hearing a name whether the person so named is male or female, and where the personal pronouns in the language are "under" and "over." "Under" is the personal pronoun appropriate for all those who are younger than thirty, while "over" is appropriate to persons older than thirty. In such a language, instead of saying such things as "Where do you think *he* is living now?" one would say such things as "Where do you think *under* is living now?"

What would one say about a cultural community that employed such a language? Clearly, one would say that they thought that for purposes of intelligible communication it was more important to know a person's age grouping than the person's height, sex, race, hair color, or parentage. (There are many actual cultures, of course, in which people are identified by names that reflect their parentage; for example, Abu ben Adam means Abu son of Adam.) I think that one would also claim that this people would not have reflected these differences in the pronominal structure of their language if they did not believe that the differences between unders and overs were such that a statement would frequently have one meaning if it were about an under and a different meaning if it were about an over. For example, in feudal times if a serf said, "My lord said to do this," that assertion was radically different from "Freeman John said to do this," since (presumably) the former had the status of a command while the latter did not. Hence the conventions of Middle English required that one refer to people in such a way as to indicate their social status. Analogously, one would not distinguish between pronominal references according to the age differences in the persons referred to were there no shift in meaning involved.

If we apply the lesson illustrated by this imaginary language to our own, I think that it should be clear that since in our language proper nouns and pronouns reflect sex rather than age, race, parentage, social status, or religion, we believe one of the most important things one can know about a person is that person's sex. (And, indeed, this is the first thing one seeks to determine about a newborn babe—our first question is almost invariably "Is it a boy or a girl?") Moreover, we would not reflect this important difference pronominally did we not also believe that statements frequently mean one thing when applied to males and something else when applied to females. Perhaps the most striking aspect of the conceptual discrimination reflected in our language is that man is, as it were, essentially human, while woman is only accidentally so.

This charge may seem rather extreme, but consider the following synonyms (which are readily confirmed by any dictionary). "Humanity" is synonymous with "mankind" but not with "womankind." "Man" can be substituted for "humanity" or "mankind" in any sentence in which the terms "mankind" or "humanity" occur without changing the meaning of the sentence, but significantly, "woman" cannot. Thus, the following expressions are all synonymous with each other: "humanity's great achievements," "mankind's great achievements," and "man's great achievements." "Woman's great achievements" is not synonymous with any of these. To highlight the degree to which women are excluded from humanity, let me point out that it is something of a truism to say that "man is a rational animal," while "woman is a rational animal" is quite debatable. Clearly, if "man" in the first assertion embraced both men and women, the second assertion would be just as much a truism as the first.[2] Humanity, it would seem, is a male prerogative. (And hence, one of the goals of women's liberation is to alter our conceptual structure so that someday "mankind" will be regarded as an improper and vestigial ellipsis for "humankind," and "man will have no special privileges in relation to "human being" that "woman" does not have.)[3]

The major question before us is, How are women conceived in our culture? I have been trying to answer this question by talking about how they are identified. I first considered pronominal identification; now I wish to turn to identification through other types of noun phrases. Methods of nonpronominal identification can be discovered by determining which terms can be substituted for "woman" in such sentences as "Who is that woman over there?" without changing the meaning of the sentence. Virtually no term is interchangeable with "woman" in that sentence for all speakers on all occasions. Even "lady," which most speakers would accept as synonymous with "woman" in that sentence, will not do for a speaker who applies the term "lady" only to those women who display manners, poise, and sensitivity. In most contexts, a large number of students in one or more of my classes will accept the following types of terms as more or less interchangeable with "woman." (An asterisk indicates interchanges acceptable to both males and females; a plus sign indicates terms restricted to black students only. Terms with neither an asterisk nor a plus sign are accepted by all males but are not normally used by females.)

→ A. NEUTRAL TERMS: *lady, *gal, *girl (especially with regard to a coworker in an office or factory, *sister, *broad (originally in the animal category, but most people do not think of the term as now meaning pregnant cow)

→ B. ANIMAL: chick, bird, fox, vixen, filly, bitch (Many do not know the literal meaning of the term. Some men and most women construe this use as pejorative; they think of "bitch" in the context of "bitchy," that is, snappy, nasty, and so forth. But a large group of men claim that it is a standard nonpejorative term of identification—which may perhaps indicate that women have come to be thought of as shrews by a large subclass of men.)

→ C. PLAYTHING: babe, doll, cuddly

→ D. GENDER (association with articles of clothing typically worn by those in the female gender role): skirt, hem

→ E. SEXUAL: snatch, cunt, ass, twat, piece (of ass, and so forth), lay, pussy (could be put in the animal category, but most users associated it with slang expression indicating the female pubic region), hammer (related to anatomical analogy between a hammer and breasts). There are many other usages, for example, "bunny," "sweat hog," but these were not recognized as standard by as many as 10 percent of any given class.

The students in my classes reported that the most frequently used terms of identification are in the neutral and animal classifications (although men in their forties claim to use the gender classifications quite a bit) and that the least frequently used terms of identification are sexual. Fortunately, however, I am not interested in the frequency of usage but only in whether the use is standard enough to be recognized as an identification among some group or other. (Recall that "brown" was not a standardized term of identification and hence we could not make sense out of "Who was the brown who planned Washington, DC?" Similarly, one has trouble with "Who was the breasts who planned Washington, DC?" but not with "Who was the babe (doll, chick, skirt, and so forth) who planned Washington, DC?"

Except for two of the animal terms, "chick" and "broad"—but note that "broad" is probably neutral today—women do not typically identify themselves in sexual terms, in gender terms, as playthings, or as animals; *only males use non-neutral terms to identify women*. Hence, it would seem that there is a male conception of women and a female conception. Only males identify women as "foxes," "babes," "skirts," or "cunts" (and since all the other nonneutral identifications are male, it is reasonable to assume that the identification of a woman as a "chick" is primarily a male conception that some women have adopted).

What kind of conception do men have of women? Clearly they think that women share certain properties with certain types of animals, toys, and playthings; they conceive of them in terms of the clothes associated with the female gender role; and, last (and, if my classes are any indication, least frequently), they conceive of women in terms of those parts of their anatomy associated with sexual intercourse, that is, as the identification "lay" indicates quite clearly, as sexual partners.

The first two nonneutral male classifications, animal and plaything, are prima facie denigrating (and I mean this in the literal sense of making one like a "nigger"). Consider the animal classification. All of the terms listed, with the possible exception of "bird," refer to animals that are either domesticated for servitude (to *man*) or hunted for sport. First, let us consider the term "bird." When I asked my students what sort of birds might be indicated, they suggested chick, canary (one member, in his forties, had suggested "canary" as a term of identification), chicken, pigeon, dove, parakeet, and hummingbird (one member). With the exception of the hummingbird, which like all the birds suggested is generally thought to be diminutive and pretty, all of the birds are domesticated, usually as pets (which reminds one that "my pet" is an expression of endearment). None of the birds were predators or symbols of intelligence or nobility (as are the owl, eagle, hawk, and falcon); nor did large but beautiful birds seem appropriate (for example, pheasants, peacocks, and swans). If one construes the bird terms (and for that matter, "filly") as applicable to women because they are thought of as beautiful, or at least pretty, *then there is nothing denigrating about them*. If, on the other hand, the common properties that underlie the metaphorical identification are domesticity and servitude, then they are indeed denigrating (as for myself, I think that both domesticity and prettiness underlie the identification). "Broad," of course, is, or at least was, clearly denigrating, since nothing renders more service to a farmer than does a pregnant cow, and cows are not commonly thought of as paradigms of beauty.

With one exception all of the animal terms reflect a male conception of women either as domesticated servants or as pets, or as both. Indeed, some of the terms reflect a conception of women first as pets and then as servants. Thus, when a pretty, cuddly little chick grows older, she becomes a very useful servant—the egg-laying hen.

"Vixen" and "fox," variants of the same term, are the one clear exception. None of the other animals with whom women are metaphorically identified are generally thought to be intelligent, aggressive, or independent—but the fox is. A chick is a soft, cuddly, entertaining, pretty, diminutive, domesticated, and dumb animal. A fox too is soft, cuddly, entertaining, pretty, and diminutive, but it is neither dependent nor dumb. It is aggressive, intelligent, and a minor predator— indeed, it preys on chicks—and frequently outsmarts ("outfoxes") men.

Thus the term "fox" or "vixen" is generally taken to be a compliment by both men and women, and compared to any of the animal or plaything terms it is indeed a compliment. Yet, considered in and of itself, the conception of a woman as a fox is not really complimentary at all, for the major connection between man and fox is that of predator and prey. The fox is an animal that men chase, and hunt, and kill for sport. If women are conceived of as foxes, then they are conceived of as prey that it is fun to hunt.

In considering plaything identifications, only one sentence is necessary. *All the plaything identifications are clearly denigrating since they assimilate women to the status of mindless or dependent objects.* "Doll" is to male paternalism what "boy" is to white paternalism.

Up to this point in our survey of male conceptions of women, every male identification, without exception, has been clearly antithetical to the conception of women as human beings (recall that "man" was synonymous with "human," while "woman" was not). Since the way we talk of things, and especially the way we identify them, is the way in which we conceive of them, any movement dedicated to breaking the bonds of female servitude must destroy these ways of identifying, and hence of conceiving of women. Only when both sexes find the terms "babe," "doll," "chick," "broad," and so forth, as objectionable as "boy" and "nigger" will women come to be conceived of as independent *human beings*.

The two remaining unexamined male identifications are gender and sex. There seems to be nothing objectionable about gender identifications per se. That is, women are metaphorically identified as skirts because in this culture skirts, like women, are peculiarly female. Indeed, if one accepts the view that the slogan "female and proud" should play the same role for the women's liberation movement that the slogan "Black is beautiful" plays for the black liberation movement, then female clothes should be worn with the same pride as Afro clothes. (Of course, one can argue that the skirt, like the cropped-down Afro, is a sign of bondage, and hence both the item of clothing and the identification with it are to be rejected—that is, cropped-down Afros are to Uncle Tom what skirts are to Uncle Mom.)

The terms in the last category are obviously sexual, and frequently vulgar. For a variety of reasons I shall consider the import and nature of these identifications in the next section.

MEN OUGHT NOT TO THINK OF WOMEN AS SEX OBJECTS ONLY.

Feminists have proposed many reforms, and most of them are clearly desirable; for example, equal opportunity for self-development, equal pay for equal work, and free daycare centers. One feminist proposal, however, is peculiarly conceptual and deeply perplexing. I call this proposal peculiarly conceptual because unlike the other reforms it is directed at getting people to think differently. The proposal is that *men should not think of women* (*and women should not think of themselves*) *as sex objects.* In the rest of this essay I shall explore this nostrum. I do so for two reasons: first, because the process of exploration should reveal the depth of the problem confronting the feminists; and second, because the feminists themselves seem to be entangled in the very concepts that obstruct their liberation

To see why I find this proposal puzzling, one has to ask what it is to think of something as a sex object.

If a known object is an object that we know, an unidentified object is an object that we have not identified, and a desired object is an object that we desire, what then is a sex object? Clearly, a sex object is an object we have sex with. Hence, to think of a woman as a sex object is to think of her as someone to have sexual relations with, and when the feminist proposes that men refrain from thinking of women in this way, *she is proposing that men not think of women as persons with whom one has sexual relations.*

What are we to make of this proposal? Is the feminist suggesting that women should not be conceived of in this way because such a conception is "dirty"? To conceive of sex and sex organs as dirty is simply to be a prude. "Shit" is the paradigm case of a dirty word. It is a dirty word because the item it designates is taboo; it is literally unclean and untouchable (as opposed to something designated by what I call a curse word, which is not untouchable but rather something to be feared—"damn" and "hell" are curse words; "piss" is a dirty word). If one claims that "cunt" (or "fuck") is a dirty word, then one holds that what this term designates is unclean and taboo; thus one holds that the terms for sexual intercourse or sexual organs are dirty, one has accepted puritanism. If one is a puritan and a feminist, then indeed one ought to subscribe to the slogan *men should not conceive of women as sexual objects.* What is hard to understand is why anyone but a puritan (or, perhaps, a homosexual) would promulgate this slogan; yet most feminists, who are neither lesbians nor puritans, accept this slogan. Why?

A word about slogans: Philosophical slogans have been the subject of considerable analysis. They have the peculiar property (given a certain seemingly sound background story) of being obviously true, yet obviously false. "Men should not conceive of women as sex objects" is, I suggest, like a philosophical slogan in this respect. The immediate reaction of any humanistically oriented person upon first hearing the slogan is to agree with it—yet the more one probes the meaning of the slogan, the less likely one is to give one's assent. Philosophical analysts attempt to separate out the various elements involved in such slogans—to render the true-false slogan into a series of statements, some of which are true, some of which are false, and others of which are, perhaps, only probable. This is what I am trying to do with the slogan in question. I have argued so far that one of the elements that seems to be implicit in the slogan is a rejection of women as sexual partners for men and that although this position might be proper for a homosexual or puritanical movement, it seems inappropriate to feminism. I shall proceed to show that at least two other interpretations of the slogan lead to inappropriate results; but I shall argue that there are at least two respects in which the slogan is profoundly correct—even if misleadingly stated.

One plausible, but inappropriate interpretation of "men ought not to conceive of women as sex objects" is that men ought not to conceive of women *exclusively* as sexual partners. The problem with this interpretation is that everyone can agree with it. Women are conceived of as companions, toys, servants, and even sisters, wives, and mothers—and hence not exclusively as sexual partners. Thus this slogan loses its revisionary impact, since even a male chauvinist could accept the slogan without changing his conceptual structure in any way—which is only to say that men do not usually identify or conceive of woman as sexual partners (recall that the sexual method of identification is the least frequently used).

Yet another interpretation is suggested by the term "object" in "sex object," and this interpretation too has a certain amount of plausibility. Men should not treat women as animate machines designed to masturbate men or as conquests that allow men to "score" for purposes of building their egos. Both of these variations rest on the view that to be treated as an object is to be treated as less than human (that is, to be treated as a machine or a score). Such relations between men and women are indeed immoral, and there are, no doubt, men who believe in "scoring." Unfortunately, however, this interpretation—although it would render the slogan quite apt—also fails because of its restricted scope. When feminists argue that men should not treat women as sex objects they are not only talking about fraternity boys and members of the Playboy Club; they are talking about all males in our society. The charge is that in our society men treat women as sex objects rather than as persons; it is this universality of scope that is lacking from the present interpretation. *Nonetheless, one of the reasons that we are prone to assent to the unrestricted charge that men treat women as sex objects is that the restricted charge is entirely correct.*

One might be tempted to argue that the charge that men treat women as sex objects is correct since such a conception underlies the most frequently used identifications, as animal and plaything; that is, these identifications indicate a sexual context in which the female is used as an object. Thus, it might be argued that the female fox is chased and slayed if she is four-legged, but chased and layed if she is two. Even if one admits the sexual context *implicit* in *some* animal and plaything identifications, one will not have the generality required, because, for the most part, the plaything and animal identifications themselves are nonsexual—most of them do not involve a sexual context. A pregnant cow, a toy doll, or a filly are hardly what one would call erotic objects. Babies do not normally excite sexual passion; and anyone whose erotic interests are directed toward chicks, canaries, parakeets, or other birds is clearly perverse. The animals and playthings to whom women are assimilated in the standard metaphorical identifications are not symbols of desire, eroticism, or passion (as, for example, a bull might be).

What is objectionable in the animal and plaything identifications is not the fact that some of these identifications reflect a sexual context but rather that regardless of the context—these identifications reflect a conception of women as mindless servants (whether animate or inanimate is irrelevant). The point is not that men ought not to think of women in sexual terms but that they ought to think of them as human beings; and the slogan *men should not think of women as sex objects* is only appropriate when a man thinking of a woman as a sexual partner automatically conceives of her as something less than human. It is precisely this antihumanism implicit in the male concept of sex that we have as yet failed to uncover—but then, of course, we have not yet examined the language we use to identify sexual acts.

OUR CONCEPTION OF SEXUAL INTERCOURSE

There are two profound insights that underlie the slogan "men ought not conceive of women as sexual objects"; both have the generality of scope that justifies the universality with which the feminists apply the slogan; neither can be put as simply as the slogan. The first is that the conception of sexual intercourse that we have in this culture is antithetical to the conception of women as human beings—as persons rather than objects. (Recall that this is congruent with the fact we noted earlier that "man" can be substituted for "humanity," while "woman" cannot.)

Many feminists have attempted to argue just this point. Perhaps the most famous defender of this view is Kate Millett,[4] who unfortunately faces the problem of trying to make a point about our conceptual structure without having adequate tools for analyzing conceptual structures.

The question Millett was dealing with was conceptual—Millett, in effect, was asking about the nature of our conception of sexual roles. She tried to answer this question by analyzing novels; I shall attempt to answer this question by analyzing the terms we use to identify coitus, or more technically, in terms that function synonymously with "had sexual intercourse with" in a sentence of the form "A had sexual intercourse with B." The following is a list of some commonly used synonyms (numerous others that are not as widely used have been omitted, for example, "diddled," "laid pipe with"):

screwed
laid
fucked
had
did it with (to)
banged
balled
humped
slept with
made love to

Now, for a select group of these verbs, names for males are the subjects of sentences with active constructions (that is, where the subjects are said to be doing the activity); and names for females require passive constructions (that is, they are the recipients of the activity—whatever is done is done to them). Thus, we would not say "Jane did it to Dick," although we would say "Dick did it to Jane." Again, Dick bangs Jane, Jane does not bang Dick; Dick humps Jane, Jane does not hump Dick. In contrast, verbs like "did it with" do not require an active role for the male; thus, "Dick did it with Jane, and Jane with Dick." Again, Jane may make love to Dick, just as Dick makes love to Jane; and Jane sleeps with Dick as easily as Dick sleeps with Jane. (My students were undecided about "laid."

Most thought that it would be unusual indeed for Jane to lay Dick, unless she played the masculine role of seducer-aggressor.)

The sentences thus form the following pairs. (Those conjoined singular noun phrases where a female subject requires a passive construction are marked with a cross. An asterisk indicates that the sentence in question is not a sentence. of English if it is taken as synonymous with the italicized sentence heading the column.)[5]

Dick had sexual intercourse with Jane
Dick screwed Jane +
Dick laid Jane +
Dick fucked Jane +
Dick had Jane +
Dick did it to Jane +
Dick banged Jane +
Dick humped Jane +
Dick balled Jane (?)
Dick did it with Jane
Dick slept with Jane
Dick made love to Jane
_____
Jane had sexual intercourse with Dick
Jane was banged by Dick
Jane was humped by Dick
*Jane was done by Dick
Jane was screwed by Dick
Jane was laid by Dick
Jane was flicked by Dick
Jane was had by Dick
Jane balled Dick (?)
Jane did it with Dick
Jane slept with Dick
Jane made love to Dick
*Jane screwed Dick
*Jane laid Dick
*Jane fucked Dick
*Jane had Dick
*Jane did it to Dick
*Jane banged Dick
*Jane humped Dick

These lists make clear that within the standard view of sexual intercourse, males, or at least names for males, seem to play a different role than females, since male subjects play an active role in the language of screwing, fucking, having, doing it, and perhaps, laying, while female subjects play a passive role.

The asymmetrical nature of the relationship indicated by the sentences marked with a cross is confirmed by the fact that the form "-ed with each other" is acceptable for the sentences not marked with a cross, but not for those that require a male subject. Thus:

> *Dick and Jane had sexual intercourse with each other*
> Dick and Jane made love to each other
> Dick and Jane slept with each other
> Dick and Jane did it with each other
> Dick and Jane balled with each other (*?)
> *Dick and Jane banged with each other
> *Dick and Jane did it to each other
> *Dick and Jane had each other
> *Dick and Jane fucked each other
> *Dick and Jane humped each other
> *(?) Dick and Jane laid each other
> *Dick and Jane screwed each other

It should be clear, therefore, that our language reflects a difference between the male and female sexual roles, and hence that we conceive of the male and female roles in different ways. The question that now arises is, what difference in our conception of the male and female sexual roles requires active constructions for males and passive for females?

One explanation for the use of the active construction for males and the passive construction for females is that this grammatical asymmetry merely reflects the natural physiological asymmetry between men and women: the asymmetry of "to screw" and "to be screwed," "to insert into" and "to be inserted into." That is, it might be argued that the difference between masculine and feminine grammatical roles merely reflects a difference naturally required by the anatomy of males and females. This explanation is inadequate. Anatomical differences do not determine how we are to conceptualize the relation between penis and vagina during intercourse. Thus one can easily imagine a society in which the female normally played the active role during intercourse, where female subjects required active constructions with verbs indicating copulation, and where the standard metaphors were terms like "engulfing"—that is, instead of saying "he screwed her," one would say "she engulfed him." It follows that the use of passive constructions for female subjects of verbs indicating copulation does not reflect differences determined by human anatomy but rather reflects those generated by human customs.

What I am going to argue next is that the passive construction of verbs indicating coitus (that is, indicating the female position) can *also* be used to indicate that a person is being harmed. I am then going to argue that the metaphor involved would only make sense if we conceive of the female role in intercourse as that of a person being harmed (or being taken advantage of).

Passive constructions of "fucked," "screwed," and "had" indicate the female role. They also can be used to indicate being harmed. Thus, in all of the following sentences, Marion plays the female role: "Bobbie fucked Marion"; "Bobbie screwed Marion"; "Bobbie had Marion"; "Marion was fucked"; "Marion was screwed"; and "Marion was had." All of the statements are equivocal. They might literally mean that someone had sexual intercourse with Marion (who played the female role); or they might mean, metaphorically, that Marion was deceived, hurt, or taken advantage of. Thus, we say such things as "I've been screwed" ("fucked," "had," "taken," and so on) when we have been treated unfairly, been sold shoddy merchandise, or conned out of valuables. Throughout this essay I have been arguing that metaphors are applied to things only if what the term *actually* applies to shares one or more properties with what the term *metaphorically* applies to. Thus, the female sexual role must have something in common with being conned or being sold shoddy merchandise. The only common property is that of being harmed, deceived, or taken advantage of. *Hence we conceive of a person who plays the female sexual role as someone who is being harmed* (that is, "screwed," "fucked," and so on).

It might be objected that this is clearly wrong, since the unsignated terms do not indicate someone's being harmed, and hence we do not conceive of having intercourse as being harmed. The point about the unsignated terms, however, is that they can take both females and males as subjects (in active constructions) and thus *do not pick out the female role*. This demonstrates that we conceive of sexual roles in such a way that only females are thought to be taken advantage of in intercourse.

The best part of solving a puzzle is when all the pieces fall into place. If the subjects of the passive construction are being harmed, presumably the subjects of the active constructions are doing harm, and, indeed, we do conceive of these subjects in precisely this way. Suppose one is angry at someone and wishes to express malevolence as forcefully as possible without actually committing an act of physical violence. If one is inclined to be vulgar one can make the sign of the erect male cock by clenching one's fist while raising one's middle finger, or by clenching one's fist and raising one's arm and shouting such things as "screw you," "up yours," or "fuck you." In other words, one of the strongest possible ways of telling someone that you wish to harm him is to tell him to assume the female sexual role relative to you. Again, to say to someone "go fuck yourself" is to order him to harm himself, while to call someone a "mother fucker" is not so much a play on his Oedipal fears as to accuse him of being so low that he would inflict the greatest imaginable harm (fucking) upon that person who is most dear to him (his mother).

Clearly, we conceive of the male sexual role as that of hurting the person in the female role—but lest the reader have any doubts, let me provide two further bits of confirming evidence: one linguistic, one nonlinguistic. One of the English terms for a person who hurts (and takes advantage of) others is the term "prick." This metaphorical identification would not make sense unless the bastard in question (that is, the person outside the bonds of legitimacy) was thought to share some characteristics attributed to things that are literally pricks. As a verb, "prick" literally means "to hurt," as in "I pricked myself with a needle"; but the usage in question is as a noun. As a noun, "prick" is a colloquial term for "penis." Thus, the question before us is what characteristic is shared by a penis and a person who harms others (or, alternatively, by a penis and by being stuck by a needle). Clearly, no physical characteristic is relevant (physical characteristics might underlie the Yiddish metaphorical attribution "schmuck," but one would have to analyze Yiddish usage to determine this); hence the shared characteristic is nonphysical; the only relevant shared nonphysical characteristic is that both a literal prick and a figurative prick are agents that harm people.

Now for the nonlinguistic evidence. Imagine two doors: in front of each door is a line of people; behind each door is a room; in each room is a bed; on each bed is a person. The line in front of one room consists of beautiful women, and on the bed in that room is a man having intercourse with each of these women in turn. One may think any number of things about this scene. One may say that the man is in heaven, or enjoying himself at a bordello; or perhaps one might only wonder at the oddness of it all. One does not think that the man is being hurt or violated or degraded—or at least the possibility does not immediately suggest itself, although one could conceive of situations where this was what was happening (especially, for example, if the man was impotent). Now, consider the other line. Imagine that the figure on the bed is a woman and that the line consists of handsome, smiling men. The woman is having intercourse with each of these men in turn. It immediately strikes one that the woman is being degraded, violated, and so forth—"that poor woman."

When one man fucks many women he is a playboy and gains status; when a woman is fucked by many men she degrades herself and loses stature.

Our conceptual inventory is now complete enough for us to return to the task of analyzing the slogan that men ought not to think of women as sex objects.

I think that it is now plausible to argue that the appeal of the slogan "men ought not to think of women as sex objects," and the thrust of much of the literature produced by contemporary feminists, turns on something much deeper than a rejection of "scoring" (that is, the utilization of sexual "conquests" to gain esteem) and yet is a call neither for homosexuality nor for puritanism.

The slogan is best understood as a call for a new conception of the male and female sexual roles. If the analysis developed above is correct, our present conception of sexuality is such that to be a man is to be a person capable of brutalizing women (witness the slogans "The marines will make a man out of you!" and "The army builds *men!*" which are widely accepted and which simply state that learning how to kill people will make a person more manly). Such a conception of manhood not only bodes ill for a society led by such men, but also is clearly inimical to the best interests of women. It is only natural for women to reject such a sexual role, and it would seem to be the duty of any moral person to support their efforts—to redefine our conceptions not only of fucking, but of the fucker (man) and the fucked (woman).

This brings me to my final point. We are a society preoccupied with sex. As I noted previously, the nature of proper nouns and pronouns in our language makes it difficult to talk about someone without indicating that person's sex. This convention would not be part of the grammar of our language if we did not believe that knowledge of a person's sex was crucial to understanding what is said about that person. Another way of putting this point is that sexual discrimination permeates our conceptual structure. Such discrimination is clearly inimical to any movement toward sexual egalitarianism and virtually defeats its purpose at the outset. (Imagine, for example, that black people were always referred to as "them" and whites as "us" and that proper names for blacks always had an "x" suffix at the end. Clearly any movement for integration as equals would require the removal of these discriminatory indicators. Thus at the height of the melting-pot era, immigrants Americanized their names: "Bellinsky" became "Bell," "Burnstein" became "Burns," and "Lubitch" became "Baker.")

I should therefore like to close this essay by proposing that contemporary feminists should advocate the utilization of neutral proper names and the elimination of gender from our language (as I have done in this essay); and they should vigorously protest any utilization of the third-person pronouns "he" and "she" as examples of sexist discrimination (perhaps "person" would be a good third-person pronoun)—for, as a parent of linguistic analysis once said, "The limits of our language are the limits of our world."

NOTES

1. The underlying techniques used in this essay were all developed (primarily by Austin and Strawson) to deal with the problems of metaphysics and epistemology. All I have done is to attempt to apply them to other areas; I should note, however, that I rely rather heavily on metaphorical identifications, and that first philosophy tends not to require the analysis of such superficial aspects of language. Note also that it is an empirical matter whether or not people do use words in a certain way. In this essay I am just going to assume that the reader uses words more or less as my students do; for I gathered the data on which words we use to identify women, and so on, simply by asking students. If the reader does not use terms as my students do, then what I say may be totally inapplicable to him.

2. It is also interesting to talk about the technical terms that philosophers use. One fairly standard bit of technical terminology is "trouser word." J. L. Austin invented this bit of jargon to indicate which term in a pair of antonyms is important. Austin called the important term a "trouser word" because "it is the use which wears the trousers." Even in the language of philosophy, to be important is to play the male role. Of course, the antifeminism implicit in the language of technical philosophy is hardly comparable to the male chauvinism embedded in commonplaces of ordinary discourse.

3. Although I thought it inappropriate to dwell on these matters in the text, it is quite clear that we do not associate many positions with females—as the following story brings out. I related this conundrum both to students in my regular courses and to students I teach in some experimental courses at a nearby community college. Among those students who had not previously heard the story, only native Swedes invariable resolved the problem; less than half of the students from an upper-class background would get it (eventually), while lower-class and black students virtually never figured it out. Radical students, women, even members of women's liberation groups fared no better than anyone else with their same class background. The story goes as follows: A little boy is wheeled into the emergency room of a hospital. The surgeon on emergency call looks at the boy and says, "I'm sorry I cannot operate on this child; he is my son." The surgeon was not the boy's father. In what relation did the surgeon stand to the child? Most students did not give any answer. The most frequent answer given was that the surgeon had fathered the boy illegitimately. (Others suggested that the surgeon had divorced the boy's mother and remarried and hence was not legally the boy's father.) Even though the story was related as a part of a lecture on women's liberation, at best only 20 percent of the written answers gave the correct and obvious answer—the surgeon was the boy's mother.

4. *Sexual Politics* (New York: Doubleday, 1971); but see also *Sisterhood Is Powerful*, ed. Robin Morgan (New York: Vintage Books, 1970).

5. For further analysis of verbs indicating copulation see "A Note on Conjoined Noun Phrases," *Journal of Philosophical Linguistics* 1, no. 2 (Evanston, IL: Great Expectations). Reprinted with "English Sentences without Overt Grammatical Subject," in *Studies Out in Left Field: Defamatory Essays Presented to James D. McCawley*, ed. Zwicky, Salus, Binnick, and Vanek (Edmonton: Linguistic Research, 1971). The puritanism in our

society is such that both of these articles are pseudoanonymously published under the name of Quang Phuc Dong; Mr. Dong, however, has a fondness for citing and criticizing the articles and theories of Professor James McCawley, Department of Linguistics, University of Chicago. Professor McCawley himself was kind enough to criticize an earlier draft of this essay. I should also like to thank G. E. M. Anscombe for some suggestions concerning this essay.

"Pricks" and "Chicks": A Postscript after Twenty-five Years

"'Pricks' and 'Chicks': A Plea for 'Persons'" is a product of a period, of personal guilt, of a strategy of reform, and of an attempt to teach philosophy. The period has passed, the guilt is gone, the reformist strategy has, for the most part, succeeded, but the essay still contains an effective tool for the analysis of conceptions of sex and gender—even though the specific terms originally analyzed are dated. In this postscript I recall the spirit of the era in which the essay was written, I try to evoke the sense of guilt that originally gave it impetus, I defend "political correctness" as strategy of moral reform, and I show how the essay can be used to teach a new generation to articulate and analyze the conceptions of sexuality and gender that inform their lives and the lives of their peers.

The period in which the essay was written was the late 1960s and early 1970s. The place was the Midwest, where I worked as a somewhat out-of-place New Yorker teaching at various state universities. Like most academics of the period, I lived a schizophrenic life split between "serious" scholarly research published in professional journals like *Noûs* and the *Review of Metaphysics*, and active participation in the "underground press" and in the reform movements reshaping American culture—civil rights, educational reform, and resistance to the war in Vietnam.

At the end of the sixties, feminism came into my life and changed it forever: Chicago feminist Marlene Dixon came to the university at which I was teaching; Her lecture, uniquely for the time, provided free baby-sitting. My wife and I both attended and left a changed couple. I realized—we both realized—that as a male I had assumed a position of privileged status that she, as a female, had been denied by virtue of her sex and by the social construction of gender roles. I discovered that I myself was by social right, however unwittingly, the very creature whom I abhorred as a matter of moral principle. We began, that night the process of rethinking and restructuring our lives.

As it happened, the restructuring process took place in another Midwestern city. I had alienated the university administration and they declined to renew my contract. In retrospect, my offenses seem innocuous: teaching a class in the city jail (student anti-war demonstrators had been arrested for picketing a military recruitment center; and the university administration had threatened to expel any student not attending class the next day, making male anti-war student pro-testers draft-eligible. Since my entire political philosophy class had been jailed, I taught the next day's class in jail, thereby protecting my students from expulsion); and acting as faculty advisor for innumerable student organizations, including the Black Athlete's Union (which went on strike to protest the inequitable treatment of African-American athletes by white coaches). Fortunately, I was well published in professional journals and I soon received a job offer from another state university. The new job was to be in Detroit, which was a move east, and hence, or so I thought at the time, a move to a more urbane and tolerant environment.

When the three of us—my wife, my young son, and I—arrived in Detroit in the fall of 1968, we were utterly unprepared for the scene that awaited us. Since I had never had an on-campus interview for my new position, we were shocked when we exited the thruway onto block after block of burned-out buildings. The inner city of Detroit was in ashes. Yet arising from the ruin of the urban riots was an oasis of white-on-white glass-and-steel buildings that housed the university at which my wife and I would soon be teaching. The rioters had burned and looted every sort of building, but the university and the nearby museums had been left unscathed. Access to education had been one of the rioters' principal demands; the unbroken windows of the gleaming university standing among the ashes symbolized this demand dramatically.

The university, however, declined to lower standards to admit those it considered unqualified, and so a number of faculty members banded together to respond to the rioters' demand for education by forming an alternative institution. I soon joined their ranks. Collectively we agreed to teach courses, initially without pay, in an open-admission proto-community college that would hold classes in abandoned storefronts, in high schools, and in factories. Working with a logician (Robert Titiev) and an African-American philosophy graduate student (Nadine Philips), I set up a modular philosophy course with three tracks: an African-American philosophy track, an ethics track, and a logic track. Students could take any two-week module in any of the tracks, and—once the institution had been accredited—would earn one "course credit" for every five modules completed (for a maximum of three course credits).

We taught the course once a week, at night, in an inner city high school with a dreadful reputation, located in a part of the city in which middle-class people, black or white, were hesitant to venture. But our students were warm and welcoming. Many were self-educated school dropouts, most had a thirst for learning. Those in my section insisted that they *not* be given a "second-rate" or "watered-down" education; they insisted on being taught "from the same books" that we used at the state university. To satisfy their insistence on parity I invited students from my regular university ethics course to attend my evening ethics track, and I had some of my evening students attend my regular university ethics course. The parity requirement also meant that I had to find a way to teach techniques of conceptual analysis to a class of forty African-American students with little formal education. So I designed an exercise that would use linguistic-conceptual analytic techniques to articulate conceptions of race: we discussed the difference between "African-American," "Black," "Colored," and "Negro" and the question of why it was insulting to call a black *man* a "boy" and a black *woman* a "girl," and so forth. Toward the end of class the techniques of analysis were challenged. Students asked me to validate the techniques by demonstrating their applicability to issues other than race. Since I had adopted the techniques from metaphysics—an area of philosophy unlikely to be illuminating to the class—I promised a demonstration of their validity at the next class meeting.

When I returned the next week I used two questions to demonstrate that techniques of linguistic-conceptual analysis could be used to articulate conceptions of sexuality and gender implicit in our ordinary language. I was soon asked to repeat this exercise, first in my regular classes and later in various feminist fora. The poet Judith McCombs Benjamin suggested that I write out the exercise as an essay that could be published in the local feminist magazine *Moving Out*. Once published, I refined the analysis as a philosophical essay "'Pricks' and 'Chicks': A Plea for 'Persons'" that I circulated in the "samizdat" circuit. This version was actually awarded a prize. Thus emboldened, I submitted the essay to several professional journals, only to have it returned immediately as unsuitable for publication.

The essay was destined to play an even larger role in my life. The state university in Detroit was as intolerant of my involvement in anti-war, civil rights, egalitarian, and feminist causes as my earlier employer had been. When I was reviewed for tenure I submitted only articles published in professional journals for assessment by the review committee, but some unnamed party called the committee's attention to the version of "'Pricks' and 'Chicks'" published in *Moving Out*. The committee decided that the essay established my untenurability. In response, I sent it to a number of leading women philosophers; many, including G. E. M. Anscombe and Ruth Barcan Marcus, wrote letters on my behalf, but to no avail.

Once again I found myself seeking a job. Determined to find a tolerant academic environment I sent copies of the essay to every hiring committee that wished to interview me. Somewhat to my surprise, a number of institutions made me offers. I accepted a position at Union College, a small private liberal arts college in upstate New York. There I began the partnership with a colleague, Fred Elliston, that culminated in the publication of the first two editions of *Philosophy and Sex*.

I outlined this history of the essay—which went on to be widely anthologized, but which also provoked a conflict with obscenity laws—to give students today some sense of the revolutionary reshaping of American culture that took place in the 1960s and 1970s. It was a time when people began the process of rethinking their received values and roles; when men and women, more often thinking and working together than not, began to reconceptualize gender and sexuality. It was an extraordinarily difficult process, made even more difficult by forces in the culture resisting the critical analysis and reassessment of the status quo.

Today it is common to deride the conceptual aspects of social reform, dismissing it with the canard "political correctness." The canard reflects a failure to appreciate the historical relationship between conceptual and sociopolitical change. Exclusionary conceptual frameworks circumscribe lives. There is thus little conceptual room for women in a world of business*men*, chair*men*, congress-*men*, fire*men*, mail*men*, police*men*—or in an academy of gentle*men* and fellows. The linguistic preference toward males explicit in this terminology accurately mirrors the social facts of life in pre-feminist American culture. One way in which feminists successfully changed these social arrangements was through a linguistic-conceptual challenge that served as the cutting edge of a political-social-economic struggle. The conceptual challenge and political change operated in tandem, as they had in the civil rights movement, in the earlier suffragette and abolitionist movements, and in the American Revolution itself. For just as "British colonial subjects" had to reconceptualize themselves as "American citizens" to rebel successfully against the British monarchy, just as the National Association for the Advancement of Colored *People* had to assert their claims as "people," rather than as a race apart, to desegregate America, feminists had to force a gender-neutral reconceptualization of the worlds of business, administration, politics, civil service—and the academy—to successfully open these worlds to women. Reconceptualization *alone* would have been insufficient to guarantee the success of any social reform or revolution, but no social or political revolution has ever succeeded without inventing a reconceptualization that delegitimates the status quo while simultaneously legitimating the reforms to which it aspires. Revolutions are conceived in the mind well before they shape the body politic.

Canards about "political correctness" are often supported by tales that parody conceptual reform. These tales presume a movement to replace words like 'fat' and 'short' with 'horizontally challenged' and 'vertically challenged'. Such tales conflate euphemisms with conceptual revisions. Euphemisms (the term originates from Greek and means "good sounds") merely substitute inoffensive terms for offensive ones. They seldom involve the reconceptualization of exploitive conceptions. Thus, while the first terms in the antonym pairs 'fat'/'thin' and 'short'/'tall' may be taken as offensive in some contexts, these terms are not integral to a conceptual framework of exclusion. There is no equivalent to the exclusionary 'business-*men*'—an expression that expressly excludes women from the workplace—in our current use of the terms 'thin' and 'tall'. One might euphemistically describe a fat person as "hefty" or a short person as "diminutive," but such a substitution involves neither a reconceptualization of a classificatory framework nor an attempt to rectify an inequality. Euphemisms generally do not change meanings, they merely say the same thing in a less offensive manner. (Note, by this standard, that "vertically challenged" does not qualify as a euphemism, since, whatever offense short people might take in being characterized as "short," that offense is unlikely to be mitigated by the substitution of the term "vertically challenged"—terminology that, by virtue of its novelty, is more likely to call attention to physical stature than the seemingly blunter 'short'.)

In striking contrast, conceptual revisions always *change* meanings. 'Business*person*' and 'chair*person*' do not have the same meaning as 'business*men*' and 'chair*men*' precisely because the latter terms expressly exclude women, whereas the former do not. Conceptual revisions differ radically from euphemisms because they aspire not to make something "sound good" to a hearer, but to replace an exploitive or exclusionary conception with a morally acceptable alternative.

Another charge characteristically directed against proponents of linguistic-conceptual reform is that it is inefficacious and thus changes linguistic traditions unnecessarily. "Sticks and stones may break my bones," the old saying goes, "but names can never hurt me." Whoever invented this silly slogan could never have been subjected to racist or sexist epithets; for the power of words to hurt exceeds those of sticks and stones. Exclusion, exploitation, even extermination all presuppose conceptual frameworks that render permissible what is normally immoral. Racism, sexism, and eliminative extermination movements (like Nazism) characteristically presuppose a linguistic-conceptual framework permitting moral people to act in ways that would otherwise be considered morally impermissible. The Nazis, for example, reconceptualized those whom they exterminated as *Gemeinschaftfremde*, or "enemies of the community," *lebensunwertes Leben*, or "life unworthy of living," and *Untermenschen*, or "subhumans." Conversely, egalitarian social reform movements succeed only if they successfully challenge such systems of conceptual exclusion, thereby extending normal moral concepts and protection to the previously excluded and exploited groups.

Names can hurt and thus changing names can alter hurtful behavior. I shall offer one particularly striking example of a conceptual revision that paved the way for social reform; a revision that has nothing whatsoever to do with race or sex, but one involving age. In his 1975 book, *Why Survive? Growing Old in America*, Dr. Robert Butler assembled a massive amount of data documenting discrimination against a group of Americans known as "old folks," "old codgers," "old hags," or, to use the epithets that epitomized the popular disdain for the elderly as useless and undesirable—"old bags" and "old farts." Butler referred to this group as "elderly" (as in "the wisdom of one's elders") and "senior citizens" (emphasizing the deference owed to "seniority" and to fellow "citizens"). Neither of these terms, however, was new to Butler's work. The term he added to the American-English lexicon was "ageism," which he defined as the "process of systematic stereotyping of and discrimination against people because they are old." The new concept "ageism" served two ends: first, it organized the disparate data about the mistreatment of the elderly into a coherent pattern of stereotyping and discrimination; second, because of the linguistic analogy to other "isms"—racism and sexism—"ageism" implicitly evoked a civil rights model.

Butler's research came to the attention of Dr. Arthur S. Flemming, Commissioner on Aging for the Department of Health, Education and Welfare and Chairman of the United States Commission on Civil Rights. Flemming quickly introduced Butler's new term into American political rhetoric. "Ageism," Flemming informed the House Education and Labor Committee in a 1975 speech, was equivalent to "racism" and "sexism" and he "hope[d] that the day will come when the Civil Rights Act will be amended to include age . . . as one of the factors that must be taken into consideration under the Civil Rights Act." Like skin color, race, sex, and handicap, age is a biophysiological fact. As testimony before the House Education and Labor Committee quickly established, this biological fact was used by businesses, private organizations, and governmental agencies to deny senior citizens access to credit, education, employment, housing, mortgage financing, and scarce medical resources, irrespective of their abilities or physical condition. Thus the biophysiological fact of old age, like that of race and sex, had become associated with negative stereotypes that effectively denied individuals the opportunity to fully function as persons.

When Martin Luther King Jr. took a stand against racism he dreamed of an America in which all persons would be judged by the content of their character, not the color of their skin. When Butler and Flemming took a stand against "ageism," they dreamed of an America in which all are judged by their ability, not the wrinkles on their face, or the date on their birth certificate. They dreamed about imposing an egalitarian moral vision upon a recalcitrant reality; for to envision all persons as equal is to accept a conceptual framework blind to a world in which everyone is different: differently abled, differently colored, differently raced, differently sexed—and differently aged. The egalitarian vision requires a conceptual framework that looks to the person underlying these biophysiological facts of race, gender, handicap—or chronological age. By the end of the year Congress accepted this vision and passed the Age Discrimination Act of 1975. The act categorically prohibited discrimination on the basis of age: "no person in the United States shall, on the basis of age, be excluded from participation in, be denied the benefits of, or be subjected to discrimination under, any program receiving Federal financial assistance."

The speed with which this particular reform moved from conception to social legislation is remarkable; it serves as apt illustration of the power of reconceptualization as an agent of reform—the power of "political correctness," so to speak.

One of the major functions of social and political philosophy is to develop tools for conceptual analysis that enable one to articulate and reconceptualize conceptual frameworks. One of the tools on the social philosopher's workbench is the set of questions that I developed in the late 1960s and early 1970s to enable my students to explore their own conceptions of race, gender, and sexual intercourse. The version of the instrument that I am currently using is divided into three parts: the first asks demographic information about the student, the second explores the language students use to identify members of the opposite sex, and the third explores the language used to characterize sexual intercourse. I typically administer the instrument twice: once to students individually, on the first day of class, and once later in the term, when I have students fill it out in small same-sex groups, subdivided further so that fraternity members are in one group, minority members in another, and so forth. After the students have reported their collective results, I then distribute a sheet tabulating the results of the survey taken on the first day of class. A lively discussion invariably follows in which we analyze the answers and unpack the metaphors implicit in the language that students use to identify members of the opposite sex, comparing the language females use for males with that used by males for females, and so forth.

A few caveats: I always warn students in advance that we will be discussing descriptions of sexual intercourse in an open and frank manner, allowing anyone who wishes to opt out of the discussion to do so. The discussion, moreover, should always be conducted in terms of what "one's friends would say," a strategy that encourages open discussion and minimizes defensiveness. On a mere technical level, it is important that students place an asterisk by the most frequently used expressions, and that the test administrator compare this with the frequency of use reported collectively, exploring differences as they emerge.

When analyzing the various ways in which students describe the situation in which "Jane and Richard had sexual intercourse after the social last night," it is important to assess whether Jane and Richard are seen as playing equally active roles, as in the expression "Jane and Richard *hooked up* last night," or whether one is playing a more active role than the other, as in the expression "Richard nailed Jane last night," or "Richard scored last night," which suggests an active male and a passive female. The "scoring" metaphor actually suggests that the female is irrelevant, except as a means to male status. Unpacking metaphors is important; thus the metaphor "nailing" not only suggests activity but activity painful to the passive partner who has been "nailed."

The expressions that students use change over time and it is interesting to supplement the exercise by comparing the current class report with reports from earlier years. At the height of the AIDS epidemic, for example, "doing the nasty" became one of the most frequently used terms for sexual intercourse. In recent years that expression has faded. "Hooked up" is now the most commonly used description by my male students; "made love" is now the most commonly used female description.

In some classes gay and lesbian students offer to discuss their language and conceptions of sexuality with the class. I always accept such offers, but, because we still live in a world that is too often inhospitable to nonheterosexuals, I never solicit them.

I always end the exercise by asking the students to envision an ideal gender sexual world and to suggest the language and metaphors that would reflect that world. My essay ends on the same note, arguing for the elimination of the generic use of 'he' as a pronoun representing someone whose sex is unspecified; as in, "one should do the best *he* can." Such male preferences violate ideals of gender egalitarianism. It is currently fashionable, in some circles, to attempt to rectify centuries of linguistic-conceptual preference toward males by using pronouns preferencing females, as in "one should do the best *she* can." Preferencing females, however, affronts ideals of gender equality as deeply as preferencing males. Ideally, one's conceptual framework should be neutral between females and males, as in "everyone should do the best they can." It is interesting to note, for example, that once gender-neutral conceptions of certain female professions were introduced (the reconceptualization of "stewardesses" as "flight attendants," for example) men gravitated to occupations that were once thought too "feminine" for them. If we would strive for a world of gender equality, we should fashion our language so that our occupations are limited only by our ambitions, efforts, and talents. For, to repeat the quotation from Wittgenstein that closed my "Plea for 'Persons'" twenty-five years ago, "the limits of our language are the limits of our world."

QUESTIONNAIRE CONCEPTIONS OF GENDER AND SEX
(copyright © Robert Baker, 1997)

Are you male or female? (Circle one)	M	F	
Your class is (Circle one):	SOPH	JR	SR
Do you live in coed housing?	Yes	No	
Single-Sex housing?	Yes	No	
Are you living in a (circle one)	Dormitory		
	Fraternity		
	Sorority		
	Student Apartment		
	Parents' Home		
	Other (explain)		

Imagine that you are having breakfast with some of your friends (all of whom are the same sex as you) on a Saturday morning. You remark that Friday night; M, a mutual acquaintance, was with someone of the opposite sex. You ask your friends "Who was that (boy/girl) M was with last night?"

1) Please list the various expressions *your friends* (all of whom are the same sex as you) might use in such a conversation with you to refer to the boy/girl; as in the sentence "The _____ M was with last night was from a local college." (For example, "The *gal/guy* M was with last night was from a local college.") Please place an asterisk, '*', after the most commonly used expressions, but do not use more than three asterisks.

2) Suppose that your friends (all of whom are the same sex as you) suspect that Jane and Richard had sexual intercourse after the social last night. Please list the words and expressions that *your friends* might use to describe this situation to you. Please place an asterisk, '*', after the most commonly used expressions, but do not use more than three asterisks.

18.

LINGUISTIC SEXES AND GENDERS

Luce Irigaray

Women's entry into the public world, the social relations they have among themselves and with men, have made cultural transformations, and especially linguistic ones, a necessity. If the male President of the Republic meets the Queen, to say *Its se sont rencontrés* (they met) borders on a grammatical anomaly.[1] Instead of dealing with this difficult question, most people wonder whether it wouldn't be better if we were governed by just men or just women, that is, by one gender alone. The rules of language have so strong a bearing on things that they can lead to such impasses. Unfortunately, there's still little appreciation of what's at stake here. Faced with the need to transform the rules of grammar, some women, even feminists—though fortunately not all—readily object that provided they have the right to use it, the masculine gender will do for them. But neutralizing grammatical gender amounts to an abolition of the difference between sexed subjectivities and to an increasing exclusion of a culture's sexuality. We would be taking a huge step backward if we abolished grammatical gender, a step our civilization can ill afford; what we do need, on the other hand, and it's essential, is for men and women to have equal subjective

From *Je, Tu, Nous: Toward a Culture of Difference* by Luce Irigaray, translated by Alison Martin. (1993) pp. 67–74. Reproduced by permission of Routledge, Inc.

rights—equal obviously meaning different but of equal value, subjective implying equivalent rights in exchange systems. From a linguistic perspective, therefore, the cultural injustices of language and its generalized sexism have to be analyzed. These are to be found in grammar, in vocabulary, in the connotations of a word's gender.

MORE OR LESS MASCULINE

For centuries, whatever has been valorized has been masculine in gender, whatever devalorized, feminine. So the sun is masculine, and the moon feminine. Yet in our cultures, *le soleil* (the sun) is thought of as the source of life, *la lune* (the moon) as ambiguous, almost harmful, except perhaps by some peasants. The attribution of masculine gender to the sun can be traced in history, and so can the attribution of the sun to the men-gods. These aren't all immutable truths but rather facts that evolve over long periods of time and at different rates of speed depending upon the culture, country, and language. The positive connotation of the masculine as word gender derives from the time of the establishment of patriarchal and phallocratic power, notably by men's appropriation of the divine. This is not a secondary matter. It is very important. Without divine power, men could not have supplanted mother-daughter relations and their attributions concerning nature and society. But man becomes God by giving himself an invisible father, a father language. Man becomes God as the Word, then as the Word made flesh. Because the power of semen isn't immediately obvious in procreation, it's relayed by the linguistic code, the *logos*. Which wants to become the all-embracing truth.

Men's appropriation of the linguistic code attempts to do at least three things:

1. prove they are fathers;
2. prove they are more powerful than mother-women;
3. prove they are capable of engendering the cultural domain as they have been engendered in the natural domain of the ovum, the womb, the body of a woman.

To guarantee loyalty to its authority, the male people consciously or unconsciously represents whatever has value as corresponding to its image and its grammatical gender. Most linguists state that grammatical gender is arbitrary, independent of sexual denotations and connotations. In fact, this is untrue. They haven't really thought about the issue. It doesn't strike them as being important.

Their personal subjectivity, their theory is content to be valorized like the masculine, passing for an arbitrary universal. A patient study of the gender of words almost always reveals their hidden sex. Rarely is this immediately apparent. And a linguist will be quick to retort that *un fauteuil* (a sofa) or *un chateau* (a castle) are not more "masculine" than *une chaise* (a chair) or *une maison* (a house). Apparently not. A degree of thought will show that the former connote greater value than the latter. While the latter are simply useful in our cultures, the others are more luxurious, ornamental, noted for their distinction as higher-class goods. A thorough analysis of all the terms of the lexicon would in this way make their secret sex apparent, signifying their adherence to an as yet uninterpreted syntax. Another example: *un ordinateur* (a computer) is of course a masculine noun and *la machine à écrire* (the typewriter) a feminine one. Value is what matters. . . . Whatever has it must be masculine. Again, *un avion* (an airplane) is superior to *une voiture* (a car), *le Boeing* to *la Caravelle*, not to mention *le Concorde*. . . . With each counterexample we find a more complex explanation: the gender could be due to the prefix or the suffix and not to the root of the word; it could depend upon the time when the term entered the lexicon and the relative value of the masculine and feminine genders then (in this respect, Italian is a less coherently sexist language than French); sometimes its determination is consequent upon the language it's borrowed from (English, for example, gives us a number of terms that become masculine in French).

GENDER AS IDENTITY OR AS POSSESSION

How is gender attributed to words? It's done on different levels and in different ways. At the most archaic level, I think there is an identification of the denominated reality with the sex of the speaking subject. *La terre* (the earth) *is* woman, *le ciel* (the sky) *is* her brother. *Le soleil* (the sun) is man, the god-man. *La lune* (the moon) is woman, sister of the man-god. And so on. Something of this first identification always remains in the gender of words. The degree to which it is explicit or hidden varies. But there is another mechanism at work apart from the identification of designated reality and gender. Living beings, the animate and cultured, become masculine; objects that are lifeless, the inanimate and uncultured, become feminine. Which means that men have attributed subjectivity to themselves and have reduced women to the status of objects, or to nothing. This is as true for actual women as it is for the gender of words. *Le moissonneur* (a harvester) is a man. But if, in line with current debate on the names of occupations, a linguist or legislator wishes to name a woman who harvests *la moissonneuse*,[2] the word is not available for a female subject: *la moissonneuse* (harvesting machine) is the tool the male harvester makes use of, or else it doesn't exist in the feminine. This state of affairs is even more ridiculous at a higher professional level where sometimes one is presented with hierarchies in the attribution of grammatical gender: *le secrétaire d'Etat/parti* (the secretary of state or a party) is masculine and *la secrétaire steno-dactylo* (the shorthand secretary) is feminine.

There is no sexed couple to create and structure the world. Men are surrounded by tools of feminine gender and by women-objects. Men don't manage the world with women as sexed subjects having equivalent rights. Only through a transformation of language will that become possible. But this transformation can only take place if we valorize the feminine gender once more. Indeed, the feminine, which was originally just different, is now practically assimilated to the nonmasculine. Being a woman is equated with not being a man. Which is what psychoanalysis calmly informs us in its theory and its practice of penis or phallus envy. Its reality only corresponds to one cultural period and one state of language. In that case, the way for women to be liberated is not by "becoming a man" or by envying what men have and their objects, but by female subjects once again valorizing the expression of their own sex and gender. That's completely different.

This confusion between liberation as equal ownership of goods and liberation as access to a subjectivity of the same value is currently upheld by several social theories and practices: psychoanalysis is one of them, but another is Marxism, to a certain extent. These discourses have been elaborated by men. They used Germanic languages. At the present time they have a relative degree of success among women in countries that speak these languages, because gender is expressed in subject-object relations. In these languages a woman can therefore have *her* (*sa*) phallus if not *her* (*sa*) penis.[3] Thus some German, English, or American women are able, for example, to demand equality in relation to the possession of goods and mark them with their gender. Having achieved this, they may abandon their right to denote gender in relation to the subject and criticize the conscious relationship made between the sexuate body and language as "materialistic," "ontological," "idealist," etc. This shows a lack of comprehension of the relations between individual bodies, social bodies, and the linguistic economy. A great deal of misunderstanding in the so-called world of women's liberation is perpetuated by this lack of comprehension. For many an Anglo-Saxon—and in general Germanic language—feminist, all she needs is her university post or to have written her book to be liberated. For them it's a question of *her* (*sa*) post and *her* (*sa*) book[4] and this appropriation of ownership seems to satisfy them. In my view, we have to be free female *subjects*. Language represents an essential tool of production for this liberation. I have to make it progress in order to have subjective rights equivalent to men, to be able to exchange language and objects with them. For one women's liberation movement, the emphasis is on equal rights in relation to the possession of goods: difference between men and women is located in the nature, the quantity, and sometimes the quality of goods acquired and possessed. For the other movement, sexual liberation means to demand access to a status of individual and collective *subjectivity* that is valid for them as women. The emphasis is on the difference of rights between male and female subjects.

THE SEX OF OCCUPATIONS

Owning a few goods equivalent to those men have doesn't solve the problem of gender for women who speak Romance languages because these goods don't bear the mark of their owner's subject. We say *mon enfant* (my child) or *mon phallus* (?) (my phallus) whether we are men or women. For valuable "objects," then, the mark of ownership is the same. As for other "objects," they are generally devalorized when they are likely to be used or appropriated by women alone. The problem of the object and its conquest cannot therefore solve the problem of inequality of sexed rights in all languages. Furthermore, I don't think it can solve it in any language. But it can just about satisfy demands, more or less immediately.

If the issue of names for occupations has been taken up so extensively, it's because such names represent an intermediary space between subject and object, object and subject. Of course, it is a matter of possessing professional status, having a job, but this cannot be possessed just like any object can. It represents a necessary, though not sufficient, part of subjective identity. In addition, this demand fits in well with the social demands already being made in the male world. Therefore, the issue is relatively easy to raise. People generally go along with it. Often its only opposition is reality as it has already been coded linguistically (so *moissonneuse* and *médecine* have become the names of objects or designate a professional discipline and are no longer names for people, and sometimes the female name for an occupation doesn't exist or designates a different job) and social resistance depending upon the level of access available for women. But in this debate about the names of occupations the issue of language's sexism has hardly been broached, and proposed solutions often tend to try to skirt around the problems it raises.

NOTES

1. Irigaray is referring to the rule of using the masculine plural in French whenever masculine and feminine are combined . . . , according primacy to the masculine, which in this case might be seen to contradict the social custom of according primacy to the one having majesty over the "ordinary" subject or citizen (even elected presidents). (Tr.)

2. The suffix *euse* designates a feminine term. (Tr.)

3. In French the possessive adjective agrees in gender (and number) with the object possessed rather than with the possessor, as in English. To illustrate the point of her companion Irigaray uses the possessive adjective for feminine singular nouns, *sa*, instead of the masculine *son*, for the masculine nouns *phallus* and *penis*.

4. University post (*poste universitaire*) and book (*livre*) are masculine, hence Irigaray here again replaces the masculine possessive adjective with the feminine one. (Tr.)

19.

WHERE IS SHE IN LANGUAGE?

Hélène Cixous

Where is she?
Activity/passivity,
Sun/Moon,
Culture/Nature,
Day/Night,
Father/Mother,
Mind/feeling,
Intelligible/perceptible,
Logos/Pathos.
Form, convex, movement, advance, seed, progress.
Matter, concave, ground—upon which the movement treads, receptacle.

Man
Woman

Originally published as Hélène Cixous, "La Jeune Née: An Excerpt," *Diacritics*, June 1977, pp. 65–68.

Always the same metaphor: we follow it, it transports us, in all its various forms, wherever there is organization of discourse. The same thread, or double strand, leads us—whether we are reading or speaking—through literature, philosophy, criticism, through centuries of representation, of reflection.

Thought has always worked by opposition.

Speech/Writing

High/Low

By dual, hierarchical oppositions. Superior/Inferior. Myths, legends, books. Philosophical systems, in every place (where) an ordering occurs, a law organizes the thinkable by oppositions (dual, irreconcilable; or sublatable, dialectical). And all the couples of oppositions are *couples*. Does that mean something? That logocentrism submits thought—all concepts, codes, values—to a system with two terms: is this in relation to "the" couple, man/woman?

Nature/History,

Nature/Art,

Nature/Spirit,

Passion/Action.

Theory of culture, theory of society, the ensemble of symbolic systems—art, religion, family, language—they all show the same patterns as they work themselves out. And the movement by which each opposition establishes itself in order to make sense is the movement by which the couple is destroyed. General battleground. Each time, a war is waged. Death is always at work.

Father/son   Relations of authority, of privilege, of force.
Logos/writing   Relations: opposition, conflict, sublation [*relève*], return.
Master/slave   Violence. Repression.

And it can be seen that the "victory" always amounts to the same thing: It's a matter of hierarchy. Hierarchization subjects the entirety of conceptual organization to man. Male privilege, which is evident in the opposition which sustains it, *activity* versus *passivity*. Traditionally, the question of sexual difference is dealt with by coupling it with the opposition: activity/passivity.

That already says a lot. If we examine the history of philosophy—insofar as philosophic discourse orders and reproduces all thought—we notice[1] that: it is marked by an absolute constant, an organizer of values, which is precisely the opposition activity/passivity.

That in philosophy woman is always on the side of passivity. Each time the question arises; when we examine kinship structures; whenever a model of the family comes into play; in fact as soon as the ontological question begins stirring; as soon as one wonders what is meant by the question "what is it"; as soon as there is any will-to-express [*vouloir-dire*]. Any will: desire, authority, you look into it, and you're led right back . . . to the father. You can even not notice that there is no place at all for woman in the process! Ultimately the world of "being" can function having foreclosed the mother. No need for a mother—so long as the maternal persists: and it is the father who then makes—is—the mother. Either woman is passive; or she does not exist. Anything else is unthinkable, unthought. Which means of course that she is not thought, that she does not enter into the oppositions, she does not form a couple with the father (who forms a couple with the son).

There is Mallarmè's tragic dream[2], this lamentation of the father on the mystery of paternity, which is wrenched from the poet by *the* grief, the sorrow of sorrows, the death of the cherished son: that dream of a marriage between the father and the son—and thus no mother. Dream of man facing death. Which always threatens him differently than it threatens woman.

"a marriage alliance, a hymen, superb And dreams of masculine
—and the life   filiation, dreams of God the father
remaining in me   going forther from himself
I will use it   into his son—and
For . . .   then no mother.
thus no mother?"

She does not exist, she *can* not be; but there must be some. Of woman, upon whom he no longer depends, he thus keeps nothing but this space, always virgin, matter subjected to the desire he wishes to imprint.

And if we examine literary history, it's the same story. Everything refers back to man, to *his* anguish, his desire to be (at) the origin. To the father. There is an intrinsic bond between the philosophical—and the literary (to the extent that it has meaning, literature is governed by philosophy)—and phallocentrism. Philosophy is constructed on the basis of the degradation of woman. Subordination of the feminine to the masculine order which then appears to be the condition necessary for the functioning of the machine.

The contestation of this solidarity of logocentrism and phallocentrism has today become urgent enough—the revelation of the fate reserved for woman and the way it's been concealed—to threaten the stability of the masculine edifice which has been passing itself off as eternal-natural; by giving rise to considerations, to hypotheses on the part of femininity which can only be disastrous for the bastion which still holds on to authority. What would become of logocentrism, of the great philosophical systems, of the world order in general if the stone upon which they have founded their church crumbled?

If one day it became glaringly apparent that the unacknowledgeable plan of logocentrism had always been to *found* phallocentrism, to ensure for the masculine order a justification equal to history, to itself?

Then all the stories would have to be told differently, the future would be incalculable, the historical forces would change, will change hands, bodies, an other thought still unthinkable will transform the functioning of every society. Now, we are living through precisely that age when the conceptual foundation of a millenary culture is in the process of being undermined by millions of a kind of mole [*taupe*] which is as yet unrecognized.

When they awaken from among the dead, from among the words, from among the laws.

Once upon a time . . .

We cannot yet say of the story which follows: "It's only a story." This tale remains true today. Most of the women who have awakened remember having slept, *having been put to sleep.*

Once upon a time . . . and still another time . . .

The beauties are sleeping, waiting for princes to come to awaken them. In their beds, in their glass coffins, in their childhood forests, as if dead. Beautiful, but passive; therefore desirable: from them emanates all mystery. It is the men who like to play with dolls. As we've known ever since Pygmalion. Their old dream: to be God the mother. The best mother, the second one, the one who gives the second birth.

She is sleeping, she is intact, eternal, absolutely helpless. He doesn't doubt that she has been waiting for him forever.

The secret of her beauty, kept for him: she has the perfection of that which is finished. Of that which hasn't begun. Nonetheless she breathes. Just enough life; not too much. Then he will kiss her. In such a way that when she opens her eyes she will see only *him*; him, taking up all the space, him-as-all.[3]

"This dream is so satisfying!" Whose is it? What wish is fulfilled by it?

He leans over her . . . Cut. It's the end of the story. Curtain. Once s/he has awakened, this would be another story altogether. Then maybe there would be two people. You never know, with women. And the voluptuous simplicity of the preliminaries would no longer take place.

Harmony, desire, achievement, research, all of these movements occur before—the arrival of woman. More precisely, before she *rises*. She lying down, he on his feet. She gets up—end of dream—what follows pertains to the socio-cultural, he keeps getting her pregnant, she spends her youth in childbirth; from bed to bed, till the age when that is no longer a woman.

"Bridebed, childbed, bed of death": so it is with the woman who makes her mark as she travels thus from bed to bed in Joyce's *Ulysses*. Excursion of Ulysses Bloom on his feet, ceaselessly wandering through Dublin. Walking, exploration. Excursion of Penelope-Everywoman: sickbed in which the mother never gets done with dying, hospital bed in which Madame Purefoy never gets done with giving birth, bed of Molly the wife, the adulteress, setting of an infinite erotic reverie, excursion of reminiscences. She wanders, but in bed. In dream. Ponders. Talks to herself. Voyage of woman: as a *body*. As if, separated from the outside world where cultural exchanges take place, apart from the social scene where history is made, she were destined to be, in the division which men set up, the nonsocial, nonpolitical, nonhuman half in the living structure, on the side of nature of course, listening tirelessly to what is happening within, to her womb, to her "house." In close touch with her appetites, her emotions.

And while he takes (for better or for worse) the risk and the responsibility of being a particle, an agent, of a public stage where transformations get played out, she represents indifference or resistance to this active tempo, she is the principle of constancy, in a certain way always the same, daily and eternal.

Man's dream: I love her, absent therefore desirable, inexistent, dependent, therefore adorable. Because she is not where she is. So long as she is not where she is. Then, how he looks at her! When she has her eyes closed; when he takes in all of her, and she is then but that form made for him: body captured in his look.

Or woman's dream? This is only a dream. I am sleeping. If I were not sleeping, he would not look for me, he would not cross his good lands and my bad lands in order to come to me. Above all don't let anyone awaken me! What anxiety! What if I must be entombed in order to attract him! And what if he kissed me? That kiss, how to want it? Do I want?

What does she want? To sleep, perchance to dream, to be loved in dream, to be approached, touched, almost—almost *jouir*. But not *jouir*: or she would wake up. But she has experienced *jouissance*[4] in dream, once upon a time. . . .

Once upon a time there was the same story, repeating through the centuries the amorous destiny of woman, its cruel and mystifying pattern. And every story, every myth tells her: "there is no place for your desire in our affairs of State." Love is a threshold affair: For us, men, who are made in order to succeed, in order to climb the social ladder, that temptation is good which urges us on, pushes us, nourishes our ambitions. But achievement is dangerous. Desire must not disappear. You, women, represent for us the eternal threat, the anti-culture. We do not remain in your homes, we are not going to linger in your beds. We roam. Entice us, provoke us, that's all we ask of you. Do not make of us spineless, feeble, feminine beings, careless about time and money. Your kind of love is death for us. A threshold affair:[5] its all in the suspense, in the "coming soon," always deferred.

What lies beyond is downfall: the both of them enslaved, domesticated, imprisoned in the family, in a social role.

By reading this story-which-ends-well, she gets to know the roads which lead to the "loss" which is her fate. And she comes tumbling after. A kiss; and off he goes. His desire, fragile, nourishing itself on lack, keeps itself alive through absence: man pursues. As if he could not manage to have what he has. Where is she, the woman in all the spaces he covers, all the scenes he stages within the literary enclosure?

There are many answers, we know them: she is in the shadows. In the shadows which he casts upon her; which she is.

Night for his day, thus it has always been fantasized. Black for his whiteness. Excluded from the space of his system, she is the repressed element which assures that the system will function.

Kept at a distance, so that he may take pleasure in the ambiguous advantages of distance, so that she may, by her very remoteness, keep alive the enigma, delight-danger, of seduction, suspended in the role of "the abductress" Helen, she is in a certain way "outside." But she cannot appropriate this "outside" (only rarely does she even desire to do so), it is his outside: the outside, so long as it is not absolutely exterior, not the unfamiliar unknown which would escape him. She dwells in a domesticated outside.

Abductress abducted from herself

—not is she the element of strangeness—within his universe which reanimates his uneasiness and his desire. She is, within his economy, the strangeness which he likes to appropriate for himself. But that's not all—there is still the "dark continent" business: she has been kept at a distance from herself, she has been allowed to see (= not-to-see) woman from the perspective of what man wants to see of her, i.e. almost nothing; she has been forbidden the possibility of the proud "inscription above my door" which stands at the threshold of *The Joyful Wisdom*. It is not she who could have exclaimed:

I inhabit my own house,
Have never limited anyone . . .

Her "own" house, her body itself, she has not been able to inhabit. It is possible in effect to imprison her, to slow down monstrously, to bring off for too long a time this triumph of Apartheid—but only for a time. It is possible to teach her, as soon as she begins to talk, and at the same time as she learns her name, that her region is dark: because you are Africa, you are black. Your continent is dark. Darkness is dangerous. In darkness you cannot see, you are afraid. Don't move because you might fall down. Above all don't go into the forest. And we have interiorized the dread of darkness. She has had no eyes for herself. She has never explored her house. Her genitals appall her still today. She has not dared to take pleasure in her body, which has been colonized. Woman is frightened and disgusted by woman.

Against women they have committed the greatest crime of all: they have led them, insidiously, violently, to hate women, to be their own enemies, to mobilize their immense power against themselves, to be the executors of man's virile task.

They have given her anti-narcissism! A narcissism in which love of self comes only from making oneself loved for what one does not have! They have fabricated the vile logic of anti-love.

The "Dark Continent" is neither dark nor unexplorable: It is still unexplored only because we have been made to believe that it was too dark to be explorable. And because they want to make us believe that what interests us is the white continent, with its monuments to the Lack. And we have believed. They have fixed us between two horrifying myths: between Medusa and the abyss. It would be enough to make half the world roar with laughter, if it were not still going on. For phallo-logocentric continuity is still there, and it is militant, reproducing the old patterns, anchored in the dogma of castration. They haven't changed anything: they have theorized their desire as reality! Let them tremble, the priests, we are going to *show* them our sexes!

Too bad for them if they fall apart upon discovering that women are not men, or that the mother doesn't have one. But doesn't that fear suit them? The worst, wouldn't it be, isn't it, in truth, that woman is not castrated, that he has only to stop listening to the Sirens (for the Sirens were men) in order for history to change direction? One has only to look the medusa in the face to see her: and she is not deadly. She is beautiful and she is laughing.

They say that there are two things which cannot be represented: death and female genitals. For they need to associate femininity with death: they get "stiff" with fear! for themselves! they need to be afraid of us. Look, the trembling Perseuses are coming towards us armed with apotropes, backwards! Pretty backs! Not a minute to lose. Let's go.

She is coming back from death's door: from forever: from "outside," from the wastelands where the witches are still alive; from beneath, beside "culture"; *from her childhood* which they have so much trouble making her forget, which they condemn to the *in pace*. Walled up, the little girls with the "ill-mannered" bodies. Preserved, untouched by themselves, in ice. Frigidified. But underneath something is stirring, wildly! What efforts they must make, the sex police, always having to begin again in order to obstruct her threatening return. On both sides, a display of force so great that the struggle, for centuries, has been immobilized in the trembling equilibrium of a deadlock.

We the precocious, we the repressed of culture, our lovely mouths clogged with gags, pollen, constricted breath; we the labyrinths, the ladders, the trampled spaces; the *volées**—we are "black" *and* we are beautiful.

NOTES

1. As all of Derrida's work crossing-detecting the history of philosophy endeavors to bring to light. In Plato, Hegel, Nietzsche a similar operation is performed, repression, foreclusion, distancing or woman. Murder which is indistinguishable from history as manifestation and representation of male power.

2. "Pour un tombeau d'Anatole" (ed. du Seuil, p. 138), tomb in which Mallarmè keeps his son, protects him, he being the mother, from death.

3. "She will awaken only at the touch of love, and before that moment she is but a dream. But in this dream existence, two stages can be distinguished: first love dreams of her, then she dreams of love." Thus muses Kierkegaard's *Seducer*.

4. *Jouissance* (verb form: *jouir*): the experience, often sexual, of intense pleasure.

5. That pleasure is preliminary, as Freud says, is a "truth," but only in part. A point of view which has in fact been upheld since the formation of the male *imaginaire*, to the extent that it is animated by the threat of castration. . . .

---

* *Voler*: To steal and to fly; thus *volées*: the robbed, those who have flown away [translator's note].

20.

SEXUAL PERVERSION

Thomas Nagel

There is something to be learned about sex from the fact that we possess a concept of sexual perversion. I wish to examine the idea, defending it against the charge of unintelligibility and trying to say exactly what about human sexuality qualifies it to admit of perversions. Let me begin with some general conditions that the concept must meet if it is to be viable at all. These can be accepted without assuming any particular analysis.

First, if there are any sexual perversions, they will have to be sexual desires or practices that are in some sense unnatural, though the explanation of this natural/unnatural distinction is of course the main problem. Second, certain practices will be perversions if anything is, such as shoe fetishism, bestiality, and sadism; other practices, such as unadorned sexual intercourse, will not be; about still others there is controversy. Third, if there are perversions, they will be unnatural sexual *inclinations* rather than just unnatural practices adopted not from inclination but for other reasons. Thus contraception, even if it is thought to be a deliberate perversion of the sexual and reproductive functions, cannot be significantly described as a *sexual* perversion. A sexual perversion must reveal itself

Journal of Philosphy 66, no. 1 (January 16, 1969): 5–17. Reprinted by permission of the *Journal of Philosophy* and the author.

in conduct that expresses an unnatural *sexual* preference. And although there might be a form of fetishism focused on the employment of contraceptive devices, that is not the usual explanation for their use.

The connection between sex and reproduction has no bearing on sexual perversion. The latter is a concept of psychological, not physiological, interest, and it is a concept that we do not apply to the lower animals, let alone to plants, all of which have reproductive functions that can go astray in various ways. (Think of seedless oranges.) Insofar as we are prepared to regard higher animals as perverted, it is because of their psychological, not their anatomical, similarity to humans. Furthermore, we do not regard as a perversion every deviation from the reproductive function of sex in humans: sterility, miscarriage, contraception, abortion.

Nor can the concept of sexual perversion be defined in terms of social disapprobation or custom. Consider all the societies that have frowned upon adultery and fornication. These have not been regarded as unnatural practices, but have been thought objectionable in other ways. What is regarded as unnatural admittedly varies from culture to culture, but the classification is not a pure expression of disapproval or distaste. In fact it is often regarded as a *ground* for disapproval, and that suggests that the classification has independent content.

I shall offer a psychological account of sexual perversion that depends on a theory of sexual desire and human sexual interactions. To approach this solution I shall first consider a contrary position that would justify skepticism about the existence of any sexual perversions at all, and perhaps even about the significance of the term. The skeptical argument runs as follows:

"Sexual desire is simply one of the appetites, like hunger and thirst. As such it may have various objects, some more common than others perhaps, but none in any sense 'natural.' An appetite is identified as sexual by means of the organs and erogenous zones in which its satisfaction can be to some extent localized, and the special sensory pleasures which form the core of that satisfaction. This enables us to recognize widely divergent goals, activities, and desires as sexual, since it is conceivable in principle that anything should produce sexual pleasure and that a nondeliberate, sexually charged desire for it should arise (as a result of conditioning, if nothing else). We may fail to empathize with some of these desires, and some of them, like sadism, may be objectionable on extraneous grounds, but once we have observed that they meet the criteria for being sexual, there is nothing more to be said on *that* score. Either they are sexual or they are not: sexuality does not admit of imperfection, or perversion, or any other such qualification—it is not that sort of affection."

This is probably the received radical position. It suggests that the cost of defending a psychological account may be to deny that sexual desire is an appetite. But insofar as that line of defense is plausible, it should make us suspicious of the simple picture of appetites on which the skepticism depends. Perhaps the standard appetites, like hunger, cannot be classed as pure appetites in that sense either, at least in their human versions.

Can we imagine anything that would qualify as a gastronomical perversion? Hunger and eating, like sex, serve a biological function and also play a significant role in our inner lives. Note that there is little temptation to describe as perverted an appetite for substances that are not nourishing: we should probably not consider someone's appetites *perverted* if he liked to eat paper, sand, wood, or cotton. Those are merely rather odd and very unhealthy tastes: they lack the psychological complexity that we expect of perversions. (Coprophilia, being already a sexual perversion, may be disregarded.) If on the other hand someone liked to eat cookbooks, or magazines with pictures of food in them, and preferred these to ordinary food—or if when hungry he sought satisfaction by fondling a napkin or ashtray from his favorite restaurant—then the concept of perversion might seem appropriate (it would be natural to call it gastronomical fetishism). It would be natural to describe as gastronomically perverted someone who could eat only by having food forced down his throat through a funnel, or only if the meal were a living animal. What helps is the peculiarity of the desire itself, rather than the inappropriateness of its object to the biological function that the desire serves. Even an appetite can have perversions if in addition to its biological function it has a significant psychological structure.

In the case of hunger, psychological complexity is provided by the activities that give it expression. Hunger is not merely a disturbing sensation that can be quelled by eating; it is an attitude toward edible portions of the external world, a desire to treat them in rather special ways. The method of ingestion: chewing, savoring, swallowing, appreciating the texture and smell, all are important components of the relation, as is the passivity and controllability of the food (the only animals we eat live are helpless mollusks). Our relation to food depends also on our size: we do not live upon it or burrow into it like aphids or worms. Some of these features are more central than others, but an adequate phenomenology of eating would have to treat it as a relation to the external world and a way of appropriating bits of that world, with characteristic affection. Displacements or serious restrictions of the desire to eat could then be described as perversions, if they undermined that direct relation between man and food which is the natural expression of hunger. This explains why it is easy to imagine gastronomical fetishism, voyeurism, exhibitionism, or even gastronomical sadism and masochism. Some of these perversions are fairly common.

If we can imagine perversions of an appetite like hunger, it should be possible to make sense of the concept of sexual perversion. I do not wish to imply that sexual desire is an appetite—only that being an appetite is no bar to admitting of perversions. Like hunger, sexual desire has as its characteristic object a certain relation with something in the external world; only in this case it is usually a person rather than an omelet, and the relation is considerably more complicated. This added complication allows scope for correspondingly complicated perversions.

The fact that sexual desire is a feeling about other persons may encourage a pious view of its psychological content—that it is properly the expression of some other attitude, like love, and that when it occurs by itself it is incomplete or subhuman. (The extreme Platonic version of such a view is that sexual practices are all vain attempts to express something they cannot in principle achieve: this makes them all perversions, in a sense.) But sexual desire is complicated enough without having to be linked to anything else as a condition for phenomenological analysis. Sex may serve various functions—economic, social, altruistic—but it also has its own content as a relation between persons.

The object of sexual attraction is a particular individual who transcends the properties that make him attractive. When different persons are attracted to a single person for different reasons—eyes, hair, figure, laugh, intelligence—we nevertheless feel that the object of their desire is the same. There is even an inclination to feel that this is so if the lovers have different sexual aims, if they include both men and women, for example. Different specific attractive characteristics seem to provide enabling conditions for the operation of a single basic feeling, and the different aims all provide expressions of it. We approach the sexual attitude toward the person through the features that we find attractive, but these features are not the objects of that attitude.

This is very different from the case of an omelet. Various people may desire it for different reasons, one for its fluffiness, another for its mushrooms, another for its unique combination of aroma and visual aspect; yet we do not enshrine the transcendental omelet as the true common object of their affections. Instead we might say that several desires have accidentally converged on the same object: any omelet with the crucial characteristics would do as well. It is not similarly true that any person with the same flesh distribution and way of smoking can be substituted as object for a particular sexual desire that has been elicited by those characteristics. It may be that they recur, but it will be a new sexual attraction with a new particular object, not merely a transfer of the old desire to someone else. (This is true even in cases where the new object is unconsciously identified with a former one.)

The importance of this point will emerge when we see how complex a psychological interchange constitutes the natural development of sexual attraction. This would be incomprehensible if its object were not a particular person, but rather a person of a certain *kind*. Attraction is only the beginning, and fulfillment does not consist merely of behavior and contact expressing this attraction, but involves much more.

The best discussion of these matters that I have seen appears in part III of Sartre's *Being and Nothingness*.[1] Sartre's treatment of sexual desire and of love, hate, sadism, masochism, and further attitudes toward others, depends on a general theory of consciousness and the body which we can neither expound nor assume here. He does not discuss perversion, and this is partly because he regards sexual desire as one form of the perpetual attempt of an embodied consciousness to come to terms with the existence of others, an attempt that is as doomed to fail in this form as it is in any of the others, which include sadism and masochism (if not certain of the more impersonal deviations) as well as several nonsexual attitudes. According to Sartre, all attempts to incorporate the other into my world as another subject, i.e., to apprehend him at once as an object for me and as a subject for whom I am an object, are unstable and doomed to collapse into one or other of the two aspects. Either I reduce him entirely to an object, in which case his subjectivity escapes the possession or appropriation I can extend to that object; or I become merely an object for him, in which case I am no longer in a position to appropriate his subjectivity. Moreover, neither of these aspects is stable; each is continually in danger of giving way to the other. This has the consequence that there can be no such thing as a *successful* sexual relation, since the deep aim of sexual desire cannot in principle be accomplished. It seems likely, therefore, that the view will not permit a basic distinction between successful or complete and unsuccessful or incomplete sex, and therefore cannot admit the concept of perversion.

I do not adopt this aspect of the theory, nor many of its metaphysical underpinnings. What interests me is Sartre's picture of the attempt. He says that the type of possession that is the object of sexual desire is carried out by "a double reciprocal incarnation" and that this is accomplished, typically in the form of a caress, in the following way: "I make myself flesh in order to impel the Other to realize *for herself* and *for me* her own flesh, and my caresses cause my flesh to be born for me in so far as it is for the Other *flesh causing her to be born as flesh*" (*Being and Nothingness*, p. 391; Sartre's italics). The incarnation in question is described variously as a clogging or troubling of consciousness, which is inundated by the flesh in which it is embodied.

The view I am going to suggest, I hope in less obscure language, is related to this one, but it differs from Sartre's in allowing sexuality to achieve its goal on occasion and thus in providing the concept of perversion with a foothold.

Sexual desire involves a kind of perception, but not merely a single perception of its object, for in the paradigm case of mutual desire there is a complex system of superimposed mutual perceptions—not only perceptions of the sexual object, but perceptions of oneself. Moreover, sexual awareness of another involves considerable self-awareness to begin with—more than is involved in ordinary sensory perception. The experience is felt as an assault on oneself by the view (or touch, or whatever) of the sexual object.

Let us consider a case in which the elements can be separated. For clarity we will restrict ourselves initially to the somewhat artificial case of desire at a distance. Suppose a man and a woman, whom we may call Romeo and Juliet, are at opposite ends of a cocktail lounge, with many mirrors on the walls which permit unobserved observation, and even mutual unobserved observation. Each of them is sipping a martini and studying other people in the mirrors. At some point Romeo notices Juliet. He is moved, somehow, by the softness of her hair and the diffidence with which she sips her martini, and this arouses him sexually. Let us say that X *senses* Y whenever X regards Y with sexual desire. (Y need not be a person, and X's apprehension of Y can be visual, tactile, olfactory, etc., or purely imaginary; in the present example we shall concentrate on vision.) So Romeo senses Juliet, rather than merely noticing her. At this stage he is aroused by an unaroused object, so he is more in the sexual grip of his body than she of hers.

Let us suppose, however, that Juliet now senses Romeo in another mirror on the opposite wall, though neither of them yet knows that he is seen by the other (the mirror angles provide three-quarter views). Romeo then begins to notice in Juliet the subtle signs of sexual arousal, heavy-lidded stare, dilating pupils, faint flush, etc. This of course intensifies her bodily presence, and he not only notices but senses this as well. His arousal is nevertheless still solitary. But now, cleverly calculating the line of her stare without actually looking her in the eyes, he realizes that it is directed at him through the mirror on the opposite wall. That is, he notices, and moreover senses, Juliet sensing him. This is definitely a new development, for it gives him a sense of embodiment not only through his own reactions but through the eyes and reactions of another. Moreover, it is separable from the initial sensing of Juliet; for sexual arousal might begin with a person's sensing that he is sensed and being assailed by the perception of the other person's desire rather than merely by the perception of the person.

But there is a further step. Let us suppose that Juliet, who is a little slower than Romeo, now senses that he senses her. This puts Romeo in a position to notice, and be aroused by, her arousal at being sensed by him. He senses that she senses that he senses her. This is still another level of arousal, for he becomes conscious of his sexuality through his awareness of its effect on her and of her awareness that this effect is due to him. Once she takes the same step and senses that he senses her sensing him, it becomes difficult to state, let alone imagine, further iterations, though they may be logically distinct. If both are alone, they will presumably turn to look at each other directly, and the proceedings will continue on another plane. Physical contact and intercourse are natural extensions of this complicated visual exchange, and mutual touch can involve all the complexities of awareness present in the visual case, but with a far greater range of subtlety and acuteness.

Ordinarily, of course, things happen in a less orderly fashion—sometimes in a great rush—but I believe that some version of this overlapping system of distinct sexual perceptions and interactions is the basic framework of any full-fledged sexual relation and that relations involving only part of the complex are significantly incomplete. The account is only schematic, as it must be to achieve generality. Every real sexual act will be psychologically far more specific and detailed, in ways that depend not only on the physical techniques employed and on anatomical details, but also on countless features of the participants' conceptions of themselves and of each other, which become embodied in the act. (It is familiar enough fact, for example, that people often take their social roles and the social roles of their partners to bed with them.)

The general schema is important, however, and the proliferation of levels of mutual awareness it involves is an example of a type of complexity that typifies human interactions. Consider aggression, for example. If I am angry with someone, I want to make him feel it, either to produce self-reproach by getting him to see himself through the eyes of my anger, and to dislike what he sees—or else to produce reciprocal anger or fear, by getting him to perceive my anger as a threat or attack. What I want will depend on the details of my anger, but in either case it will involve a desire that the object of that anger be aroused. This accomplishment constitutes the fulfillment of my emotion, through domination of the object's feelings.

Another example of such reflexive mutual recognition is to be found in the phenomenon of meaning, which appears to involve an intention to produce a belief or other effect in another by bringing about his recognition of one's intention to produce that effect. (That result is due to H. P. Grice,[2] whose position I shall not attempt to reproduce in detail.) Sex has a related structure: it involves a desire that one's partner be aroused by the recognition of one's desire that he or she be aroused.

It is not easy to define the basic types of awareness and arousal of which these complexes are composed, and that remains a lacuna in this discussion. In a sense, the object of awareness is the same in one's own case as it is in one's sexual awareness of another, although the two awarenesses will not be the same, the difference being as great as that between feeling angry and experiencing the anger of another. All stages of sexual perception are varieties of identification of a person with his body. What is perceived is one's own or another's *subjection* to or *immersion* in his body, a phenomenon which has been recognized with loathing by St. Paul and St. Augustine, both of whom regarded "the law of sin which is in my members" as a grave threat to the dominion of the holy will.[3] In sexual desire and its expression the blending of involuntary response with deliberate control is extremely important. For Augustine, the revolution launched against him by his body is symbolized by erection and the other involuntary physical components of arousal. Sartre too stresses the fact that the penis is not a prehensile organ. But mere involuntariness characterizes other bodily processes as well. In sexual desire the involuntary responses are combined with submission to spontaneous impulses: not only one's pulse and secretions but one's actions are taken over by the body; ideally, deliberate control is needed only to guide the expression of those impulses. This is to some extent also true of an appetite like hunger, but the takeover there is more localized, less pervasive, less extreme. One's whole body does not become saturated with hunger as it can with desire. But the most characteristic feature of a specifically sexual immersion in the body is its ability to fit into the complex of mutual perceptions that we have described. Hunger leads to spontaneous interactions with food; sexual desire leads to spontaneous interactions with other persons, whose bodies are asserting their sovereignty in the same way, producing involuntary reactions and spontaneous impulses in *them*. These reactions are perceived, and the perception of them is perceived, and that perception is in turn perceived; at each step the domination of the person by his body is reinforced, and the sexual partner becomes more possessible by physical contact, penetration, and envelopment.

Desire is therefore not merely the perception of a preexisting embodiment of the other, but ideally a contribution to his further embodiment, which in turn enhances the original subject's sense of himself. This explains why it is important that the partner be aroused, and not merely aroused, but aroused by the awareness of one's desire. It also explains the sense in which desire has unity and possession as its object: physical possession must eventuate in creation of the sexual object in the image of one's desire, and not merely in the object's recognition of that desire, or in his or her own private arousal.

Even if this is a correct model of the adult sexual capacity, it is not plausible to describe as perverted every deviation from it. For example, if the partners in heterosexual intercourse indulge in private heterosexual fantasies, thus avoiding recognition of the real partner, that would, on this model, constitute a defective sexual relation. It is not, however, generally regarded as a perversion. Such examples suggest that a simple dichotomy between perverted and unperverted sex is too crude to organize the phenomena adequately.

Still, various familiar deviations constitute truncated or incomplete versions of the complete configuration, and may be regarded as perversions of the central

264 PHILOSOPHY AND SEX

impulse. If sexual desire is prevented from taking its full interpersonal form, it is likely to find a different one. The concept of perversion implies that a normal sexual development has been turned aside by distorting influences. I have little to say about this causal condition. But if perversions are in some sense unnatural, they must result from interference with the development of a capacity that is there potentially.

It is difficult to apply this condition, because environmental factors play a role in determining the precise form of anyone's sexual impulse. Early experiences in particular seem to determine the choice of a sexual object. To describe some causal influences as distorting and others as merely formative is to imply that certain general aspects of human sexuality realize a definite potential, whereas many of the details in which people differ realize an indeterminate potential, so that they cannot be called more or less natural. What is included in the definite potential is therefore very important, although the distinction between definite and indeterminate potential is obscure. Obviously a creature incapable of developing the levels of interpersonal sexual awareness I have described could not be deviant in virtue of the failure to do so. (Though even a chicken might be called perverted in an extended sense if it had been conditioned to develop a fetishistic attachment to a telephone.) But if humans will tend to develop some version of reciprocal interpersonal sexual awareness unless prevented, then cases of blockage can be called unnatural or perverted.

Some familiar deviations can be described in this way. Narcissistic practices and intercourse with animals, infants, and inanimate objects seem to be stuck at some primitive version of the first stage of sexual feeling. If the object is not alive, the experience is reduced entirely to an awareness of one's own sexual embodiment. Small children and animals permit awareness of the embodiment of the other, but present obstacles to reciprocity, to the recognition by the sexual object of the subject's desire as the source of his (the object's) sexual self-awareness. Voyeurism and exhibitionism are also incomplete relations. The exhibitionist wishes to display his desire without needing to be desired in return; he may even fear the sexual attentions of others. A voyeur, on the other hand, need not require any recognition by his object at all: certainly not a recognition of the voyeur's arousal.

On the other hand, if we apply our model to the various forms that may be taken by two-party heterosexual intercourse, none of them seem clearly to qualify as perversions. Hardly anyone can be found these days to inveigh against oral-genital contact, and the merits of buggery are urged by such respectable figures as D. H. Lawrence and Norman Mailer. In general, it would appear that any bodily contact between a man and a woman that gives them sexual pleasure is a possible vehicle for the system of multilevel interpersonal awareness that I have claimed is the basic psychological content of sexual interaction. Thus a liberal platitude about sex is upheld.

The really difficult cases are sadism, masochism, and homosexuality. The first two are widely regarded as perversions and the last is controversial. In all three cases the issue depends partly on causal factors: do these dispositions result only when normal development has been prevented? Even the form in which this question has been posed is circular, because of the word "normal." We appear to need an independent criterion for a distorting influence, and we do not have one.

It may be possible to class sadism and masochism as perversions because they fall short of interpersonal reciprocity. Sadism concentrates on the evocation of passive self-awareness in others, but the sadist's engagement is itself active and requires a retention of deliberate control which may impede awareness of himself as a bodily subject of passion in the required sense. De Sade claimed that the object of sexual desire was to evoke involuntary responses from one's partner, especially audible ones. The infliction of pain is no doubt the most efficient way to accomplish this, but it requires a certain abrogation of one's own exposed spontaneity. A masochist on the other hand imposes the same disability on his partner as the sadist imposes on himself. The masochist cannot find a satisfactory embodiment as the object of another's sexual desire, but only as the object of his control. He is passive not in relation to his partner's passion but in relation to his nonpassive agency. In addition, the subjection to one's body characteristic of pain and physical restraint is of a very different kind from that of sexual excitement: pain causes people to contract rather than dissolve. These descriptions may not be generally accurate. But to the extent that they are, sadism and masochism would be disorders of the second stage of awareness—the awareness of oneself as an object of desire.

Homosexuality cannot similarly be classed as a perversion on phenomenological grounds. Nothing rules out the full range of interpersonal perceptions between persons of the same sex. The issue then depends on whether homosexuality is produced by distorting influences that block or displace a natural tendency to heterosexual development. And the influences must be more distorting than those which lead to a taste for large breasts or fair hair or dark eyes. These also are contingencies of sexual preference in which people differ, without being perverted.

The question is whether heterosexuality is the natural expression of male and female sexual dispositions that have not been distorted. It is an unclear question, and I do not know how to approach it. There is much support for an aggressive-passive distinction between male and female sexuality. In our culture the male's arousal tends to initiate the perceptual exchange, he usually makes the sexual approach, largely controls the course of the act, and of course penetrates, whereas the woman receives. When two men or two women engage in intercourse they cannot both adhere to these sexual roles. But a good deal of deviation from them occurs in heterosexual intercourse. Women can be sexually aggressive and men passive, and temporary reversals of role are not uncommon in heterosexual exchanges of reasonable length. For these reasons it seems to be doubtful that homosexuality must be a perversion, though like heterosexuality it has perverted forms.

Let me close with some remarks about the relation of perversion to good, bad, and morality. The concept of perversion can hardly fail to be evaluative in some sense, for it appears to involve the notion of an ideal or at least adequate sexuality which the perversions in some way fail to achieve. So, if the concept is viable, the judgment that a person or practice or desire is perverted will constitute a sexual evaluation, implying that better sex, or a better specimen of sex, is possible. This in itself is a very weak claim, since the evaluation might be in a dimension that is of little interest to us. (Though, if my account is correct, that will not be true.)

Whether it is a moral evaluation, however, is another question entirely—one whose answer would require more understanding of both morality and perversion than can be deployed here. Moral evaluation of acts and of persons is a rather special and very complicated matter, and by no means all our evaluations of persons and their activities are moral evaluations. We make judgments about people's beauty or health or intelligence which are evaluative without being moral. Assessments of their sexuality may be similar in that respect.

Furthermore, moral issues aside, it is not clear that unperverted sex is necessarily *preferable* to the perversions. It may be that sex which receives the highest marks for perfection *as sex* is less enjoyable than certain perversions; and if enjoyment is considered very important, that might outweigh considerations of sexual perfection in determining rational preference.

That raises the question of the relation between the evaluative content of judgments of perversion and the rather common *general* distinction between good and bad sex. The latter distinction is usually confined to sexual acts, and it would seem, within limits, to cut across the other: even someone who believed, for example, that homosexuality was a perversion could admit a distinction between better and worse homosexual sex, and might even allow that good homosexual sex could be better sex than not very good unperverted sex. If this is correct, it supports the position that if judgments of perversion are viable at all, they represent only one aspect of the possible evaluation of sex, even *qua sex*. Moreover it is not the only important aspect: sexual deficiencies that evidently do not constitute perversions can be the object of great concern.

Finally, even if perverted sex is to that extent not so good as it might be, bad sex is generally better than none at all. This should not be controversial: it seems to hold for other important matters, like food, music, literature, and society. In the end, one must choose from among the available alternatives, whether their availability depends on the environment or on one's own constitution. And the alternatives have to be fairly grim before it becomes rational to opt for nothing.

Notes

1. *L'Être et le Néant* (Paris: Gallimard, 1943), translated by Hazel E. Barnes (New York: Philosophical Library, 1956).

2. "Meaning," *Philosophical Review* 66, no. 3 (July 1957): 377–88.

3. See Rom. 7:23; and the *Confessions*, bk. 8, part 5.

21.

SEXUAL USE AND WHAT TO DO ABOUT IT

Internalist and Externalist Sexual Ethics

Alan Soble

I begin (in section 1) by describing the hideous nature of sexuality, that in virtue of which sexual desire and activity are morally suspicious, or at least what we have been told about the moral foulness of sex by, in particular, Immanuel Kant.[1] A problem arises because acting on one's sexual desire, given Kant's metaphysics of sex, apparently conflicts with the Categorical Imperative, especially its Second Formulation (section 2). I then propose a typology of possible solutions to this problem and critically discuss recent philosophical ethics of sex that fall into the typology's various categories (sections 3 and 4). I conclude (section 5) with remarks about Kant's own solution to this sex problem.

1. THE NATURE OF SEX

On Kant's view, a person who sexually desires another person objectifies that other, both before and during sexual activity.[2] This can occur in several ways. Certain types of manipulation and deception (primping, padding, making an overly good

© 2001, Alan Soble. Reprinted, with the permission of, and thanks to, Michael Goodman, the journal's editor, and Alan Soble, from *Essays in Philosophy* 2:2 (June 2001). The journal can be accessed at http://www.humboldt.edu/~essays/.

first impression) seem required prior to engaging in sex, or are so common as to appear part of the nature of human sexual interaction.³ The other's body, his or her lips, thighs, buttocks, and toes, are desired as the arousing parts they are, distinct from the person. As Kant says (about the genitals, apparently):

> sexuality is not an inclination which one human being has for another as such, but is an inclination for the sex of another. . . . [O]nly her sex is the object of his desires. . . . [A]ll men and women do their best to make not their human nature but their sex more alluring.⁴

Further, both the body and the compliant actions of the other person are tools (a means) that one uses for one's own sexual pleasure, and to that extent the other person is a fungible, functional thing. Sexual activity itself is a strange activity, not only by manifesting uncontrollable arousal and involuntary movements of the body, but also with its yearning to master, dominate, and even consume the other's body. During the sexual act, then, a person both loses control of himself and loses regard for the humanity of the other. Sexual desire is a threat to the other's personhood, but the one who is under the spell of sexual desire also loses hold of his or her own personhood. The person who desires another depends on the whims of that other for satisfaction, and becomes as a result a jellyfish, vulnerable to the other's demands and manipulations.⁵ Merely being sexually aroused by another person can be experienced as coercive; similarly, a person who proposes an irresistible sexual offer may be exploiting another who has been made weak by sexual desire.⁶ Moreover, a person who willingly complies with another person's request for a sexual encounter voluntarily makes an object of himself or herself. As Kant puts it, "For the natural use that one sex makes of the other's sexual organs is *enjoyment*, for which one gives oneself up to the other. In this act a human being makes himself into a thing."⁷ And, for Kant, because those engaged in sexual activity make themselves into objects merely for the sake of sexual pleasure, both persons reduce themselves to animals. When

> a man wishes to satisfy his desire, and a woman hers, they stimulate each other's desire; their inclinations meet, but their object is not human nature but sex, and each of them dishonours the human nature of the other. They make of humanity an instrument for the satisfaction of their lusts and inclinations, and dishonour it by placing it on a level with animal nature.⁸

Finally, the power of the sexual urge makes it dangerous.⁹ Sexual desire is inelastic, relentless, the passion most likely to challenge reason and make us succumb to *akrasia*, compelling us to seek satisfaction even when doing so involves the risks of dark-alley gropings, microbiologically filthy acts, slinking around the

White House, or getting married impetuously. Sexually motivated behavior easily destroys our self-respect.

The sexual impulse or inclination, then, is morally dubious and, to boot, a royal pain. Kant made this point in more general terms, claiming that humans would be delighted to be free of such promptings:

> Inclinations . . . as sources of needs, are so far from having an absolute value to make them desirable for their own sake that it must rather be the universal wish of every rational being to be wholly free from them.[10]

I am not sure I believe all these claims about the nature of sexuality, but that is irrelevant for my purpose, since many philosophers, with good reason, have taken them seriously. In some moods I might reply to Kant by muttering a Woody Allen type of joke: "Is sex an autonomy-killing, mind-numbing, sub-human passion? Yes, but only when it's good." In this essay, however, I want to examine how sexual acts could be moral, if this description is right.

2. Sex and the Second Formulation

Michael Ruse has explained in a direct way how a moral problem arises in acting on sexual desire:

> The starting point to sex is the sheer desire of a person for the body of another. One wants to feel the skin, to smell the hair, to see the eyes—one wants to bring one's own genitals into contact with those of the other. . . . This gets danger-ously close to treating the other as a means to the fulfillment of one's own sexual desire—as an object, rather than as an end.[11]

We should add, to make Ruse's observation more comprehensively Kantian, that the desire to be touched, to be thrilled by the touch of the other, to be the object of someone else's desire, is just as much "the starting point" that raises the moral problem.

Because this sex problem arises from the intersection of a Kantian view of the nature of sexuality and Kantian ethics, let us review the Second Formulation: "Act in such a way that you always treat humanity, whether in your own person or in the person of any other, never simply as a means, but always at the same time as an end." Or "man . . . *exists* as an end in himself, *not merely as a means* for arbitrary use by this or that will: he must in all his actions, whether they are directed to himself or to other rational beings, always be viewed *at the same time as an end*."[12] So the question arises: how can sexual desire be expressed and satisfied without merely using the other or treating the other as an object, and without treating the self as an object? How can sexual activity be planned and carried out while "at the same time" treating the other and the self as persons, while treating their "humanity" as an end, while confirming their autonomy and rationality? Of course, the Second Formulation directs us not to treat ourselves and others *merely* as means or objects. It is permissible to treat another and ourselves as a means as long as we are also treated as persons or our humanity is treated as an end. How can this be done?

A person's providing free and informed consent to an action or to interactions with other persons is, in general for Kant, a necessary but not sufficient condition for satisfying the Second Formulation. In addition, for Kant, treating someone as a person at least includes taking on the other's ends as if they were one's own ends. Thus Kant writes in the *Groundwork*, "the ends of a subject who is an end in himself must, if this conception is to have its *full* effect in me, be also, as far as possible, *my* ends."[13] And I must take on the other's ends for their own sake, not because that is an effective way to advance my own goals in using the other. It is further required, when I treat another as a means, that the other can take on my ends, my purpose, in so using him or her as a means. Kant likely expressed this condition in the *Groundwork*: "the man who has a mind to make a false promise to others will see at once that he is intending to make use of another man *merely as a means* to an end he does not share. For the man whom I seek to use for my own purposes by such a promise cannot possibly agree with my way of behaving to him, and so cannot himself share the end of [my] action."[14] Given Kant's metaphysics of sexuality, can *all* these requirements of the Second Formulation of the Categorical Imperative be satisfied in *any* sexual interaction? That is the Kantian sex problem.

But it should noted that even though, in general, Kant advances these two conditions in addition to free and informed consent—I must take on your ends, and you must be able to take on my ends—Kant apparently relaxes his standard for some situations, allowing one person to use another just with the free and informed consent of the used person, as long as one allows the used person to *retain* personhood or one does *not interfere* with his or her retaining personhood. This weaker variation on how to satisfy the Second Formulation may be important in Kant's account of the morality of work-for-hire and of sexual relations, as I discuss below (sections 4a and 5).[15]

I now proceed to display a conceptual typology of various solutions to the Kantian sex problem, and discuss critically whether, or to what extent, solutions that occupy different logical locations in the typology conform with the Second Formulation. There are five types of solution: behavioral internalist, psychological internalist, thin externalist, thick minimalist externalist, and thick extended externalist. I will define and discuss examples of each type in that order.

3. INTERNALIST SOLUTIONS TO THE SEX PROBLEM

Internalist solutions to the sex problem advise us to modify the character of sexual activity so that persons engaged in it satisfy the Second Formulation. For internalists, restraints on how sexual acts are carried out, or restraints on the natural expression of the impulse, must be present. Consent, then, is necessary for the morality of sexual acts, but not sufficient. Note that one might fix a sexual act internally so that qua sexual act the act is unobjectionable, but it still might be wrong for other reasons, for example, it might be adulterous. There are two internalisms: *behavioral* internalism, according to which the physical components of sexual acts make the moral difference, and *psychological* internalism, according to which certain attitudes must be present during sexual activity.

3a. Behavioral Internalism

Alan Goldman defines "sexual desire" as the "desire for contact with another person's body and for the pleasure which such contact produces. . . . The desire for another's body is . . . the desire for the pleasure that physical contact brings."[16] Since sexual desire is a desire for one's own self-interested pleasure, it is understandable that Goldman senses a Kantian problem with sexual activity. Thus Goldman writes that sexual activities "invariably involve at different stages the manipulation of one's partner for one's own pleasure" and thereby, he notes, seem to violate the Second Formulation—which, on Goldman's truncated rendition, "holds that one ought not to treat another as a means to such private ends."[17] The sex problem is one that Goldman must deal with from a Kantian perspective, because he firmly rejects a utilitarian view of sexual morality. But Goldman reminds us that from a Kantian perspective, "using other individuals for personal benefit," in sex or in other interactions, is "immoral only when [the acts] are one-sided, when the benefits are not mutual."[18] As a solution to the sex problem, then, Goldman proposes that

> Even in an act which by its nature "objectifies" the other, one recognizes a partner as a subject with demands and desires by yielding to those desires, by allowing oneself to be a sexual object as well, by giving pleasure or ensuring that the pleasures of the act are mutual.[19]

This sexual moral principle—make sure that you provide sexual pleasure to your partner—seems plausible enough. And because, for Goldman, consent is a necessary condition but not sufficient for the morality of a sexual act (one must go beyond consent, attempting to ensure that the other experiences sexual pleasure), and if providing sexual pleasure for your partner is a way to make the other person's ends your own ends, Goldman's proposal seems at least in spirit consistent with the Second Formulation.[20]

But let us ask: *why* might one sexually please the other? (Pleasing the other person can be done, as Goldman recognizes, by actively doing something to or for the other, or by allowing the other person to treat us as an object, so that they do things to us as we passively acquiesce.) One answer is suggested by a form of sexual egoism or hedonism: pleasing the other is *necessary for or contributes to one's own pleasure.* How so? By inducing the other, through either the other's sexual arousal or gratitude, to act to furnish pleasure to oneself. Or because sexually pleasing the other satisfies one's desire to exert power or influence over the other. Or because in providing pleasure to the other we get pleasure by witnessing the effects of our exertions.[21] Or by inducing the other to hold us in an esteem that may heighten our arousal. ("You are *so* good," the other moans.) Or because while giving pleasure to the other person we identify with his or her arousal and pleasure, which identification increases our own arousal and pleasure.[22] Or because pleasing the other alleviates or prevents guilt feelings, or doing so makes us feel good that we have kept a promise. I am sure readers can supplement this list of self-serving reasons for providing sexual pleasure to the other person.

Another answer is that providing pleasure to the other can *and should* be done just for the sake of pleasing the other, just because you know the other person has sexual needs and desires and has hopes for their satisfaction. The sexual satisfaction of the other is to be taken as an end in itself, as something valuable in its own right, not as something that has instrumental value. It follows, as a corollary, that in some circumstances you must be willing and ready to please the other person sexually when doing so does not contribute to your own satisfaction or even runs counter to it. (The last scenario is the kind of case Kant likes to focus on in the *Groundwork*, cases that single out the motive of benevolence or duty from motives based on inclination.)

By the way, according to the Marquis de Sade, sexual desire is absolutely egoistic; it is concerned only with its own satisfaction, not caring a whit about the pleasure of the other. This Kantian claim is compatible, in principle, with one's getting sexual pleasure by providing sexual pleasure to the other, when providing that pleasure is a mechanism for increasing one's pleasure. Sade, however, does not take the thesis in that direction. Instead, Sade asserts that the pleasure of the other is an impediment to or a distraction from one's own sexual pleasure, that allowing the other to pursue his or her pleasure at the same time is to undermine one's own pleasure.[23] I think we can acknowledge some truth here: when both persons attempt to satisfy their own sexual desire at the same time, their frantic grabbings sometimes result in sexually incongruous bodies and movements. The sexual satisfaction of one person often requires the passive acquiescence of the other, an abandonment to what the first one wants and how he or she wants it—in Goldman's language, one must sometimes allow the other to treat oneself as an object. Romantically perfect sexual events are hard to come by.

To return to Goldman's proposal: I have categorized Goldman as a behavioral internalist because all he insists on, in order to make sexual activity morally permissible from a Kantian perspective, is the *behavior* of providing pleasure for the other person. Goldman never claims that providing pleasure be done with a benevolent *motive* or purity of purpose. But this feature of his proposal is exactly why it fails, in its *own* terms. If providing pleasure to the other is just a mechanism for attaining or improving one's own pleasure, providing pleasure to the other *continues to treat the other merely as a means.* Since giving pleasure to the other is instrumental in obtaining my pleasure, giving pleasure has not at all succeeded in internally *fixing* the nature of the sexual act. Providing pleasure can be a genuine internalist solution, by changing the nature of the sexual act, only if providing pleasure is an unconditional giving; otherwise objectification, instrumentality, and use remain.

Goldman's proposal thus fails to accommodate his own Kantian commitments. When Kant claims that we must treat the other as a person by taking on his or her ends as our own—by providing sexual pleasure, if that is his or her end—Kant does not mean that as a hypothetical, as if taking on the other's ends were a mechanism for getting the other person to allow us to treat him or her as a means.[24] We must not take on the other's ends as our own simply because doing so is useful for us in generating our own pleasure or achieving our own sexual goals. Attitude, for Kant, is also morally important, not only behavior, even if that behavior has the desired and beneficial effects for the other person. Sharing the ends of the other person means viewing those ends as valuable in their own right. Further, for Kant, we may take on the ends of the other as our own only if the other's ends are themselves morally permissible: I may "make the other's ends my ends provided only that these are not immoral."[25] Given the objectification and use involved in sexual activity, as conceded by Goldman, the moral permissibility of the end of seeking sexual pleasure by means of another person has not yet been established for *either* party. We are not to make the other's ends our own ends if the other's ends are not, in themselves, already morally permissible, and whether the sexual ends of the other person *are* permissible is precisely the question at issue. Thus, to be told by Goldman that it is morally permissible for one person to objectify another in sexual activity if the other also objectifies the first, with the first's allowance, does not answer the question. Goldman's internalist solution attempts to change the nature of the sexual act, from what it is essentially to what it might be were we to embrace *slightly* better bedroom behavior—by avoiding raw selfishness. But this really doesn't go far enough to fix or change the nature of sexual activity, if all that is required is that both parties must add the giving of pleasure to an act that is by its nature, and remains, self-centered. Finally (and *perhaps* most important; see section 5), Goldman ignores, in Kant's statement of the Second Formulation, that we must also respect the humanity *in one's own person.* To make oneself voluntarily an object for the sake of the other person's sexual pleasure, as Goldman recommends, only multiplies the use, and does not eliminate it, and so apparently violates that prescription.

Goldman has, in effect, changed the problem from one of sexual objectification and use to one of distributive justice.[26] Sex is morally permissible, on his view, if the pleasure is mutual; the way to make sexual activity moral is to make it nonmorally good for both participants. Use and objectification remain, but they are permissible, on his view, because the objectification is reciprocal and the act is mutually beneficial. Even though in one sense Goldman makes sexual activity moral by making it *more* nonmorally good, for the *other* party, he also makes sexual activity moral by making it *less* nonmorally good, for the *self,* since one's sexual urgings must be restrained. What goes morally wrong in sexual activity, for Goldman, is that only one person might experience pleasure (or lopsidedly) and only one might bear the burden of providing it. This is what Goldman means, I think, by saying that "one-sided" sexual activity is immoral. The benefits of receiving pleasure, and the burdens of the restraint of seeking pleasure and of providing it to the other, must be passed around to everyone involved in the encounter. This is accomplished, for Goldman, by an equal or reciprocal distribution of being used as an object.

Suppose, instead, that both parties are expected to inject *unconditional* giving into an act that is essentially self-centered. Then both parties must buckle down more formidably, in order to restrain their impulses for their own pleasure and to provide pleasure to the other. But if altruistic giving were easy, given our natures, there would be less reason for thinking, to begin with, that sexual desire tends to use the other person in a self-centered way. To the extent that the sexual impulse is self-interested, as Goldman's definitions make clear, it is implausible that sexual urges could be controlled by a moral command to provide pleasure unconditionally. The point is not only that a duty to provide pleasure unconditionally threatens the nonmoral goodness of sexual acts, that it reduces the sexual excitement and satisfaction of both persons. Fulfilling such a duty, if we assume Goldman's account of sexual desire, may be impossible or unlikely.[27] Kant might have seen this point, for his own solution to the sex problem (see section 5) was not that persons engaged in sexual activity should unconditionally provide sexual pleasure for each other.

3b. Psychological Internalism

We have seen that if Goldman is to be able to fix the sexual act internally, to change its nature, he needs to insist not merely on our performing behaviors that produce pleasure for the other, but on our producing pleasure for a certain reason. In this way, we move from behavioral to psychological internalism, which claims that sexual acts must be accompanied and restrained by certain attitudes, the presence of which ensure the satisfaction of the Second Formulation.

At one point in her essay "Defining Wrong and Defining Rape," Jean Hampton lays out a view that is similar to Goldman's, in which the occurrence of mutual pleasure alone solves the sex problem:

> when sex is as much about pleasing another as it is about pleasing oneself, it certainly doesn't involve using another as a means and actually incorporates the idea of respect and concern for another's needs.[28]

Providing sexual pleasure to the other person, then, seems to satisfy Kant's Second Formulation. But Hampton goes beyond Goldman in attempting to understand the depth or significance of the sexual experience:

> one's humanity is perhaps never more engaged than in the sexual act. But it is not only present in the experience; more important, it is "at stake" in the sense that each partner puts him/herself in a position where the behavior of the other can either confirm it or threaten it, celebrate it or abuse it.[29]

This point is surely Kantian: sex is metaphysically and psychologically dangerous.[30] Hampton continues:

> If this is right, then I do not see how, for most normal human beings, sexual passion is heightened if one's sexual partner behaves in a way that one finds personally humiliating or that induces in one shame or self-hatred or that makes one feel like a "thing." . . . Whatever sexual passion is, such emotions seem antithetical to it, and such emotions are markers of the disrespect that destroys the morality of the experience. . . . [W]hat makes a sexual act morally right is also what provides the groundwork for the experience of emotions and pleasures that make for "good sex."[31]
>
> If the wrongness of the act is a function of its diminishing nature, then that wrongness can be present even if, ex ante, each party consented to the sex. So . . . consent is *never by itself* that which makes a sexual act morally right. . . . Lovemaking is a set of experiences . . . which includes attitudes and behaviors that are different in kind from the attitudes and behaviors involved in morally wrongful sex.[32]

Hampton's thesis, then, as I understand it, is that sexual activity must be accompanied by certain humanity-affirming attitudes or emotions that manifest themselves in the sexual activity itself. Attitudes and emotions that repudiate humanity, that are disrespectful, are morally wrong and (because) destructive of mutual pleasure.[33] Hampton's psychological internalism seems fairly consistent with Kant's Second Formulation: for Hampton, consent may be a necessary condition but it is not sufficient for behaving morally or respectfully toward another person sexually; giving pleasure to the other person, taking on their sexual ends, is required; and *why* the persons produce pleasure for each other is morally relevant. But Kant would still object to Hampton's view, even though he might well admit that she is on the right track. The willingness to provide, selflessly, sexual pleasure for the other, for Kant, does not erase the fundamentally objectifying nature of sexual activity. And the nonmarital (even if humanity-affirming) sexual activity that is in principle justifiable by Hampton's criterion would be rejected by Kant as immoral.

It seems to follow from Hampton's view that casual sex, in which both parties are just out to satisfy their own randiness, is morally wrong, along with prostitution, since these sexual acts are not likely to be, in some robust sense, humanity-affirming. And sadomasochistic sexual acts would seem to be morally wrong, on her view, because they likely involve what Hampton sees as humanity-denying attitudes. Yet casual sex and prostitution, as objectifying and instrumental as they can be, and sadomasochistic sexual acts, as humiliating to one's partner as they can be, still often produce tremendous sexual excitement and pleasure—contrary to what Hampton implies. For this reason I perceive a problem in Hampton's position. She believes, as does Goldman, that morally permissible sex involves mutual sexual pleasing, that the morality of sexual activity then depends on its nonmoral goodness, and, further, that disrespectful attitudes destroy this mutual pleasure or nonmoral goodness. But is the expression of disrespectful attitudes morally wrong exactly because these attitudes destroy the other's sexual pleasure or, instead, just because they are disrespectful? This question is important regarding Hampton's assessment of sadomasochism. For if her argument is that disrespectful attitudes that occur during sexual encounters are morally wrong exactly because they are disrespectful, then sadomasochistic sexual activities are morally wrong even if they do, contra Hampton's intuition, produce pleasure for the participants. (If so, Hampton may be what I later call an "externalist.") But if her argument is that disrespectful attitudes are wrong because or when they destroy the mutuality of the pleasure, or the pleasure of the experience for the other person, then sadomasochism does not turn out to be morally wrong. (And, in this case, Hampton remains an internalist.)

Perhaps Hampton means that sexual activity is morally permissible only when it is *both* mutually pleasure-producing *and* incorporates humanity-affirming attitudes. This dual test for the morality of sexual encounters prohibits casual sex between strangers, prostitution, as well as sadomasochistic sexuality, no matter how sexually satisfying these activities are. In Hampton's essay, however, I could find no clear criterion of "humanity-affirming" behavior and attitudes other than "provides mutual pleasure." This is exactly why Hampton does have trouble denying the permissibility of sadomasochism. Consider what the lesbian sadomasochist Pat Califia has said about sadomasochism: "The things that seem beautiful, inspiring, and life-affirming to me seem ugly, hateful, and ludicrous to most other people."[34] As far as I can tell, Califia means "provides sexual pleasure" by "life-affirming." If so, no disagreement in principle exists between Hampton and Califia, if Hampton means "provides pleasure" by "humanity-affirming." What Hampton does not take seriously, indeed what she rejects, is Califia's observation that brutal behaviors and humiliating attitudes that occur or are expressed during sexual activity can, even for "normal" people, make for mutually exciting and pleasurable sex.

4. EXTERNALIST SOLUTIONS TO THE SEX PROBLEM

According to *externalism*, morality requires that we place restraints on when sexual acts are engaged in, with whom sexual activity occurs, or on the conditions under which sexual activities are performed. Properly setting the background context in which sexual acts occur enables the persons to satisfy the Second Formulation. One distinction among externalisms is that between *minimalist* externalism, which claims that morality requires that only the context of the sexual activity be set, and the sexual acts may be whatever they turn out to be, and *extended* externalism, which claims that setting the context will also affect the character of the sexual acts. Another distinction among externalisms is that between *thin* externalism, according to which free and informed consent is both necessary and sufficient for the moral permissibility of sexual acts (with a trivial ceteris paribus clause), and *thick* externalism, which claims that something beyond consent is required for the morality of sexual activity.

4a. Thin Externalism

I begin my discussion of externalism by examining a theory of sexual morality proposed by Thomas Mappes, who argues that only weak contextual constraints are required for satisfying Kantian worries about sexual activity.[35] According to Mappes, the giving of free and informed consent by the persons involved in a sexual encounter is both a necessary condition and sufficient for the morality of their sexual activity, for making permissible the sexual use of one person by another person.[36] Consent is not sufficient for the morality of sexual acts *simpliciter*, because even though a sexual act might be morally permissible qua sexual act, it still might be, for example, adulterous. Mappes's position is a thin minimalist externalism. Indeed, thin externalism, defined as making consent both necessary and sufficient, must also be minimalist. This criterion of the morality of sexual activity is contentless, or fully procedural: it does not evaluate the form or the nature of the sexual act (for example, what body parts are involved, or in what manner the sexual acts are carried out), but only the antecedent and concurrent conditions or context in which the sexual acts take place. In principle, the acts engaged in need not even produce (mutual) sexual pleasure for the consenting participants, an implication that differs from Goldman's behavioral internalism.[37]

Mappes, while developing his theory of sexual ethics, begins by repeating a point made frequently about Kantian ethics:

> According to a fundamental Kantian principle, it is morally wrong for A to use B *merely as a means* (to achieve A's ends). Kant's principle does not rule out A using B as a means, only A using B *merely* as a means, that is, in a way incompatible with respect for B as a person.

Then Mappes lays out his central thesis:

> A immorally uses B if and only if A intentionally acts in a way that violates the requirement that B's involvement with A's ends be based on B's voluntary informed consent.[38]

For Mappes, the presence of free and informed consent—there is no deception and no coercive force or threats—satisfies the Second Formulation, since each person's providing consent ensures that the persons involved in sexual activity with each other are not *merely* or *wrongfully* using each other as means. Mappes intends that this principle be applied to any activity, whether sexual or otherwise; he believes, along with Goldman, that sexual activity should be governed by moral principles that apply in general to human behavior.[39]

Having advanced this interpretation of what it takes to satisfy the Second Formulation in sexual matters, Mappes spends almost all his essay discussing various situations that might, or might not, involve violating the free and informed consent criterion taken as stating a necessary condition for the morality of sexual activity. Mappes discusses what sorts of actions count as deceptive, coercive (by force or threat), or exploitative, in which case sexual activity made possible by such maneuvers would be morally wrong. Some of these cases are intriguing, as anyone familiar with the literature on the meaning and application of the free and informed consent criterion in the area of medical ethics knows. But, putting aside for now the important question of the suffi- ciency of consent, not everyone agrees that in sexual (or other) contexts free and informed consent is absolutely necessary. Jeffrie Murphy, for one, has raised some doubts:

> "Have sex with me or I will find another girlfriend" strikes me (assuming normal circumstances) as a morally permissible threat, and "Have sex with me and I will marry you" strikes me (assuming the offer is genuine) as a morally permissible offer. . . . We negotiate our way through most of life with schemes of threats and offers . . . and I see no reason why the realm of sexuality should be utterly insulated from this very normal way of being human.[40]

Both "Have sex with me or I will find another girlfriend" and "Marry me or I will never sleep with you again (or at all)" seem to be coercive yet permissible threats,[41] but sexual activity obtained by the employment of these coercions involves immoral use, on Mappes's criterion. Further, it is not difficult to imagine circumstances in which deception in sexual contexts is not morally wrong (even if we ignore the universal and innocuous practice of deceptive physical primping: the use of cosmetics and suggestive clothing).[42] Mappes claims that my *withholding* information from you, information that I believe would influ- ence your decision as to whether to have sexual relations with me, is deception that makes any subsequent sexual activity between us morally wrong.[43] But if I withhold the fact that I have an extraordinarily large or minuscule penis, and withholding that fact about my sexual anatomy plays a role in your eventually agreeing to engage in sex with me, it is not obviously true that my obtaining sex through this particular deception-by-omission is morally wrong. I suspect that what such cases tend to show is that we cannot rely comprehensively on a con- sent criterion to answer all (or perhaps any of) our pressing questions about sexual morality.[44] Does the other person have a *right* to know the size of my penis while deliberating whether to have sex with me? What types of coercive threat do we have a *right* to employ in trying to achieve our goals? These significant ques- tions cannot be answered by a free and informed consent criterion; they also sug- gest that reading the Second Formulation such that consent by itself can satisfy the Second Formulation is questionable.

Indeed, Mappes provides little reason for countenancing his unKantian notion that the presence of free and informed consent is a sufficient condition for the satisfaction of the Second Formulation, for not treating another person merely as a means or not wrongfully using him or her. He does write that "respect for persons entails that each of us recognize the rightful authority of other persons (as rational beings) to conduct their individual lives as they see fit,"[45] which suggests the following kind of argument: Allowing the other's consent to control when the other may be used for my sexual or other ends is to respect that person by taking his or her autonomy, his or her ability to reason and make choices, seriously, while not to allow the other to make the decision about when to be used for my sexual or other ends is disrespectfully paternalistic. If the other's consent is acknowledged to be sufficient, that shows that I respect his or her choice of ends, sexual or otherwise; or that even if I do not respect his or her particular choice of ends, at least I thereby show respect for his or her ends—making capacity or for his or her being a self-determining agent. And taking the other's consent as a sufficient condition can be a way of taking on his or her sexual or other ends as my own ends, as well as his or her taking on my sexual or other ends in my proposing to use him or her. According to such an argument, perhaps the best way to read Kant's Second Formulation is as a pronouncement of moral libertarianism—or a quasi-libertarianism that also, as Mappes does, pays careful moral attention and scrutiny to situations that are ripe for exploitation.[46]

Even if the argument makes some Kantian sense, Mappes's sexual principle seems to miss the point. The Kantian problem about sexuality is not, or is not only, that one person might make false promises, engage in deception, or employ force or threats against another person in order to gain sex. The problem of the objectification and use of both the self and the other arises for Kant even in those cases, or especially in those cases, in which both persons give perfectly free and informed consent. Thin externalism does not get to the heart of *this* problem. Perhaps no liberal philosophy that borders on moral libertarianism could even sense it as a problem; at any rate, no minimalist externalism could. The only sexual objectification that Mappes considers in his essay is that which arises with coercion, most dramatically in rape.[47] Nothing in his essay deals with what Kant and other philosophers discern as the intrinsically objectifying nature of sexuality itself. As Goldman does, Mappes assimilates sexual activity to all other human activities, all of which should be governed by the same moral principles. Whether Mappes's proposal works will depend, then, in part on whether sex is not so different from other joint human activities that free and informed consent is not too weak a criterion in this area of life.

It is an interesting question why free and informed consent does not, for Kant, solve the sex problem. It seems so obvious, to many today, that Mappes's consent criterion solves the sex problem that we wonder what Kant was up to in his metaphysical critique of sexuality. Kant's rejection of Mappes's solution suggests that Kant perceived deeper problems in sexual desire and activity than Mappes and Goldman acknowledge. In the *Lectures on Ethics*, Kant apparently accepts a Mappesian consent criterion regarding work-for-hire, but rejects it for sexual activity:

> Man [may], of course, use another human being as an instrument for his serv-
> ices; he [may] use his hands, his feet, and even all his powers; he [may] use him
> for his own purposes with the other's consent. But there is no way in which a
> human being can be made an Object of indulgence for another except through
> sexual impulse.[48]

For Kant, it seems that using another person in a work-for-hire situation is permissible, just with free and informed consent, as long as one does not undermine
or deny the worker's humanity in any other way. But Kant finds something problematic about sexual interaction that does not exist during, say, a tennis game
between two people (or in a work-for-hire situation), while Mappes sees no
moral difference between playing tennis with someone and playing with their
genitals, as long as free and informed consent is present. This disagreement
between those philosophers who view sexual activity as something or as
somehow special, and those philosophers who lump all human interactions
together, requires further philosophical thought.[49]

4b. Thick Externalism

Let us see if thick externalism, according to which more stringent contextual
constraints, in addition to free and informed consent, are required for the
morality of sexual activity, offers anything more substantial in coming to grips
with the Kantian sex problem. My central example is Martha Nussbaum's essay
"Objectification," in which Nussbaum submits that the Kantian sex problem is
solved if sexual activity is confined to the context of an abiding, mutually
respectful, and mutually regarding relationship. However, Nussbaum advances
both a thick minimalist externalism and a thick extended externalism. Thus, in
her long and complex essay, we can find at least two theses: (1) a background
context of an abiding, mutually respectful and regarding relationship makes noxious objectification during sexual activity morally *permissible*; and (2) a background context of an abiding, mutually respectful and regarding relationship
turns what might have been noxious objectification into something *good* or even
"wonderful," a valuable type of objectification in which autonomy is happily
abandoned—a thesis she derives from her reading of D. H. Lawrence.

4b-1. Thick Minimalist Externalism

In several passages of Nussbaum's essay, she proposes a thick minimalist externalism, according to which sexual objectification is morally permissible in the context of an abiding, mutually respectful relationship. To start, consider this modest statement of her general thesis:

> If I am lying around with my lover on the bed, and use his stomach as a pillow, there seems to be nothing at all baneful about this [instrumental objectification], provided that I do so with his consent . . . and without causing him pain, provided, as well, that I do so in the context of a relationship in which he is generally treated as more than a pillow. This suggests that what is problematic is not instrumentalization per se but treating someone *primarily* or *merely* as an instrument [for example, as a pillow]. The overall context of the relationship thus becomes fundamental.[50]

We can modify this passage so that Nussbaum's general point about permissible instrumental objectification-in-context can be applied more directly to the sex problem:

> If I am lying around with my lover on the bed, and use his penis for my sexual satisfaction, there seems to be nothing at all baneful about this instrumental objectification, provided that I do so with his consent . . . and without causing him pain, provided, as well, that I do so in the context of a relationship in which he is generally treated as more than a penis. This suggests that what is problematic is not instrumentalization per se but treating someone *primarily* or *merely* as an instrument [for example, as a penis]. The overall context of the relationship thus becomes fundamental.

Other passages in Nussbaum's essay also express her thick minimalist externalism: "where there is a loss in subjectivity in the moment of lovemaking, this can be and frequently is accompanied by an intense concern for the subjectivity of the partner *at other moments.*"[51] Again: "When there is a loss of autonomy in sex, the context . . . can be . . . one in which, on the whole, autonomy is respected and promoted"[52] And "denial of autonomy and denial of subjectivity are objectionable if they persist throughout an adult relationship, but *as phases* in a relationship characterized by mutual regard they can be all right, or even quite wonderful."[53]

One of Nussbaum's theses, then, is that a loss of autonomy, subjectivity, and individuality in sex, and the reduction of a person to his or her sexual body or its parts, in which the person is or becomes a tool or object, are morally acceptable if they occur within the background context of a psychologically healthy and morally sound relationship, an abiding relationship in which one's personhood—one's autonomy, subjectivity, and individuality—is generally respected and acknowledged. This solution to the sex problem seems plausible. It confirms the common (even if sexually conservative) intuition that one difference between morally permissible sexual acts and those that are wrongful because they are merely mutual use is the difference between sexual acts that occur in the context of a loving or caring relationship and those that occur in the absence of love, mutual care, or concern. Further, it appeals to our willingness to tolerate, exculpate, or even bless (as the partner's own private business) whatever nastiness that occurs in bed between two people *as long as* the rest, and the larger segment, of their relationship is morally sound. The lovers may sometimes engage in objectifying sexual games, by role-playing boss and secretary, client and prostitute, or teacher and student (phases of their relationship in which autonomy, subjectivity, and individuality might be sacrificed), since *outside* these occasional sexual games, they do display respect and regard for each other and abidingly support each other's humanity.

But this solution to the sex problem is inconsistent with Kant's Second Formulation, for that moral principle requires that a person be treated as an end *at the same time* he or she is being treated as a means.[54] On Nussbaum's thick minimalist externalism, small, sexually vulgar chunks of a couple's relationship, small pieces of noxious sexual objectification, are morally permissible in virtue of the larger or more frequent heavenly chunks of mutual respect that comprise their relationship. But it is not, in general, right (except, perhaps, for some utilitarians) that my treating you badly today is either *justified* or *excusable* if I treated you admirably the whole day yesterday and will treat you more superbly tomorrow and the next day. As Nussbaum acknowledges, Kant insists that we ought not to treat someone *merely* as means, instrumentally, or as an object, but by that qualification Kant does not mean that treating someone as a means, instrumentally, or as an object at *some* particular time is morally permissible as long as he or she is treated with respect as a full person at *other* particular times.[55] That Nussbaum's thick minimalist externalist solution to Kant's sex problem violates the Second Formulation in this way is not the fault of the details of her account of the proper background context; the problem arises whether the background context is postulated to be one of abiding mutual respect and regard, or love, or marriage, or something else. Any version of thick minimalist externalism violates Kant's prescription that someone who is treated as a means must be treated *at the same time* as an end. Thick minimalist externalism, in any version, fails because, unlike behavioral or psychological internalism, it makes no attempt to improve or fix the nature of sexual activity itself. It leaves sexual activity exactly as it was or would be, as essentially objectifying or instrumental, although it claims that even when having this character, it is morally permissible.

4b-2. Thick Extended Externalism

Thick extended externalism tries to have it both ways: to justify sexual activity when it occurs within the proper context *and* to fix the nature of the sexual acts that occur in that context. So Nussbaum's second proposal would seem to stand a better chance of conforming with the Second Formulation. In explaining the thesis that sexual objectification can be a wonderful or good thing in the proper context, Nussbaum says that in Lawrence's *Lady Chatterley's Lover,*

> both parties put aside their individuality and become identified with their bodily organs. They see one another in terms of those organs. And yet Kant's suggestion that in all such focusing on parts there is denial of humanity seems quite wrong. . . . The intense focusing of attention on the bodily parts seems an *addition*, rather than a subtraction.[56]

Nussbaum means that being reduced to one's body or its parts is an addition to one's personhood, not a subtraction from it, *as long as* the background context of an abiding, mutually respectful and regarding relationship exists, as she assumes it did between Constance Chatterley and Oliver Mellors. Nussbaum is claiming that sexual objectification, the reduction of a person to his or her flesh, and the loss of individuality and autonomy in sexual activity,[57] can be a wonderful or good aspect of life and sexuality. Being reduced to one's flesh, to one's genitals, supplements, or is an expansion or extension of, one's humanity, as long as it happens in a psychologically healthy and morally sound relationship.[58]

Nussbaum goes so far in this reasoning as to make the astonishing assertion that "In Lawrence, being treated as a cunt is a permission to expand the sphere of one's activity and fulfillment."[59] In the ablutionary context of an abiding relationship of mutual regard and respect, it is permissible and good for persons to descend fully to the level of their bodies, to become "cock" and "cunt," to become identified with their genitals, because in the rest of the relationship they are treated as *whole* persons. Or, more precisely, the addition of the objectification of being sexually reduced to their flesh *makes* their personhoods whole (it is, as Nussbaum writes, not a "subtraction"), as if without such a descent into their flesh they would remain partial, incomplete persons. This is suggested when Nussbaum writes, "Lawrence shows how a kind of sexual objectification . . . how the very surrender of autonomy in a certain sort of sex act can free energies that can be used to make the self *whole and full.*"[60] I suppose it is a metaphysical truth of some sort that to be whole and full (to be all that I can be, as the US Army, following J. S. Mill, used to promise in its television advertisements), I must realize all my potential. But some of this potential, it is not unreasonable to think, should not be realized, just because it would be immoral or perversely and stupidly imprudent to do so. Shall I, a professor of philosophy, fulfill my humanity by standing on street corners in the French Quarter and try homosexual tricking? Recall Kant: I may take on the other's ends only if those ends are themselves moral. Similarly, I may supplement or try to attain the fullness of my humanity only in ways that are moral. And whether adding to my personhood the identification of myself with my genitals is moral is precisely the question at issue. Merely because reducing myself to my genitals is an "expansion" of myself and of my "sphere of . . . activity" does little to justify it.

In any event, one implication of Nussbaum's requirement of a background context of an abiding, mutually respectful relationship worries me, whether this background context is part of a thick minimalist or a thick extended externalism: casual sex turns out to be morally wrong. In the sexual activity that transpires between strangers or between those who do not have much or any mutual regard for each other, sexual objectification and instrumentalization make those sexual acts wrong, because there is no background context of the requisite sort that would either justify the sexual objectification or transform it into something good. Casual sex is a descent to the level of the genitals with nothing for the persons to hang on to, nothing that would allow them to pull themselves back up to personhood when their sexual encounter is over. (This is, in effect, what Kant claims about prostitution and concubinage.)[61] Nussbaum explicitly states this sexually conservative trend in her thought, and does not seem to consider it a weakness or defect of her account. Sounding like Kant, she writes:

> For in the absence of any narrative history with the person, how can desire attend to anything else but the incidental, and how can one do more than use the body of the other as a tool of one's own states? . . . Can one really treat someone with . . . respect and concern . . . if one has sex with him in the anonymous spirit? . . . [T]he instrumental treatment of human beings, the treatment of human beings as tools of the purposes of another, is always morally problematic; if it does not take place in a larger context of regard for humanity, it is a central form of the morally objectionable.[62]

Now, it is one thing to point out that Nussbaum's thick externalism is inimical to casual sex, or sex in the "anonymous spirit," for many would agree with her. Yet there is another point to be made. If noxious sexual objectification is permissible or made into something good only in the context of an abiding, mutually respectful relationship, then it is morally impermissible to engage in sexual activity in getting a relationship *underway*. The two persons may not engage in sexual activity early in their acquaintance, before they know whether they will come to have such an abiding and respectful relationship, because the sexual objectification of that premature sex could not be redeemed or cleansed—the requisite background context is missing. But, as some of us know, engaging in sexual activity, even when the persons do not know each other very well, often reveals to them important information about whether to pursue a relationship, whether to attempt to ascend to the abiding level. This is another aspect of Nussbaum's conservative turn: the persons must *first* have that abiding, mutually respectful relationship before engaging in sexual activity.[63] It would be unconvincing to argue, in response, that sexual objectification in the early stages of their relationship is morally permissible, after all, because that sexual activity might contribute to the formation of an abiding, mutually respectful and regarding relationship that does succeed, later, in eliminating or cleansing the sexual objectification of the couple's sexual activity. That argument simply repeats in another form the dubious claim that morally bad phases or segments of a relationship are justified or excused in virtue of the larger or more frequent morally good segments of that relationship.

Let me close my discussion of Nussbaum's proposals by examining what she writes about sadomasochism. In response to her own question, "can sadomasochistic sexual acts ever have a simply Lawrentian character, rather than a more sinister character?" Nussbaum replies:

> There seems to be no . . . reason why the answer . . . cannot be "yes." I have no very clear intuitions on this point, . . . but it would seem that some narrative depictions of sadomasochistic activity do plausibly attribute to its consensual form a kind of Lawrentian character in which the willingness to be vulnerable to the infliction of pain . . . manifests a more complete trust and receptivity than could be found in other sexual acts. Pat Califia's . . . short story ["Jessie"] is one example of such a portrayal.[64]

This is unconvincing (it also sounds more like a Hamptonian psychological internalism than a thick externalism). Califia describes in this lesbian sadomasochistic short story a first sexual encounter between two *strangers*, women, who meet at a party, an encounter about which neither knows in advance whether it will lead to a narrative history or an abiding relationship between them. In the sexual encounter described by Califia, there is no background context of an abiding, let alone mutually respectful and regarding, relationship. This means that the nature of their sexual activity *as sadomasochism* is irrelevant; the main point is that each woman, as a stranger to the other, must, on Nussbaum's own account, be merely using each other in the "anonymous spirit." Something Califia writes in "Jessie" makes a mockery of Nussbaum's proposal:

> I hardly know you—I don't know if you play piano, I don't know what kind of business it is you run, I don't know your shoe size—but I know you better than anyone else in the world.[65]

If Nussbaum wants to justify sadomasochistic sexual acts, she must say that, *in the context of an abiding, mutually regarding and respectful relationship*, either (1) sadomasochistic sexuality is permissible, no matter how humiliating or brutal the acts are to the participants (thick minimalist externalism), or (2) sadomasochistic sexuality is permissible because, in this background context, it can be a good or wonderful thing, an expansion of the couple's humanity (thick expanded externalism). In either case, appealing to Califia's "Jessie" is of no help at all.

5. KANT'S SOLUTION

To satisfy (or provoke) the reader's curiosity about Kant, and to stimulate further research on the topic, I conclude by making some preliminary remarks about Kant's own solution to the sex problem. These remarks must be preliminary, because this topic requires a separate, lengthy essay on its own right.[66]

Kant argues in both the earlier *Lectures on Ethics* and the later *Metaphysics of Morals* that sexual activity is morally permissible only within the context of a heterosexual, lifelong, and monogamous marriage, a contractual marriage formalized in law. Hence Kant advances a thick externalism. (I will soon suggest that his externalism is also minimalist.) Kant barely argues in these texts, or argues weakly, that marriage must be lifelong and heterosexual.[67] But Kant's argument that the only permissible sexual activity is married sexual activity is distinctive and presented forcefully. In the *Metaphysics of Morals*, for example, Kant writes:

> There is only one condition under which this is possible: that while one person is acquired by the other *as if it were a thing*, the one who is acquired acquires the other in turn; for in this way each reclaims itself and restores its personality. But acquiring a member of a human being [i.e., access to or possession of the other's genitals and associated sexual capacities] is at the same time acquiring the whole person, since a person is an absolute unity. Hence it is not only admissible for the sexes to surrender and to accept each other for enjoyment under the condition of marriage, but it is possible for them to do so *only* under this condition.[68]

Kant's idea seems to be that sexual activity, with its essential sexual objectification, is morally permissible only in marriage, because only in marriage can each of the persons engage in sexual activity *without losing* their own personality—their personhood or humanity. In a marriage of a Kantian type, each person is "acquired" by the other person (along with his or her genitals and sexual capacities) as if he or she were an object, and hence, by being acquired, loses his or her humanity (autonomy, individuality). But because the acquisition in marriage is reciprocal, each person *regains* his or her personhood (and hence does not lose it, after all). When I "surrender" myself to you, and you thereby acquire me, but you also "surrender" yourself to me, and I thereby acquire you, which "you" includes the "me" that you have acquired, we each surrender but then re-acquire ourselves. (I think this means that the "I do"s must be said simultaneously.)

There are many puzzles in Kant's solution.[69] One is that Kant does not explicitly state in laying out his solution that through such a reciprocal surrender and acquisition the persons in some robust sense treat each other as persons or acknowledge each other's humanity as an end, in bed or otherwise. That is, after laying out his relentless criticism of sexual desire and activity, Kant never poses the question, "How might two people, married or not, treat themselves and each other as persons during sexual activity?" Kant is notorious for being stingy with examples, but why here? In fact, in only one place that I could find, a mere footnote in the *Metaphysics of Morals*, does Kant use the language of the Second Formulation to speak about marriage:

> if I say "my wife," this signifies a special, namely a rightful, relation of the possessor to an object as a *thing* (even though the object is also a person). Possession (*physical* possession), however, is the condition of being able to *manage* . . . something as a thing, even if this must, in another respect, be treated at the same time as a person.[70]

But neither in the footnote nor in the text does Kant explain what "in another respect" being treated as a person amounts to. The language of the Second Formulation is plainly here, in the footnote, including the crucial "at the same time," but not its substance. Further, in the text, Kant refrains from using the language of the Second Formulation:

> What is one's own here does not . . . mean what is one's own in the sense of property in the person of another (for a human being cannot have property in himself, much less in another person), but means what is one's own in the sense of usufruct . . . to make direct use of a person *as of* a thing, as a means to my end, but still *without infringing* upon his personality.[71]

Kant is asserting, I think, that it is permissible in *some* contexts to use another person as a means or treat as an object, merely with the other's free and informed consent, as long as one does not violate the humanity of the other in some other way, as long as one allows him or her otherwise to retain intact his or her personhood. The reciprocal surrender and acquisition of Kantian marriage, which involves a contractual free and informed agreement to exchange selves, *prevents* this (possibly extra) denial or loss of personhood. But this moral principle is far removed from the Second Formulation as Kant usually articulates and understands it.

Kant, I now submit, advances an externalism that is minimalist: the objectification and instrumentality that attach to sexuality remain even in marital sexual activity. Hence not even Kant abides by the "at the same time" requirement of the Second Formulation in his solution to the sex problem. Nussbaum, for one, seems to recognize Kant's minimalism when she writes, "sexual desire, according to his analysis, drives out every possibility of respect. This is so even in marriage."[72] Raymond Belliotti, by contrast, finds thick extended externalism in Kant:

> Kant suggests that two people can efface the wrongful commodification inherent in sex and thereby redeem their own humanity only by mutually exchanging "rights to their whole person." The *implication* is that a deep, abiding relationship of the requisite sort ensures that sexual activity is not separated from personal interaction which honors individual dignity.[73]

But the "implication" is something Belliotti illicitly reads into Kant's texts. Kant nowhere says that in marriage, which is for him a contractual relationship characterized by mutual acquisition of persons as if they were objects (hardly a "deep, abiding relationship"), sexual activity "honors individual dignity." Belliotti reads Kant as if Kant were Nussbaum. When Kant asserts in the *Metaphysics of Morals* that sexual activity is permissible only in marriage, he speaks about the *acquisition* or *possession* of the other person by each spouse, and never mentions love, altruism, or benevolence. For similar reasons, Robert Baker and Frederick Elliston's view must be rejected. They claim that, according to Kant, "marriage transubstantiates immoral sexual intercourse into morally permissible human copulation by transforming a manipulative masturbatory relationship into one of altruistic unity."[74] But Kant never says anything about "altruism" in his account of marriage or of sexual activity in marriage; nowhere, for example, does he claim that the persons come to treat each other as ends and respect their humanity in sexual activity by unconditionally providing sexual pleasure to each other. Indeed, Kant writes in the *Metaphysics of Morals* that "benevolence . . . deter[s] one from carnal enjoyment."[75] Further, both these readings of Kant are insensitive to the sharp contrast between Kant's glowing account of male friendship, in both the *Lectures on Ethics* and the *Metaphysics of Morals*, as a morally exemplary and fulfilling balance of love and respect, and Kant's dry account of heterosexual marriage, which makes marriage look like a continuation, or culmination, of the battle of the sexes. Kant never says about marriage, for example, anything close to this: "Friendship . . . is the union of two persons through equal mutual love and respect. . . . [E]ach participat[es] and shar[es] sympathetically in the other's well-being through the morally good will that unites them."[76]

Of course, the virtue of Belliotti's reading, and that of Baker and Elliston, is that if sexual activity can indeed be imbued with Kantian respect or "altruism," then the "at the same time" requirement of the Second Formulation is satisfied. But there is good evidence that Kant's own view is minimalist. For example, when Kant writes in the *Lectures on Ethics* that

> If . . . a man wishes to satisfy his desire, and a woman hers, they stimulate each other's desire; their inclinations meet, but their object is not human nature but sex, and each of them dishonours the human nature of the other. They make of humanity an instrument for the satisfaction of their lusts and inclinations, and dishonour it by placing it on a level with animal nature.[77]

He intends this description to apply to sexual activity even in marriage, and not only to casual sex, prostitution, or concubinage. This point is confirmed by Kant's letter to C. G. Schütz, who had written to Kant to complain about Kant's similar treatment of sexuality in the later *Metaphysics of Morals*. To this objection offered by Schütz, "You cannot really believe that a man makes an object of a woman just by engaging in marital cohabitation with her, and vice versa," Kant concisely replies: "if the cohabitation is assumed to be *marital*, that is, *lawful*, . . . the authorization is already contained in the concept."[78] Note that Kant does not deny that objectification still occurs in marital sex; he simply says it is permissible, or authorized. Schütz makes the point another way: "married people do not become *res fungibiles* just by sleeping together," to which Kant replies: "An enjoyment of this sort involves at once the thought of this person as merely *functional*, and that in fact is what the reciprocal use of each other's sexual organs by two people *is*."[79] "Is," that is, even in marriage.

Further, that marriage is designed and defined by Kant to be only about sexuality, about having access to the other person's sexual capacities and sexual body parts—for enjoyment or pleasure, not necessarily for reproduction—also suggests that his solution is minimalist. Consider Kant's definition of marriage in the *Metaphysics of Morals*: "Sexual union in accordance with principle is *marriage* (*matrimonium*), that is, the union of two persons of different sexes for lifelong possession of each other's sexual attributes."[80] There is no suggestion in this definition of marriage that Belliottian human, individual dignity will make its way into marital sexual activity (quite the contrary). Howard Williams tartly comments, about Kant's notion of marriage, that "sex, for Kant, seems simply to be a form of mutual exploitation for which one must pay the price of marriage. He represents sex as a commodity which ought only to be bought and sold for life in the marriage contract."[81] If sexual activity in marriage is, for Kant, a commodity, it has hardly been cleansed of its essentially objectionable qualities. Kant's view of marriage has much in common with St. Paul's (see 1 Corinthians 7), in which each person has power over the body of the other spouse, and each spouse has a "conjugal debt" to engage in sexual activity with the other nearly on demand.[82] That marriage is defined by Kant to be only about access to sex is what is astounding, even incomprehensible, to the contemporary mind, and may explain why modern philosophers are quick to attribute to Kant more congenial solutions to the sex problem.

Finally, a commonly neglected aspect of the Second Formulation, that one must *also* treat the humanity in one's own person as an end, is important in understanding Kant's solution to the sex problem. Duties to self are important for Kant, a fact overlooked by those philosophers (for example, Mappes and Goldman) who emphasize the treat-the-other-as-an-end part of the Second Formulation. Notice the prominence of Kant's discussion of the duties to self in the *Lectures on Ethics.* They are elaborately discussed early in the text, well before Kant discusses moral duties to others, and Kant in the *Lectures* launches into his treatment of sexuality immediately after he concludes his account of duties to self in general and before he, finally, gets around to duties to others. Allen Wood is one of the few commentators on Kant who, I think, gets this right:

> He thinks sexual intercourse is "a degradation of humanity" because it is an act in which "people *make themselves* into an object of enjoyment, and hence into a thing" (VE 27:346). He regards sex as permissible only within marriage, and even there it is in itself "a merely animal union." (MS 6:425)[83]

Kant does make it clear that a duty to treat the humanity in one's own person as an end is his primary concern in restricting sexual activity to marriage:

> there ar[ises] from one's duty to oneself, that is, to the humanity in one's own person, a right (*ius personale*) of both sexes to acquire each other as persons *in the manner of things* by marriage.[84]

For Kant, then, the crux of the argument about sex and marriage does not turn on a duty to avoid sexually objectifying the other, but to avoid the sexual objectification of the self. It would be an ironic reading of Kant to say that he claims that *my right to use you* in sexual activity in marriage arises from *my duty to myself.* What Kant is saying, without irony, is that as a result of the duty toward myself, I cannot enter into sexual relations with you unless I preserve my personhood; you, likewise, cannot enter into sexual relations with me unless you are able to preserve your own personhood. Each of us can accomplish that goal only by mutual surrender and acquisition, the exchange of rights to our persons and to our genitals and sexual capacities that constitutes marriage. It is not the right to use you sexually that is my goal, although I do gain that right. My goal is to preserve my own personhood in the face of the essentially objectifying nature of sexuality. But preserving my own personhood, as admirable as that might be, is not the same thing as treating you with dignity (or altruism) during marital sexual activity. Kant has still done nothing to accomplish that—nor, if I am right, was that his intention.

6. METAPHILOSOPHICAL FINALE

Howard Williams has made a shrewd observation about Kant's solution to the sex problem:

> [A]n important premise of Kant's argument is that sexual relations necessarily involve treating oneself and one's partner as things. . . . [T]o demonstrate convincingly that marriage is the only ethically desirable context for sex, Kant ought to start from better premises than these.[85]

Let me explain what is interesting here. Bernard Baumrin argues that if we want to justify sexual activity *at all*, we should start our philosophizing by conceding the worst: "I begin . . . by admitting the most damaging facts . . . that any theory of sexual morality must countenance," viz., that "human sexual interaction is essentially manipulative—physically, psychologically, emotionally, and even intellectually."[86] Starting with premises about sexuality any less ugly or more optimistic would make justifying sexual activity too easy. Williams's point is that if we want to justify the specific claim that sex is *permissible only in marriage*, starting with Kantian premises about the nature of sex makes *that* task too easy. If sex is in its essence wholesome, or if, as in Mappes and Goldman, sexual activity does not significantly differ from other activities that involve human interaction, then it becomes easier both to justify sexual activity and to justify sex outside of marriage. Those, including many Christian philosophers and theologians, who assume the worst about sexuality to begin with, gain an advantage in defending the view that sexuality must be restricted to matrimony.[87] This tactic is copied in a milder way by Nussbaum and Hampton, who reject casual sex. The convincing intellectual trick would be to assume the *best* about sex, that it is by its nature wholesome, and then argue, *anyway*, that it should be restricted to lifelong, monogamous matrimony and that casual sex is morally wrong.[88] Perhaps the liberals Baumrin and Goldman are trying to pull off the reverse trick, in that they admit the worst about sexuality and still come out with a permissive sexual morality. But in admitting the worst, how do they avoid concluding, with Kant, that sexual activity is permissible only in the restrictive conditions of marriage? Perhaps they succeed, or think they do, only by reading the Second Formulation in a very narrow or an easily satisfied way.[89]

The topics in this paper are developed in Alan Soble, "Comments on 'Good Sex on Kantian Grounds, or A Reply to Alan Soble,' or A Reply to Joshua Schulz," *Essays in Philosophy* 8, no. 2 (June 2007); http://www.humboldt.edu/~essays/soblereply.html

NOTES

1. Immanuel Kant's views on sexuality are presented mainly in his *Lectures on Ethics* [ca. 1780], trans. Louis Infield (Indianapolis, IN: Hackett, 1963), pp. 162–71, and in *The Metaphysics of Morals* [1797], trans. Mary Gregor (Cambridge: Cambridge University Press, 1996), pp. 61–64, 126–28, 178–80. There is also much on sex, gender, and marriage in his *Anthropology from a Pragmatic Point of View*, trans. Mary J. Gregor (The Hague: Martinus Nijhoff, 1974). Part of the sex section from the *Lectures on Ethics* is reprinted in this volume, pp. 199–205. ["This volume" in these notes refers to my *The Philosophy of Sex*, 4th edition (Lanham, MD: Rowman and Littlefield, 2002).]

2. For more on the Kantian view of the nature of sex, see my discussion of metaphysical sexual pessimism in "The Fundamentals of the Philosophy of Sex," in this volume, pp. xxi–xxiv.

3. See Bernard Baumrin, "Sexual Immorality Delineated," in *Philosophy and Sex*, 2nd ed., ed. Robert Baker and Frederick Elliston (Amherst, NY: Prometheus Books, 1984), pp. 300–11, pp. 300–302.

4. Kant, *Lectures on Ethics*, p. 164; in this volume, p. 200.

5. "In desire you are compromised in the eyes of the object of desire, since you have displayed that you have designs which are vulnerable to his intentions" (Roger Scruton, *Sexual Desire: A Moral Philosophy of the Erotic* [New York: Free Press, 1986], p. 82).

6. See Virginia Held, "Coercion and Coercive Offers," in J. Roland Pennock and John W. Chapman, eds., *Coercion: Nomos VIX* (Chicago: Aldine, 1972), pp. 49–62; at p. 58: "A person unable to spurn an offer may act as unwillingly as a person unable to resist a threat. Consider the distinction between rape and seduction. In one case constraint and threat are operative, in the other inducement and offer. If the degree of inducement is set high enough in the case of seduction, there may seem to be little difference in the extent of coercion involved. In both cases, persons may act against their own wills." I think we do recognize that a sexual offer may be a powerful, even overwhelming, inducement. Whether a person is able to resist depends at least on his or her nature (desires, needs) and what is being offered.

7. Kant, *Metaphysics of Morals*, p. 62.

8. Kant, *Lectures*, p. 164; in this volume, p. 200. Kant also suggests that sexuality can reduce humans *below* the level of animals; animals in their instinctual innocence do not and

cannot use each other sexually. See Kant, *Lectures*, pp. 122–23: "In the case of animals inclinations are already determined by subjectively compelling factors; in their case . . . disorderliness is impossible. But if man gives free rein to his inclinations, he sinks lower than an animal because he then lives in a state of disorder which does not exist among animals."

9. For Adam Smith, "the passion by which nature unites the two sexes . . . [is] the most furious of the passions" (*The Theory of Moral Sentiments* [New York: Augustus M. Kelley, 1966], part 1, sect. 2, chap. 1, p. 33).

10. Kant, *Groundwork of the Metaphysic of Morals*, trans. H. J. Paton (New York: Harper Torchbooks, 1964), pp. 95–96 (AK 4:428). Marcia W. Baron, in *Kantian Ethics Almost without Apology* (Ithaca, NY: Cornell University Press, 1995), pp. 199–204, and H. J. Paton, well before her, in *The Categorical Imperative: A Study in Kant's Moral Philosophy* (New York: Harper and Row, 1967), pp. 55–57, point out that in his later works Kant retracts or softens this judgment. Baron's discussion is more complete and especially enlightening.

11. Michael Ruse, *Homosexuality: A Philosophical Inquiry* (Oxford: Basil Blackwell, 1988), p. 185.

12. Kant, *Groundwork*, p. 96 (429); p. 95 (428).

13. Ibid., p. 98 (430); see also *Metaphysics*, p. 199.

14. Kant, *Groundwork*, p. 97 (429). See Christine Korsgaard, "Creating the Kingdom of Ends: Reciprocity and Responsibility in Personal Relations," *Philosophical Perspectives* 6, *Ethics* (1992), pp. 305–32 at p. 309: "respect gets its most positive and characteristic expression at precisely the moments when we must act together. . . . If my end requires your act for its achievement, then I must let you make it your end too. . . . Thus I must make your ends and reasons mine, and I must choose [my ends] in such a way that they can be yours."

15. C. E. Harris Jr. seems to have this weaker version of the Second Formulation in mind when he claims that we are permitted to use another person in our transactions or interactions with him or her (e.g., a post office worker, doctor, professor) and long as, beyond using these persons for our purposes, we "do nothing to negate [their] status as a moral being," "do not deny him his status as a person," or "do not obstruct [their] humanity." Harris applies this principle to casual sex: as long as "neither person is overriding the freedom of the other or diminishing the ability of the other to be an effective goal-pursuing agent," it is permissible (*Applying Moral Theories*, 4th ed. [Belmont, CA: Wadsworth, 2002], pp. 153–54, 164).

16. Goldman, "Plain Sex," in this volume, pp. 39–55, at p. 40.

17. Ibid., p. 51. Kant would have said "subjective," "discretionary," or "arbitrary" ends, instead of Goldman's "private" ends, but he would be making the same point.

18. Ibid.

19. Ibid.

20. David Archard's position is similar to Goldman's. See his *Sexual Consent* (Boulder, CO: Westview, 1998), p. 41 (italics added):

> If Harry has sex with Sue solely for the purpose of deriving sexual gratification from the encounter and with no concern for what Sue might get out of it, if Harry pursues this end single-mindedly and never allows himself to think of

how it might be for Sue, then Harry treats Sue merely as a means to his ends. If, *by contrast*, Harry derives pleasure from his sex with Sue but also strives to attend to Sue's pleasure and conducts the encounter in a way that is sensitive to her needs, then Harry does not treat Sue merely as a means.

That the sexual relationship between Sue and Harry is consensual does not mean that neither one of them is treating the other merely as a means.

21. See Hobbes: "the delight men take in delighting, is not sensual, but a pleasure or joy of the mind consisting in the imagination of the power they have so much to please" ("Human Nature, or the Fundamental Elements of Policy," in *The English Works of Thomas Hobbes*, vol. IV, ed. Sir William Molesworth [Germany: Scientia Verlag Aalen, 1966], chap. 9, sect. 15, p. 48).

22. See Thomas Nagel, "Sexual Perversion," in this volume, pp. 13–15.

23. Marquis de Sade, *Justine, Philosophy in the Bedroom, and Other Writings*, trans. Richard Seaver and Austryn Wainhouse (New York: Grove Press, 1965), in *Philosophy in the Bedroom*, pp. 343–44.

24. The conditionality of giving pleasure is inherent in Baumrin's approach: "the crucial element in creating specifically sexual rights and duties is the desire to use another as a means for a certain kind of end and the willingness to offer oneself to that person as an inducement" ("Sexual Immorality Delineated," p. 304). One person in effect says to the other: "I wish to use you as an instrument for my sexual purposes and therefore undertake to make myself the instrument of your sexual purposes to the extent that you accept my proposal" (pp. 303–304; italics omitted).

25. Kant, *Metaphysics*, p. 199.

26. See my discussion, "Orgasmic Justice," in *Sexual Investigations* (New York: New York University Press, 1996), pp. 53–57.

27. Requiring that persons inject unconditional giving into sexual activity is incompatible with the letter and spirit of Goldman's "Plain Sex," which is in part devoted to undermining restrictive in favor of permissive sexual ethics. Casual sex in which there are no commitments, consensual sex between perfect strangers, and prostitution, which liberal sexual ethics usually permit, would seem to be the least likely situations in which to find altruistic sexual giving, although it is not impossible.

28. Hampton, "Defining Wrong and Defining Rape," in Keith Burgess-Jackson, ed., *A Most Detestable Crime: New Philosophical Essays on Rape* (New York: Oxford University Press, 1999), pp. 118–56, at p. 147.

29. Ibid., p. 147.

30. It is interesting that Hampton makes this Kantian point about the dangerous nature of sex, because she also criticizes what she takes to be Kant's overly pessimistic metaphysics of sex; see ibid., pp. 146–47.

31. Ibid., pp. 147–48.

32. Ibid., p. 150.

33. A similar view is advanced by Alan Donagan, in *The Theory of Morality* (Chicago: University of Chicago Press, 1977), who praises "life-affirming and nonexploitative" sexuality. By contrast, "sexual acts which are life-denying in their imaginative significance, or

are exploitative, are impermissible." He rejects, specifically, sadomasochism, prostitution, and casual sex (p. 107; italics omitted).

34. Califia, "Introduction," *Macho Sluts* (Los Angeles: Alyson Books, 1988), p. 9.

35. Mappes's Kantian theory of sexual ethics can be understood as a solution to the Kantian sex problem, for he concedes that "the domain of sexual interaction seems to offer ample opportunity for 'using' another person" (from Mappes's introductory essay to chapter 4, "Sexual Morality," in *Social Ethics: Morality and Social Policy*, 6th ed., ed. Thomas A. Mappes and Jane S. Zembaty (New York: McGraw-Hill, 2002), pp. 157–64, at p. 160; or see the 4th edition (1992), p. 192; or the 5th (1997), p. 153).

36. For another Kantian consent view, see Raymond Belliotti, "A Philosophical Analysis of Sexual Ethics," *Journal of Social Philosophy* 10, no. 3 (1979): 8–11.

37. I interpret Baumrin's theory of sexual ethics as an amalgam of Mappes's thin externalism and Goldman's behavioral internalism. For Baumrin, consent is both necessary and sufficient for the morality of sexual activity, as in Mappes; but Baumrin also thinks that each person consents, in particular, to be the instrument for the sexual satisfaction of the other, as in Goldman ("Sexual Immorality Delineated," p. 304).

38. Mappes, "Sexual Morality and the Concept of Using Another Person."

39. Goldman, "Plain Sex," in this volume, pp. 49–51.

40. Murphy, "Some Ruminations on Women, Violence, and the Criminal Law," in Jules Coleman and Allen Buchanan, eds., *In Harm's Way: Essays in Honor of Joel Feinberg* (Cambridge: Cambridge University Press, 1994), pp. 209–30, at p. 218.

41. Alan Wertheimer argues that "Have sexual relations with me or I will dissolve our dating relationship" is *not* "a coercive proposal" (although it *might* still be wrong); see his "Consent and Sexual Relations," in *Legal Theory* 2 (1996), Special Issue: Sex and Consent, Part 1: 105–106.

42. I found this interesting passage in Rex Stout's Nero Wolfe mystery novel *Before Midnight* (New York: Bantam, 1955): "a bill which . . . had been introduced into the English Parliament in 1770 . . . ran[:] All women of whatever age, rank, profession, or degree, whether virgins, maids, or widows, that shall, from and after this Act, impose upon, seduce, and betray into matrimony, any of His Majesty's subjects, by the scents, paints, cosmetic washes, artificial teeth, false hair, Spanish wool, iron stays, hoops, high heeled shoes, bolstered hips, shall incur the penalty of the law in force against witchcraft and like misdemeanors and the marriage, upon conviction, shall stand null and void" (p. 54; italics omitted). Stout doesn't say whether the bill passed.

43. Mappes, "Sexual Morality and the Concept of Using Another Person."

44. This is the thrust of Wertheimer's "Consent and Sexual Relations."

45. Mappes, "Sexual Morality and the Concept of Using Another Person."

46. Mappes's free and informed consent test seems to imply that prostitution is permissible if the prostitute is not exploited, taken advantage of in virtue of her economic needs. Baumrin's consent view seems to imply that prostitution is permissible, because either party may "discharge" the other's duty of providing sexual satisfaction ("Sexual Immorality Delineated," p. 303; see also p. 305). But Goldman's position on prostitution is unclear. He does not advance a mere free and informed consent test, but lays it down that each person must make a sexual object of himself or herself for the sake of the

pleasure of the other, or must provide sexual pleasure to the other so that their activity is mutually pleasurable. That seems to condemn prostitution, unless the client provides pleasure for the prostitute, or unless the prostitute's pleasure in receiving money makes their encounter "mutual" enough for Goldman.

47. Mappes, "Sexual Morality and the Concept of Using Another Person."

48. Kant, *Lectures*, p. 163; in several places I replaced "can" in Infield's translation with "may"; Kant's point is moral, not about natural or conceptual possibility.

49. The "New Natural Law" philosophers (as well as the old ones) emphasize the difference that *only* in (hetero)sexuality can a new life be generated by a procreative sexual act. For example, see John Finnis's contribution to "Is Homosexual Conduct Wrong? A Philosophical Exchange," in *New Republic* 209, no. 20 (1993); and his "Law, Morality, and 'Sexual Orientation,'" *Notre Dame Law Review* 69, no. 5 (1994): 1049–76, at pp. 1066ff.

50. Martha C. Nussbaum, "Objectification," *Philosophy and Public Affairs* 24, no. 4 (Autumn 1995): 249–91. In a slightly revised version of "Objectification," which appears in Nussbaum's *Sex and Social Justice* (New York: Oxford University Press, 1999), pp. 213–39, she changed "without causing him pain" to "without causing him unwanted pain" (p. 223).

51. Ibid.

52. Ibid.

53. Ibid.

54. "The words 'at the same time' . . . must not be overlooked: they are absolutely essential to Kant's statement" of the Second Formulation (Paton, *The Categorical Imperative*, p. 165).

55. There is a similar problem of Kant exegesis in Baumrin's "Sexual Immorality Delineated." He claims that what is morally wrong, for Kant, is treating a person in *every* respect as a means. What is permissible, for Baumrin (or Baumrin's Kant), then, is treating a person as a means as long as the person is treated in (at least and perhaps only) *one* respect *not* as a means (p. 300). What this means and whether it is compatible with the Second Formulation are unclear. Note that Baumrin's rendition of the Second Formulation (he quotes the translation of Lewis White Beck) does not include the phrase "at the same time" (p. 310, note 1).

56. Nussbaum, "Objectification" (italics added).

57. Nussbaum could cite Scott Tucker: "one reason so many of us like sex so much is because we can selectively entrust ourselves to annihilation, and rise with new life from our graves and beds. . . . Of course, not all sex is like this; not all sex should be; plenty of sex is companionable, habitual, and self-possessed" ("Gender, Fucking, and Utopia: An Essay in Response to John Stoltenberg's *Refusing to Be a Man*," *Social Text* 27 [1990]: 3–34, at p. 30).

58. By contrast, for Roger Scruton, the reduction of a person to flesh, as occurs in masturbation, is obscene; "masturbation involves a concentration on the body and its curious pleasures" (*Sexual Desire: A Moral Philosophy of the Erotic* [New York: Free Press, 1986], p. 319). See also p. 139: in obscenity and perversion, "we suffer that dangerous shift of attention which is the mark of original sin—the shift from the embodied person to the dominating and dissolving body."

59. Nussbaum, "Objectification." It is interesting to consider that "though cunt was a standard term until the 16th century, it then became regarded as so vulgar as to be taboo through the 20th century. . . . Only when the word began to be used by writers such as D. H. Lawrence and James Joyce did the taboo begin to crumble" (Alan Richter, *Dictionary of Sexual Slang* [New York: John Wiley, 1993], p. 59). Maybe Lawrence et al. killed the taboo surrounding the *use* of the word "cunt," but they did little to destroy its sharp negative connotations, as when we call a woman (or a man), disparagingly, a "cunt," or when we say that a man (or a woman) treats a woman as a "cunt."

60. Nussbaum, "Objectification" (italics added).

61. Kant, *Lectures*, pp. 165–66.

62. Nussbaum, "Objectification." I am not able to explore here the tension between Nussbaum's rejecting sexuality in the "anonymous spirit" and her legal and moral defense of prostitution, as presented in "'Whether From Reason or Prejudice.' Taking Money for Bodily Services," *Sex and Social Justice*, pp. 276–98. See my discussion of Nussbaum in *Pornography, Sex, and Feminism* (Amherst, NY: Prometheus Books, 2002), pp. 72–78, 163–74.

63. Contrast, on the value of premarital sex for women, the essay by the conservative feminist Sidney Callahan ("Abortion and the Sexual Agenda: A Case for Prolife Feminism"), in *Abortion and Catholicism*, ed. Jung and Shannon, pp. 128–40, and the essay by the liberal feminist Ellen Willis ("Abortion: Is a Woman a Person?"), in *Powers of Desire: The Politics of Sexuality*, ed. Ann Snitow, Christine Stansell, and Sharon Thompson, 471–76 (New York: Monthly Review Press, 1983).

64. Nussbaum, "Objectification." Nussbaum mistakenly calls Califia's short story "Jenny."

65. Califia, "Jessie," in *Macho Sluts*, pp. 28–62, at p. 60. This was said by the top, Jessie, to her bottom, Liz, the morning after their sexual encounter.

66. Some important accounts of Kant on sexuality are provided by Vincent M. Cooke, "Kant, Teleology, and Sexual Ethics," *International Philosophical Quarterly* 31, no. 1 (1991): 3–13; Onora O'Neill, "Between Consenting Adults," in her *Constructions of Reason: Explorations of Kant's Practical Philosophy* (Cambridge: Cambridge University Press, 1989), pp. 105–25; Susan Meld Shell, *The Embodiment of Reason: Kant on Spirit, Generation, and Community* (Chicago: University of Chicago Press, 1996) and *The Rights of Reason: A Study of Kant's Philosophy and Politics* (Toronto: University of Toronto Press, 1980); Irving Singer, *The Nature of Love, vol. 2: Courtly and Romantic* (Chicago: University of Chicago Press, 1984); Keith Ward, *The Development of Kant's View of Ethics* (Oxford: Basil Blackwell, 1972); and others referred to in the notes below. (What follows in section 5 of this essay is an addition to the version published in *Essays in Philosophy*, and makes it more "whole.")

67. Kant's philosophical objections to homosexuality and, a fortiori, to homosexual marriage, are examined critically in my "Kant and Sexual Perversion," *Monist* 86, no. 1 (2003), forthcoming.

68. Kant, *Metaphysics*, p. 62. See *Lectures*, p. 167.

69. On problems with the notion of a metaphysical "union" of two-into-one, and the implications of such a union for the fate of individual autonomy and genuine benevo-

lence, see my "Union, Autonomy, and Concern," in *Love Analyzed*, ed. Roger Lamb (Belmont, CA: Westview Press, 1997), pp. 65–92. The ideas I would like to develop is that a Kantian marriage union destroys the autonomy that lies at the heart of Kantian humanity or personhood and also logically prevents the spouses from being genuinely benevolent to each other, as required by the Second Formulation's insistence on showing respect for the other.

70. Kant, *Metaphysics*, p. 126.

71. Ibid., p. 127; italics added.

72. Nussbaum, "Objectification."

73. Belliotti, *Good Sex: Perspectives on Sexual Ethics* (Lawrence: University Press of Kansas, 1993), p. 100; italics added.

74. Baker and Elliston, "Introduction," *Philosophy and Sex*, 1st ed. (Amherst, NY: Prometheus Books, 1975), pp. 8–9; 2nd ed. (Amherst, NY: Prometheus Books, 1984), pp. 17–18. Or see the "Introduction" in Robert B. Baker, Kathleen J. Wininger, and Frederick A. Elliston, eds., *Philosophy and Sex*, 3rd ed. (Amherst, NY: Prometheus Books, 1998), p. 23.

75. Kant, *Metaphysics*, p. 180. In her earlier translation of the *Metaphysics*, Gregor rendered this line "benevolence . . . stop[s] short of carnal enjoyment" (*The Doctrine of Virtue: Part II of the Metaphysic of Morals* [New York: Harper Torchbooks, 1964], p. 90).

76. Kant, *Metaphysics*, p. 215. There are maybe two lines in the *Lectures* that might be construed as supporting a "love" or "altruism" reading of his solution to the sex problem. These lines might explain why Robert Trevas, Arthur Zucker, and Donald Borchert (*Philosophy of Sex and Love: A Reader* [Upper Saddle River, NJ: Prentice-Hall, 1997], p. 129) claim that, *for Kant,*

> If . . . we give our whole selves to each other, we become committed to concern for each other's total well-being and overall happiness. Indeed, we find ourselves treating each other as "ends" and not simply as "means."

But on the basis of Kant's slender statement that in marriage one person obtains "the right to dispose over the [other] person as a whole—over the welfare and happiness and generally over all the circumstances of that person" (*Lectures*, pp. 166–67), we cannot conclude that Kant meant that in exchanging their selves the spouses thereby become concerned for each other's well-being or treat each other as ends. Similarly, in the statement "one devotes one's person to another, one devotes not only sex but the whole person; the two cannot be separated. . . . [O]ne yields one's person, body and soul, for good and ill in every respect, so that the other has complete rights over it" (*Lectures*, p. 167), Kant does not say that love or altruism overcomes mere use. Any hint of altruism in the "devotes" that occurs in this passage is erased by the closing "so that the other has complete rights over it," which reasserts the acquisition or possession of Kantian marriage. Even if Kant thought that marriage should include love, this does not mean that he thought that the love in marriage is that which makes sexual activity permissible; nor does it mean that he thought that love in marriage fixed the nature of the sexual act, from something objectifying to something not objectifying.

77. Ibid., p. 164.

78. Kant, *Philosophical Correspondence: 1759–99*, trans. Arnulf Zweig (Chicago: University of Chicago Press, 1967), letter dated July 10, 1797, p. 235.

79. Ibid., pp. 235–36; italics added to "is."

80. Kant, *Metaphysics*, p. 62.

81. Williams, *Kant's Political Philosophy* (New York: St. Martin's Press, 1983), p. 117.

82. For some hints of Kant's indebtedness to Paul, see *Metaphysics*, pp. 179–80.

83. Wood, *Kant's Ethical Thought* (Cambridge: Cambridge University Press, 1999), p. 2; italics added. Here is the line in the *Metaphysics* to which Wood refers ("MS 6:425") at the end: "even the permitted bodily union of the sexes in marriage . . . [is] a union which is in itself merely an animal union" (p. 179). This is more evidence that Kant's solution is minimalist.

84. Kant, *Metaphysics*, p. 64.

85. Williams, *Kant's Political Philosophy*, p. 117.

86. Baumrin, "Sexual Immorality Delineated," pp. 300, 301.

87. Mary Geach (a daughter of Peter Geach and Elizabeth Anscombe), for example, claims, in the manner of Augustine and Jerome, that Christianity "encourages men and women to recognize the whoredom in their own souls. It is a decline from Christianity to see oneself as better than a prostitute if one is . . . given to masturbatory fantasies, or if one defiles ones [*sic*] marriage with contraception." Geach, not surprisingly, limits sexual activity to marriage ("Marriage: Arguing to a First Principle in Sexual Ethics," in *Moral Truth and Moral Tradition: Essays in Honour of Peter Geach and Elizabeth Anscombe*, ed. Luke Gormally [Dublin: Four Courts Press, 1994], pp. 177–93, at p. 178).

88. But what wholesome definition of the sexual impulse could there be, that would soften the sex problem—that sexual desire essentially wants only to please the other for the other's sake? That metaphysical optimism would be a convenient account of the nature of human sexuality, in which *eros* is already by its nature perfectly moral and would not need marriage, or anything else (not even consent?), to improve or restrain it. Maybe, then, a nasty metaphysical account of sexuality is *required* if one wants to argue that only in marriage is sexual activity morally permissible.

89. An early, short, and rough version of this essay (titled "Kant on Sex") was presented at a meeting of the Society for the Philosophy of Sex and Love, held with the Central Division meetings of the American Philosophical Association, New Orleans, May 8, 1999. I thank, for their assistance, Laura D. Kaplan, who was in the audience during the presentation, and Natalie Brender, the commentator on my paper. Another version of this essay (titled "Sexual Use") was presented at Washburn University (Topeka, Kansas) as the Keynote Lecture of the 54th Mountain-Plains Philosophy Conference, October 13, 2000. I thank the audience for its questions and, especially, Russell Jacobs and the other organizers of the Conference for their kind invitation and generous hospitality. I am also grateful for Edward Johnson's many useful suggestions at various stages in the essay's history.

22.

WHY HOMOSEXUALITY
IS ABNORMAL*

Michael Levin

1. INTRODUCTION

This paper defends the view that homosexuality is abnormal and hence undesirable—not because it is immoral or sinful, or because it weakens society or
hampers evolutionary development, but for a purely mechanical reason. It is a
misuse of bodily parts. Clear empirical sense attaches to the idea of *the use of*
such bodily parts as genitals, the idea that they are *for* something, and consequently to the idea of their misuse. I argue on grounds involving natural selection that misuse of bodily parts can with high probability be connected to
unhappiness. I regard these matters as prolegomena to such policy issues as the
rights of homosexuals, the rights of those desiring not to associate with homosexuals, and legislation concerning homosexuality, issues which I shall not
discuss systematically here. However, I do in the last section draw a seemingly

Reprinted from *Monist* 67, no. 2 (April 1984). Copyright © 1984, *Monist*, LaSalle, IL 61301. Reprinted by
permission.

*Arthur Caplan, R. M. Hare, Michael Slote, Ed Erwin, Steven Goldberg, Ed Sagarin, Charles Win-
nick, Robert Gary, Thomas Nagel, David Benfield, Michael Green, and my wife, Margarita, all commented
helpfully on earlier drafts of this paper, one of which was read to the New York chapter of the Society for
Philosophy and Public Policy. My definition of naturalness agrees to some extent with Gary's (1978), and
I have benefited from seeing an unpublished paper by Michael Ruse.

evident corollary from my view that homosexuality is abnormal and likely to lead to unhappiness.

I have confined myself to male homosexuality for brevity's sake, but I believe that much of what I say applies mutatis mutandis to lesbianism. There may well be significant differences between the two: the data of Bell and Weinberg, for example, support the popular idea that sex per se *is* less important to women and in particular lesbians than it is to men. On the other hand, lesbians are generally denied motherhood, which seems more important to women than is fatherhood—normally denied homosexual males—to men. . . . Overall, it is reasonable to expect general innate gender differences to explain the major differences between male homosexuals and lesbians.

Despite the publicity currently enjoyed by the claim that one's "sexual preference" is nobody's business but one's own, the intuition that there is something unnatural about homosexuality remains vital. The erect penis fits the vagina, and fits it better than any other natural orifice; penis and vagina seem made for each other. This intuition ultimately derives from, or is another way of capturing, the idea that the penis is not *for* inserting into the anus of another man—that so using the penis is not the way it is *supposed*, even *intended*, to be used. Such intuitions may appear to rest on an outmoded teleological view of nature, but recent work in the logic of functional ascription shows how they may be explicated, and justified, in suitably naturalistic terms. . . . Furthermore, when we understand the sense in which homosexual acts involve a misuse of genitalia, we will see why such misuse is bad and not to be encouraged. . . . Clearly, the general idea that homosexuality is a pathological violation of nature's intent is not shunned by scientists. Here is Gadpille (1972):

> The view of cultural relativity seems to be without justification. Cultural judgment is collective human caprice, and whether it accepts or rejects homosexuality is irrelevant. Biological intent . . . is to differentiate male and female both physiologically and psychologically in such a manner as to insure species survival, which can be served only through heterosexual union.

Gadpille refers to homosexuality as "an abiological maladaptation." The novelty of the present paper is to link adaptiveness and normality via the notion of happiness.

But before turning to these issues, I want to make four preliminary remarks. The first concerns the explicitness of my language in the foregoing paragraph and the rest of this paper. Explicit mention of bodily parts and the frank description of sexual acts are necessary to keep the phenomenon under discussion in clear focus. Euphemistic vagary about "sexual orientation" or "the gay lifestyle" encourage one to slide over homosexuality without having to face or even acknowledge what it really is. Such talk encourages one to treat "sexual preference" as if it were akin to preference among flavors of ice cream. Since unusual taste in ice cream is neither right nor wrong, this usage suggests, why should unusual taste in sex be regarded as objectionable? Opposed to this usage is the unblinkable fact that the sexual preferences in question are such acts as mutual fellation. Is one man's taste for pistachio ice cream really just like another man's taste for fellation? Unwillingness to call this particular spade a spade allows delicacy to award the field by default to the view that homosexuality is normal. Anyway, such delicacy is misplaced in a day when "the love that dare not speak its name" is shouting its name from the rooftops.[1]

My second, related, point concerns the length of the present paper, which has a general and a specific cause. The general cause is that advocates of an unpopular position—as mine is, at least in intellectual circles—assume the burden of proof. My view is the one that needs defending, my presuppositions the ones not widely shared. I would not have entertained so many implausible and digressive objections had not so many competent philosophers urged them on me with great seriousness. Some of these objections even generate a dialectic among themselves. For example, I have to defend my view on two sociobiological fronts—against the view that what is innate is polymorphous sexuality shaped by culture, and against the incompatible view that not only are the details of sexual behavior innate, but homosexuality is one such behavior, and hence "normal."

The third point is this. The chain of intuitions I discussed earlier has other links, links connected to the conclusion that homosexuality is bad. They go something like this: Homosexual acts involve the use of the genitals for what they aren't for, and it is a *bad* or at least *unwise* thing to use a part of your body for what it isn't for. Calling homosexual acts "unnatural" is intended to sum up this entire line of reasoning. "Unnatural" carries disapprobative connotations, and any explication of it should capture this. One can, stipulatively or by observing the ordinary usage of biologists, coin an evaluatively neutral use for "normal," or "proper function," or any cognate thereof. One might for example take the normal use of an organ to be what the organ is used for 95 percent of the time. But there is a normative dimension to the concept of abnormality that all such explications miss. To have anything to do with our intuitions—even if designed to demonstrate them groundless—an explication of "abnormal" must capture the analytic truth that the abnormality of a practice is a reason for avoiding it. If our ordinary concept of normality turns out to be ill-formed, so that various acts are at worst "abnormal" in some nonevaluative sense, this will simply mean that, as we ordinarily use the expression, *nothing is abnormal.* (Not that anyone really believes this—people who deny that cacophagia or necrophilia is abnormal do so only to maintain the appearance of consistency.) . . .

2. ON "FUNCTION" AND ITS COGNATES

To bring into relief the point of the idea that homosexuality involves a misuse of bodily parts, I will begin with an uncontroversial case of misuse, a case in which the clarity of our intuitions is not obscured by the conviction that they are untrustworthy. Mr. Jones pulls all his teeth and strings them around his neck because he thinks his teeth look nice as a necklace. He takes pureéd liquids supplemented by intravenous solutions for nourishment. It is surely natural to say that Jones is misusing his teeth, that he is not using them for what they are for, that indeed the way he is using them is incompatible with what they are for. Pedants might argue that Jones's teeth are no longer part of him and hence that he is not misusing any bodily parts. To them I offer Mr. Smith, who likes to play "Old MacDonald" on his teeth. So devoted is he to this amusement, in fact, that he never uses his teeth for chewing—like Jones, he takes nourishment intravenously. Now, not only do we find it perfectly plain that Smith and Jones are misusing their teeth, we predict a dim future for them on purely physiological grounds; we expect the muscles of Jones's jaw that are used for—that *are* for—chewing to lose their tone, and we expect this to affect Jones's gums. Those parts of Jones's digestive tract that are for processing solids will also suffer from disuse. The net result will be deteriorating health and perhaps a shortened life. Nor is this all. Human beings enjoy chewing. Not only has natural selection selected in muscles for chewing and favored creatures with such muscles, it has selected in a tendency to find the use of those muscles reinforcing. Creatures who do not enjoy using such parts of their bodies as deteriorate with disuse, will tend to be selected out. Jones, product of natural selection that he is, descended from creatures who at least tended to enjoy the use of such parts. Competitors who didn't simply had fewer descendants. So we expect Jones sooner or later to experience vague yearnings to chew something, just as we find people who take no exercise to experience a general listlessness. Even waiving for now my apparent reification of the evolutionary process, let me emphasize how little anyone is tempted to say "each to his own" about Jones or to regard Jones's disposition of his teeth as simply a deviation from a statistical norm. This sort of case is my paradigm when discussing homosexuality. . . .

3. APPLICATIONS TO HOMOSEXUALITY

The application of this general picture to homosexuality should be obvious. There can be no reasonable doubt that one of the functions of the penis is to introduce semen into the vagina. It does this, and it has been selected in because it does this. . . . Nature has consequently made this use of the penis rewarding. It is clear enough that any proto-human males who found unrewarding the insertion of penis into vagina have left no descendants. In particular, proto-human males who enjoyed inserting their penises into each other's anuses have left no descendants. This is why homosexuality is abnormal, and why its abnormality counts prudentially against it. Homosexuality is likely to cause unhappiness because it leaves unfulfilled an innate and innately rewarding desire. And should the reader's environmentalism threaten to get the upper hand, let me remind him again of an unproblematic case. Lack of exercise is bad and even abnormal not only because it is unhealthy but also because one feels poorly without regular exercise. Nature made exercise rewarding because, until recently, we had to exercise to survive. Creatures who found running after game unrewarding were eliminated. Laziness leaves unreaped the rewards nature has planted in exercise, even if the lazy man cannot tell this introspectively. If this is a correct description of the place of exercise in human life, it is by the same token a correct description of the place of heterosexuality.

It hardly needs saying, but perhaps I should say it anyway, that this argument concerns tendencies and probabilities. Generalizations about human affairs being notoriously "true by and large and for the most part" only, saying that homosexuals are bound to be less happy than heterosexuals must be understood as short for "Not coincidentally, a larger proportion of homosexuals will be unhappy than a corresponding selection of the heterosexual population." There are, after all, genuinely jolly fat men. To say that laziness leads to adverse affective consequences means that, because of our evolutionary history, the odds are relatively good that a man who takes no exercise will suffer adverse affective consequences. Obviously, some people will get away with misusing their bodily parts. Thus, when evaluating the empirical evidence that bears on this account, it will be pointless to cite cases of well-adjusted homosexuals. I do not say they are nonexistent; my claim is that, of biological necessity, they are rare. . . .

Utilitarians must take the present evolutionary scenario seriously. The utilitarian attitude toward homosexuality usually runs something like this: even if homosexuality is in some sense unnatural, as a matter of brute fact homosexuals take pleasure in sexual contact with members of the same sex. As long as they don't hurt anyone else, homosexuality is as great a good as heterosexuality. But the matter cannot end here. Not even a utilitarian doctor would have words of praise for a degenerative disease that happened to foster a certain kind of pleasure (as sore muscles uniquely conduce to the pleasure of stretching them). A utilitarian doctor would presumably try just as zealously to cure diseases that feel good as less pleasant degenerative diseases. A pleasure causally connected with great distress cannot be treated as just another pleasure to be toted up on the felicific scoreboard. Utilitarians have to reckon with the inevitable consequences of pain-causing pleasure.

Similar remarks apply to the question of whether homosexuality is a "disease." A widely quoted pronouncement of the American Psychiatric Association runs:

> Surely the time has come for psychiatry to give up the archaic practice of classifying the millions of men and women who accept or prefer homosexual object choices as being, by virtue of that fact alone, mentally ill. The fact that their alternative life-style happens to be out of favor with current cultural conventions must not be a basis in itself for a diagnosis.

Apart from some question-begging turns of phrase, this is right. One's taste for mutual anal intercourse is nothing "in itself" for one's psychiatrist to worry about, any more than a life of indolence is anything "in itself" for one's doctor to worry about. In fact, in itself there is nothing wrong with a broken arm or an occluded artery. The fact that my right ulna is now in two pieces is just a fact of nature, not a "basis for diagnosis." But this condition is a matter for medical science anyway, because it will lead to pain. Permitted to persist, my fracture will provoke increasingly punishing states. So if homosexuality is a reliable sign of present or future misery, it is beside the point that homosexuality is not "by virtue of that fact alone" a mental illness. High rates of drug addiction, divorce, and illegitimacy are in themselves no basis for diagnosing social pathology. They support this diagnosis because of what else they signify about a society which exhibits them. Part of the problem here is the presence of germs in paradigm diseases, and the lack of a germ for homosexuality (or psychosis). I myself am fairly sure that a suitably general and germ-free definition of "disease" can be extruded from the general notion of "function" . . . , but however that may be, whether homosexuality is a disease is a largely verbal issue. If homosexuality is a self-punishing maladaptation, it hardly matters what it is called.

4. EVIDENCE AND FURTHER CLARIFICATION

I have argued that homosexuality is "abnormal" in both a descriptive and a normative sense because—for evolutionary reasons—homosexuals are bound to be unhappy. In Kantian terms, . . . it is possible for homosexuality to be unnatural even if it violates no cosmic purpose or such purposes as we retrospectively impose on nature. What is the evidence for my view? For one thing, by emphasizing homosexual unhappiness, my view explains a ubiquitous fact in a simple way. The fact is the universally acknowledged unhappiness of homosexuals. Even the staunchest defenders of homosexuality admit that, as of now, homosexuals are not happy. (Writers even in the very recent past, like Lord Devlin, could not really believe that anyone could publicly advocate homosexuality as intrinsically good: see Devlin, p. 87.) . . .

The usual environmentalist explanation for homosexuals' unhappiness is the misunderstanding, contempt, and abuse that society heaps on them. But this not only leaves unexplained why society has this attitude, it sins against parsimony by explaining a nearly universal phenomenon in terms of variable circumstances that have, by coincidence, the same upshot. Parsimony urges that we seek the explanation of homosexual unhappiness in the nature of homosexuality itself, as my explanation does. Having to "stay in the closet" may be a great strain, but it does not account for all the miseries that writers on homosexuality say is the homosexual's lot.

Incorporating unhappiness into the present evolutionary picture also smooths a bothersome ad-hocness in some otherwise appealing analyses of abnormality. Many writers define abnormality as compulsiveness. On this conception, homosexuality is abnormal because it is an autonomy-obstructing compulsion. Such an analysis is obviously open to the question, What if an autonomous homosexual comes along? To that, writers like van den Haag point out that homosexuality is, in fact, highly correlated with compulsiveness. The trouble here is that the definition in question sheds no light on why abnormal, compulsive, traits are such. The present account not only provides a criterion for abnormality, it encapsulates an explanation of *why* behavior abnormal by its lights is indeed compulsive and bound to lead to unhappiness.

One crucial test of my account is its prediction that homosexuals will continue to be unhappy even if people altogether abandon their "prejudice" against homosexuality. This prediction, that homosexuality being unnatural homosexuals will still find their behavior self-punishing, coheres with available evidence. It is consistent with the failure of other oppressed groups, such as American Negroes and European Jews, to become warped in the direction of "cruising," sado-masochism, and other practices common in homosexual life (see McCracken, 1979). It is consistent as well with the admission by even so sympathetic an observer of homosexuality as Rechy (1977) that the immediate cause of homosexual unhappiness is a taste for promiscuity, anonymous encounters, and humiliation. It is hard to see how such tastes are related to the dim view society takes of them. Such a relation would be plausible only if homosexuals courted multiple anonymous encounters faute de mieux, longing all the while to settle down to some sort of domesticity: But, again, Europeans abhorred Jews for centuries, but this did not create in Jews a special weakness for anonymous, promiscuous sex. Whatever drives a man away from women, to be fellated by as many different men as possible, seems independent of what society thinks of such behavior. It is this behavior that occasions misery, and we may expect the misery of homosexuals to continue.

In a 1974 study, Weinberg and Williams found no difference in the distress experienced by homosexuals in Denmark and the Netherlands, and in the United States, where they found public tolerance of homosexuality to be lower. This would confirm rather strikingly that homosexual unhappiness is endogenous, unless one says that Weinberg's and Williams's indices for public tolerance and distress—chiefly homosexuals' self-reports of "unhappiness" and "lack of faith in others"—are unreliable. Such complaints, however, push the social causation theory toward untestability. Weinberg and Williams themselves cleave to the hypothesis that homosexual unhappiness is entirely a reaction to society's attitudes, and suggest that a condition of homosexual happiness is positive endorsement by the surrounding society. It is hard to imagine a more flagrantly ad hoc hypothesis. Neither a Catholic living among Protestants nor a copywriter working on the great American novel in his off hours asks more of society than tolerance in order to be happy in his pursuits.

It is interesting to reflect on a natural experiment that has gotten under way in the decade since the Weinberg-Williams study. A remarkable change in public opinion, if not private sentiment, has occurred in America. For whatever reason —the prodding of homosexual activists, the desire not to seem like a fuddy-duddy—various organs of opinion are now hard at work providing a "positive image" for homosexuals. Judges allow homosexuals to adopt their lovers. The Unitarian Church now performs homosexual marriages. Hollywood produces highly sanitized movies like *Making Love* and *Personal Best* about homosexuality. Macmillan strongly urges its authors to show little boys using cosmetics. Homosexuals no longer fear revealing themselves, as is shown by the prevalence of the "clone look." Certain products run advertising obviously directed at the homosexual market. On the societal reaction theory, there ought to be an enormous rise in homosexual happiness. I know of no systematic study to determine if this is so, but anecdotal evidence suggests it may not be. The homosexual press has been just as strident in denouncing pro-homosexual movies as in denouncing Doris Day movies. Especially virulent venereal diseases have very recently appeared in homosexual communities, evidently spread in epidemic proportions by unabating homosexual promiscuity. One selling point for a presumably serious "gay rights" rally in Washington, DC, was an "all-night disco train" from New York to Washington. What is perhaps most salient is that, even if the changed public mood results in decreased homosexual unhappiness, the question remains of why homosexuals in the recent past, who suffered greatly for being homosexuals, persisted in being homosexuals.

310 PHILOSOPHY AND SEX

But does not my position also predict—contrary to fact—that any sexual activity not aimed at procreation or at least sexual intercourse leads to unhappiness? First, I am not sure this conclusion is contrary to the facts properly understood. It is universally recognized that, for humans and the higher animals, sex is more than the insertion of the penis into the vagina. Foreplay is necessary to prepare the female and, to a lesser extent, the male. Ethologists have studied the elaborate mating rituals of even relatively simple animals. Sexual intercourse must therefore be understood to include the kisses and caresses that necessarily precede copulation, behaviors that nature has made rewarding. What my view does predict is that exclusive preoccupation with behaviors normally preparatory for intercourse is highly correlated with unhappiness. And, so far as I know, psychologists do agree that such preoccupation or "fixation" with, e.g., cunnilingus, is associated with personality traits independently recognized as disorders. In this sense, sexual intercourse really is virtually necessary for well-being. Only if one is antecedently convinced that "nothing is more natural than anything else" will one confound foreplay as a prelude to intercourse with "foreplay" that leads nowhere at all. One might speculate on the evolutionary advantages of foreplay, at least for humans: by increasing the intensity and complexity of the pleasures of intercourse, it binds the partners more firmly and makes them more fit for child-rearing. In fact, such analyses of sexual perversion as Nagel's (1969), which correctly focus on the interruption of mutuality as central to perversion, go wrong by ignoring the evolutionary role and built-in rewards of mutuality. They fail to explain why the interruption of mutuality is disturbing.[2]

It should also be clear that my argument permits gradations in abnormality. Behavior is the more abnormal, and the less likely to be rewarding, the more its emission tends to extinguish a genetic cohort that practices it. The less likely a behavior is to get selected out, the less abnormal it is. Those of our ancestors who found certain aspects of foreplay reinforcing might have managed to reproduce themselves sufficiently to implant this strain in us. There might be an equilibrium between intercourse and such not directly reproductive behavior. It is not required that any behavior not directly linked to heterosexual intercourse lead to maximum dissatisfaction. But the existence of these gradations provides no entering wedge for homosexuality. As no behavior is more likely to get selected out than rewarding homosexuality—except perhaps an innate tendency to suicide at the onset of puberty—it is extremely unlikely that homosexuality can now be unconditionally reinforcing in humans to any extent.

Nor does my position predict, again contrary to fact, that celibate priests will be unhappy. My view is compatible with the existence of happy celibates who deny themselves as part of a higher calling which yields compensating satisfactions. Indeed, the very fact that one needs to explain how the priesthood can compensate for the lack of family means that people do regard heterosexual mating as the natural or "inertial" state of human relations. The comparison between priests and homosexuals is in any case inapt. Priests do not simply give up sexual activity without ill-effect; they give it up for a reason. Homosexuals have hardly given up the use of their sexual organs, for a higher calling or anything else. Homosexuals continue to use them, but, unlike priests, they use them for what they are not for.

I have encountered the thought that by my lights female heterosexuality must be abnormal, since according to feminism women have been unhappy down the ages. The datum is questionable, to say the least. Feminists have offered no documentation whatever for this extravagant claim; their evidence is usually the unhappiness of the feminist in question and her circle of friends. Such attempts to prove female discontent in past centuries as Greer's (1979) are transparently anachronistic projections of contemporary feminist discontent onto inappropriate historical objects. An objection from a similar source runs that my argument, suitably extended, implies the naturalness and hence rewardingness of traditional monogamous marriage. Once again, instead of seeing this as a *reductio*, I am inclined to take the supposed absurdity as a truth that nicely fits my theory. It is not a theoretical contention but an observable fact that women enjoy motherhood, that failure to bear and care for children breeds unhappiness in women, and that the role of "primary caretaker" is much more important for women than men. However, there is no need to be dogmatic. This conception of the family is in extreme disrepute in contemporary America. Many women work and many marriages last less than a decade. Here we have another natural experiment about what people find reinforcing. My view predicts that women will on the whole become unhappier if current trends continue. Let us see.

Not directly bearing on the issue of happiness, but still empirically pertinent, is animal homosexuality. I mentioned earlier that the overwhelmingly heterosexual tendencies of animals in all but such artificial and genetically irrelevant environs as zoos cast doubt on sheer polymorphous sexuality as a sufficiently adaptive strategy. By the same token, it renders implausible the claim in Masters and Johnson (1979) that human beings are born with only a general sex drive, and that the objects of the sex drive are *entirely* learned. If this were so, who teaches male tigers to mate with female tigers? Who teaches male primates to mate with female primates? In any case, the only evidence Masters and Johnson cite is the entirely unsurprising physiological similarity between heterosexual and homosexual response. Plainly, the inability of the penile nerve endings to tell what is rubbing them has nothing to do with the innateness of the sexual object. The inability of a robin to tell twigs from clever plastic lookalikes is consistent with an innate nest-building instinct.

The work of Beach (1976) is occasionally cited (e.g., in Wilson, 1978) to document the existence of animal homosexuality and to support the contention that homosexuality has some adaptive purpose, but Beach in fact notes certain important disanalogies between mammalian homosexual behavior in the wild and human homosexuality. Citing a principle of "stimulus-response complementarity," he remarks that a male chimpanzee will mount another male if the latter emits such characteristically female behavior as display of nether parts. Male homosexual humans, on the other hand, are attracted to maleness. More significantly, the male chimpanzee's mounting is unaccompanied by erection, thrusting or, presumably, intromission. Beach suggests that this display-mounting sequence may be multipurpose in nature, signaling submission and dominance when it occurs between males. In the same vein, Barash (1979: 60) cites male-male rape in *Xylocanis maculipennis*, but here the rapist's sperm is deposited in the rape victim's storage organs. This is a smart evolutionary move . . . but it is not comparable in its effects to homosexuality in humans. . . .

5. On Policy Issues

Homosexuality is intrinsically bad only in a prudential sense. It makes for unhappiness. However, this does not exempt homosexuality from the larger categories of ethics—rights, duties, liabilities. Deontic categories apply to acts which increase or decrease happiness or expose the helpless to the risk of unhappiness.

If homosexuality is unnatural, legislation which raises the odds that a given child will become homosexual raises the odds that he will be unhappy. The only gap in the syllogism is whether legislation which legitimates, endorses, or protects homosexuality does increase the chances that a child will become homosexual. If so, such legislation is prima facie objectionable. The question is not whether homosexual elementary school teachers will molest their charges. Pro-homosexual legislation might increase the incidence of homosexuality in subtler ways. If it does, and if the protection of children is a fundamental obligation of society, legislation which legitimates homosexuality is a dereliction of duty. I am reluctant to deploy the language of "children's rights," which usually serves as one more excuse to interfere with the prerogatives of parents. But we do have obligations to our children, and one of them is to protect them from harm. If, as some have suggested, children have a right to protection from a religious education, they surely have a right to protection from homosexuality. So protecting them limits somebody else's freedom, but we are often willing to protect quite obscure children's rights at the expense of the freedom of others. There is a movement to ban TV commercials for sugar-coated cereals, to protect children from the relatively trivial harm of tooth decay. Such a ban would restrict the freedom of advertisers, and restrict it even though the last clear chance of avoiding the harm, and thus the responsibility, lies with the parents who control the TV set. I cannot see how one can consistently support such legislation and also urge homosexual rights, which risk much graver damage to children in exchange for increased freedom for homosexuals. (If homosexual behavior is largely compulsive, it is falsifying the issue to present it as balancing risks to children against the freedom of homosexuals.) The right of a homosexual to work for the Fire Department is not a negligible good. Neither is fostering a legal atmosphere in which as many people as possible grow up heterosexual.

It is commonly asserted that legislation granting homosexuals the privilege or right to be firemen endorses not homosexuality, but an expanded conception of human liberation. It is conjectural how sincerely this can be said in a legal order that forbids employers to hire whom they please and demands hours of paperwork for an interstate shipment of hamburger. But in any case legislation "legalizing homosexuality" cannot be neutral because passing it would have an inexpungeable speech-act dimension. Society cannot grant unaccustomed rights and privileges to homosexuals while remaining neutral about the value of homosexuality. Working from the assumption that society rests on the family and its consequences, the Judaeo-Christian tradition has deemed homosexuality a sin and withheld many privileges from homosexuals. Whether or not such denial was right, for our society to grant these privileges to homosexuals *now* would amount to declaring that it has rethought the matter and decided that homosexuality is not as bad as it had previously supposed. And unless such rethinking is a direct response to new empirical findings about homosexuality, it can only be a revaluing. Someone who suddenly accepts a policy he has previously opposed is open to the same interpretation: he has come to think better of the policy. And if he embraces the policy while knowing that this interpretation will be put on his behavior, and if he knows that others know that he knows they will so interpret it, he is acquiescing in this interpretation. He can be held to have intended, meant, this interpretation. A society that grants privileges to homosexuals while recognizing that, in the light of generally known history, this act can be interpreted as a positive reevaluation of homosexuality, is signaling that it now thinks homosexuality is all right. Many commentators in the popular press have observed that homosexuals, unlike members of racial minorities, can always "stay in the closet" when applying for jobs. What homosexual rights activists really want, therefore, is not access to jobs but legitimation of their homosexuality. Since this is known, giving them what they want will be seen as conceding their claim to legitimacy. And since legislators know their actions will support this interpretation, and know that their constituencies know they know this, the

Gricean effect or symbolic meaning of passing anti-discrimination ordinances is to declare homosexuality legitimate (see Will, 1977).

Legislation permitting frisbees in the park does not imply approval of frisbees for the simple reason that frisbees are new; there is no tradition of banning them from parks. The legislature's action in permitting frisbees is not interpretable, known to be interpretable, and so on, as the reversal of long-standing disapproval. It is because these Gricean conditions are met in the case of abortion that legislation—or rather judicial fiat-permitting abortions and mandating their public funding are widely interpreted as tacit approval. Up to now, society has deemed homosexuality so harmful that restricting it outweighs putative homosexual rights. If society reverses itself, it will in effect be deciding that homosexuality is not as bad as it once thought.

NOTES

1. "Sexual preference" typifies the obfuscatory language in which the homosexuality debate is often couched. "Preference" suggests that sexual tastes are voluntarily chosen, whereas it is a commonplace that one cannot decide what to find sexually stimulating. True, we talk of "preferences" among flavors of ice cream even though one cannot choose what flavor of ice cream to like; such talk is probably a carryover from the voluntariness of *ordering* ice cream. "Sexual preference" does not even sustain this analogy, however, since sex is a forced choice for everyone except avowed celibates, and especially for the relatively large number of homosexuals who cruise regularly.

2. Nagel attempts to meet these counterexamples in effect by accepting such consequences of the classical analysis as that the beat of the heart is sometimes for diagnosis. The only reply to this sort of defense is that this is *not* what people mean. Met with such a reply, many philosophers feel impelled to say, "Well, it ought to be what you mean." This invitation to change the subject is attractive or relevant only if we haven't meant anything the first time around. If a coherent thought can be found behind our initial words which maximizes coherence with all hypothetical usages, it is *that thought* we were expressing and whose articulation was the aim of the analytic exercise.

BIBLIOGRAPHY

Barash, D. *The Whispering Within.* New York: Harper & Row, 1979.

Beach, F. "Cross-Species Comparisons and the Human Heritage." *Archives of Sexual Behavior* 5 (1976): 469–85.

Bell, A., and M. Weinberg. *Homosexualities.* New York: Simon and Schuster, 1978.

Devlin, P. *The Enforcement of Morals.* Oxford: Oxford University Press, 1965.

Gadpille, W. "Research into the Physiology of Maleness and Femaleness: Its Contribution to the Etiology and Psychodynamics of Homosexuality." *Archives of General Psychiatry* (1972): 193–206.

Gary, R. "Sex and Sexual Perversion." *Journal of Philosophy* 74 (1978): 189–99.

Greer, G. *The Obstacle Race.* New York: Farrar, Strauss & Giroux, 1979.

Masters, W., and V. Johnson. *Homosexuality in Perspective.* Boston: Little, Brown and Company, 1979.

McCracken, S. "Replies to Correspondents." *Commentary*, April 1979.

Mossner, E. *The Life of David Hume*, 1st. ed. New York: Nelson & Sons, 1954.

Nagel, E. "Sexual Perversion." *Journal of Philosophy* 66 (1969): 5–17. This discussion can be found elsewhere in the present volume.

———. "Teleology Revisited." *Journal of Philosophy* 74 (1977): 261–301.

Rechy, J. *The Sexual Outlaw.* New York: Grove Press, 1977.

Weinberg, M., and C. Williams. *Male Homosexuals: Their Problems and Adaptations.* Oxford: Oxford University Press, 1974.

Will, G. "How Far Out of the Closet?" *Newsweek.* May 30, 1977, p. 92.

Wilson, E. *On Human Nature.* Cambridge, MA: Harvard University Press, 1978.

———. *Sociobiology: The New Synthesis.* Cambridge, MA: Harvard University Press, 1975.

23.

AN ESSAY ON "PAEDERASTY"

Jeremy Bentham

Introduction to Bentham's Essay

I have been tormenting myself for years to find, if possible, a sufficient ground for treating them [homosexuals] with the severity with which they are treated at this time of day by all European nations: but upon the principle of utility I can find none.

Had these words been penned by a famous social philosopher of the 1980s, they would be noteworthy but not exceptional; written by a social philosopher of the 1880s, they would have been both noteworthy and exceptional; but since the passage was written by a famous English social philosopher of the 1780s, Jeremy Bentham, and since it prefaces what appears to be the first philosophical treatment of homosexuality in the English language, the passage is extraordinary indeed.

Bentham and his fellow utilitarians sought a rational standard against which they could measure the customs and laws of their society. The device they hit upon was the calculus of utility. To employ the calculus one had to conceptualize the social world in terms of acts that were morally neutral in and of themselves, but which acquired value in terms of their consequences. Acts were then held to be moral

Jeremy Bentham, "An Essay on 'Paederasty'" from the *Journal of Homosexuality* (New York: Haworth Press, Summer-Fall 1978). Originally written by Bentham c.1785.

insofar as their consequences were conducive to human happiness, and immoral insofar as their effects militated against happiness and/or promoted pain, suffering, or any other form of human misery.

The utilitarian project was to measure all customs and laws in terms of the calculus of utility—including, as it turned out, those relating to "unnatural" sexual acts. Bentham appraised the moral nature of these acts and the laws that criminalize them in three different sets of writings dated ca. 1774, ca. 1785, and 1814–1816. In each case, when the sexual acts in themselves were regarded as morally neutral and appraised only in terms of their consequences he found that, except in cases of homosexual rape, the most certain consequence of a homosexual act was the pleasure experienced by the participants. There was, therefore, a strong prima facie case both against the moral opprobrium with which homosexuality was customarily viewed and against imposing criminal sanctions on homosexual acts. (According to some scholars more than sixty people were hanged for "sodomy" and other homosexual acts in England during the years 1806–1835.) Bentham carefully examined all of the purported negative consequences of homosexual intercourse suggested by his nonutilitarian contemporaries—Blackstone, Montesquieu, and Voltaire—for example, its supposed tendency to corrupt and debilitate practitioners, its effects on population, and so on. Weighing these conjectured effects against the historical data supplied by Greek homosexuality, Bentham concluded that since the net consequences of homosexual sex appear not to be harmful, utilitarians must reject the proscription and criminalization of homosexuality.

Like most of Bentham's writings, his work on homosexuality was not published in his lifetime. The first publication of any of this material occurred in 1931 when C. K. Ogden published some of the 1814–1816 materials as an appendix to his 1931 edition of Bentham's Theory of Legislation. *The essay on "Paederasty" was not published until 1978, when it appeared in the Fall and Summer editions of the* Journal of Homosexuality. *Louis Compton, a professor of English at the University of Nebraska, had rediscovered these materials among Bentham's papers and transcribed the manuscript (whose page numbers are given in square brackets).[1] Although the style of Bentham's writings reflects the period in which they were written, the thought is remarkably contemporary; the essay is undoubtedly one of the most significant publications in the recent literature on philosophy and sex.—**R.B.***

To what class of offences shall we refer these irregularities of the venereal appetite which are styled unnatural? . . . I have been tormenting myself for years to find if possible a sufficient ground for treating them with the severity with which they are treated at this time of day by all European nations: but upon the principle of utility I can find none.

. . . In settling the nature and tendency of this offence we shall for the most part have settled the nature and tendency of all the other offences that come under this disgusting catalogue.

PAEDERASTY: DOES IT PRODUCE ANY PRIMARY MISCHIEF?

1. As to any primary mischief, it is evident that it produces no pain in anyone. On the contrary it produces pleasure, and that a pleasure which, by their perverted taste, is by this supposition preferred to that pleasure which is in general reputed the greatest. The partners are both willing. If either of them be unwilling, the act is not that which we have here in view: it is an offence totally different in its nature of effects: it is a personal injury; it is a kind of rape.

AS A SECONDARY MISCHIEF WHETHER THEY PRODUCE ANY ALARM IN THE COMMUNITY

2. As to any secondary mischief, it produces not any pain of apprehension. For what is there in it for any body to be afraid of? By the supposition, those only are the objects of it who choose to be so, who find a pleasure, for so it seems they do, in being so.

WHETHER ANY DANGER

3. As to any danger exclusive of pain, the danger, if any, must consist in the tendency of the example. But what is the tendency of this example? To dispose others to engage in the same practises: but this practise for anything that has yet appeared produces not pain of any kind to anyone.

REASONS THAT HAVE COMMONLY BEEN ASSIGNED

Hitherto we have found no reason for punishing it at all: much less for punishing it with the degree of severity with which it has been commonly punished. Let us see what force there is in the reasons that have been commonly assigned for punishing it.

Whether Against the Security of the Individual

Sir W. Blackstone [argues that paederasty] is not only an offence against the peace, but it is of that division of offences against the peace which are offences against security. According to the same writer, if a man is guilty of this kind of filthiness, for instance, with a cow, as some men have been known to be, it is an offence/against somebody's security. He does not say whose security, for the law makes no distinction in its ordinances, so neither does this lawyer or any other English lawyer in his comments make any distinction between this kind of filthiness when committed with the consent of the patient and the same kind of filthiness when committed against his consent and by violence. It is just as if a man were to make no distinction between concubinage and rape.

Whether it Debilitates—Montesquieu

The reason that Montesquieu gives for reprobating it is the weakness which he seems to suppose it to have a tendency to bring upon those who practise it. (*Esp. des Loix*, L. 12, ch. 6. 11) This, if it be true in fact, is a reason of a very different complexion from any of the preceding and it is on the ground of this reason as being the most plausible one that I have ranked the offence under its present head. As far as it is true in fact, the act ought to be regarded in the first place as coming within the list of offences against one's self, of offences of imprudence: in the next place, as an offence against the state, an offence the tendency of which is to diminish the public force. If, however, it tends to weaken a man it is not any single act that can in any sensible degree have that effect. It can only be the habit: the act thus will become obnoxious as evidencing the existence, in probability, of the habit. This enervating tendency, be it what it may, if it is to be taken as a ground for treating the / [192] practise in question with a degree of severity which is not bestowed upon the regular way of gratifying the veneral appetite, must be greater in the former case than in the latter. Is it so? If the affirmative can be shown it must be either by arguments a priori drawn from considerations of the nature of the human frame or from experience. Are there any such arguments from physiology? I have never heard of any: I can think of none.

What Says History?

What says historical experience? The result of this can be measured only upon a large scale or upon a very general survey. Among the modern nations it is comparatively but rare. In modern Rome it is perhaps not very uncommon; in Paris probably not quite so common; in London still less frequent; in Edinburgh or Amsterdam you scarce hear of it two or three times in a century. In Athens and in ancient Rome in the most flourishing periods of the history of those capitals, regular intercourse between the sexes was scarcely much more common. It was upon the same footing throughout Greece; everybody practised it; nobody was ashamed of it. They might be ashamed of what they looked upon as an excess in it, or they might be ashamed of it as a weakness, as a propensity that had a tendency to distract men from more worthy and important occupations, / just as a man with us might be ashamed of excess or weakness in his love for women. In itself one may be sure they were not ashamed of it. . . .

What is remarkable is that there is scarce a striking character in antiquity, not one that in other respects men are in use to cite as virtuous, of whom it does not appear by one circumstance or another, that / he was infected with this inconceivable propensity. . . .

Many moderns, and among others Mr. Voltaire, dispute the fact, but that intelligent philosopher sufficiently intimates the ground of his incredulity—if he does not believe it, it is because he likes not to believe it. What the ancients called love in such a case was what we call Platonic, that is, was not love but friendship. But the Greeks knew the difference between love and friendship as well as we— they had distinct terms to signify them by: it seems reasonable therefore to suppose that when they say love they mean love, and that when they say friendship only they mean friendship only. And with regard to Xenophon and his master, Socrates, and his fellow-scholar Plato, it seems more reasonable to believe them to have been addicted to this taste when they or, any of them tell us so in express terms than to trust to the interpretations, however ingenious and however well-intended, of any men who write at this time of day, when they tell us it was no such thing. / Not to insist upon Agesilaus and Xenophon, it appears by one circumstance or another that Themistocles, Aristides, Epaminondas, Alcibiades, Alexander and perhaps the greatest number of the heroes of Greece were infected with this taste. Not that the historians are at the pains of informing us so expressly, for it was not extraordinary enough to make it worth their while, but it comes out collaterally in the course of the transactions they have occasion to relate.

It appears then that this propensity was universally predominant among the ancient Greeks and Romans, among the military as much as any. The ancient Greeks and Romans, however, are commonly reputed as / a much stouter as well as a much braver people than the stoutest and bravest of any of the modern nations of Europe. They appear to have been stouter at least in a very considerable degree than the French in whom this propensity is not very common and still more than the Scotch in whom it is still less common, and this although the climate even of Greece was a great deal warmer and in that respect more enervating than that of modern Scotland.

If then this practise was in those ancient warm countries attended with any enervating effects, they were much more than counteracted by the superiority of [illegible] in the exertions which were then required by the military education over and above those which are now called forth by ordinary labour. But if there be any ground derived from history for attributing to it any such enervating effects it is more than I can find.

WHETHER IT ENERVATES THE PATIENT MORE THAN THE AGENT

Montesquieu however seems to make a distinction—he seems to suppose these enervating effects to be exerted principally upon the person who is the patient in such a business. This distinction does not seem very satisfactory in any point of view. Is there any reason for supposing it to be a fixed one? Between persons of the same age actuated by the same incomprehensible desires would not the parts they took in the business be convertible? Would not the patient / be the agent in his turn? If it were not so, the person on whom he supposes these effects to be the greatest is precisely the person with regard to whom it is most difficult to conceive whence those consequences should result. In the one case there is exhaustion which when carried to excess may be followed by debility: in the other case there is no such thing.

WHAT SAYS HISTORY?

In regard to this point too in particular, what says history? As the two parts that a man may take in this business are so naturally convertible however frequently he may have taken a passive part, it will not ordinarily appear. According to the notions of the ancients, there was something degrading in the passive part which was not in the active. It was ministering to the pleasure, for so we are obliged to call it, of another without participation, it was making one's self the property of another man, it was playing the woman's part: it was therefore unmanly. (*Paedicabo vos et irrumabo, Antoni* [sic] *pathice et cinaede Furi.* [Carm. 16] Catullus. J.B.) On the other hand, to take the active part was to make use of another for one's pleasure, it was making another man one's property, it was preserving the manly, the commanding character. Accordingly, Solon in his laws prohibits slaves from bearing an active part where the passive is borne by a freeman. In the few instances in which we happen to hear of a person's taking the passive part there is nothing to favour / the above-mentioned hypothesis. The beautiful Alcibiades, who in his youth, says Cornelius Nepos, after the manner of the Greeks, was beloved by many, was not remarkable either for weakness or for cowardice: at least, [blank] did not find it so. The Clodius whom Cicero scoffs at for his servile obsequiousness to the appetite of Curio was one of the most daring and turbulent spirits in all Rome. Julius Caesar was looked upon as a man of tolerable courage in his day, notwithstanding the complaisance he showed in his youth to the King of Bithynia, Nicomedes, Aristotle, the inquisitive and observing Aristotle, whose physiological disquisitions are looked upon as some of the best of his works—Aristotle, who if there had been anything in this notion had every opportunity and inducement to notice and confirm it—gives no intimation of any such thing. On the contrary he sits down very soberly to distribute the male half of the species under two classes: one class having a natural propensity, he says, to bear a passive part in such a business, as the other have to take an active part. (*Probl.* Sect. 4 art. 27: The former of these propensities he attributes to a peculiarity of organization, analogous to that of women. The whole passage is abundantly obscure and shows in how imperfect a state of anatomical knowledge was his time. J.B.) This observation it must be confessed is not much more satisfactory than that other of the same philosopher when he speaks of two sorts of men—the one born to be masters, the other to be slaves. If however there had appeared any reason for supposing this practise, either with regard to the passive or the active part of it, to have had any remarkable effects in the way of debilitation upon those who were addicted to it, he would have hardly said so much / [194] upon the subject without taking notice of that circumstance.

WHETHER IT HURTS THE POPULATION?

A notion more obvious, but perhaps not much better founded than the former is that of its being prejudicial to population. Mr. Voltaire appears inclined in one part of his works to give some countenance to this opinion. He speaks of it as a vice which would be destructive to the human race if it were general. "How did it come about that a vice which would destroy mankind if it were general, that an infamous outrage against nature . . . ?" (*Questions sur l'Encyclop.* "Amour Socratique." J.B.)

A little further on, speaking of Sextus Empiricus who would have us believe that this practise was "recommended" in Persia by the laws, he insists that the effect of such a law would be to annihilate the human race if it were literally observed. "No," says he, "it is not in human nature to make a law that contradicts and outrages nature, a law that would annihilate mankind if it were observed to the letter." This consequence however is far enough from being a necessary one. For a law of the purport he represents to be observed, it is sufficient that this unprolific kind of venery be practised; it is not necessary that it should be practised to the exclusion of that which is prolific. Now that there should ever be wanting such a measure of the regular and ordinary inclination of desire for the proper object / as is necessary for keeping up the numbers of mankind upon their present footing is a notion that stands warranted by nothing that I can find in history. To consider the matter a priori [?], if we consult Mr. Hume and Dr. Smith, we shall find that it is not the strength of the inclination of the one sex for the other that is the measure of the numbers of mankind, but the quantity of subsistence which they can find or raise upon a given spot. With regard to the mere object of population, if we consider the time of gestation in the female sex we shall find that much less than a hundredth part of the activity a man is capable of exerting in this way is sufficient to produce all the effect that can be produced by ever so much more. Population therefore cannot suffer till the inclination of the male sex for the female be considerably less than a hundredth part as strong as for their own. Is there the least probability that [this] should ever be the case? I must confess I see not any thing that should lead us to suppose it. Before this can happen the nature of the human composition must receive a total change and that propensity which is commonly regarded as the only one of the two that is natural must have become altogether an unnatural one.

I have already observed that I can find nothing in history to countenance the notion I am examining. On the contrary the country in which the prevalence of this practise / is most conspicuous happens to have been remarkable for its populousness. The bent of popular prejudice has been to exaggerate this populousness: but after all deductions [are] made, still it will appear to have been remarkable. It was such as, notwithstanding the drain of continual wars in a country parcelled out into paltry states as to be all of it frontier, gave occasion to the continued necessity of emigration.

This reason however well grounded soever it were in itself could not with any degree of consistency be urged in a country where celibacy was permitted, much less where it was encouraged. The proposition which (as will be shown more fully by and by) is not at all true with respect to paederasty, I mean that were it to prevail universally it would put an end to the human race, is most evidently and strictly true with regard to celibacy. If then merely out of regard to population it were right that paederasts should be burnt alive, monks ought to be roasted alive by a slow fire. If a paederast, according to the monkish canonist Bermondus, destroys the whole human race Bermondus destroyed it I don't know how many thousand times over. The crime of Bermondus is I don't know how many times worse than paederasty.

WHETHER IT ROBS WOMEN

A more serious imputation for punishing this practise [is] that the effect of it is to produce in the male sex an indifference to the female, and thereby defraud the latter of their rights. This, as far as it holds good in point of fact, is in truth a serious imputation. The interest of the female part of the species claim just as much attention, and not a whit more, on the part of the legislator, as those of the male. A complaint of this sort, it is true, would not come with a very good grace from a modest woman; but should the woman be stopped from making complaint in such a case it is the business of the men to make it for them. This then as far as it holds good in point of fact is in truth a very serious imputation: how far it does it will be proper to enquire.

In all European countries and such others on which we bestow the title of civilized, this propensity, which in the male sex is under a considerable degree of restraint, is under an incomparably greater restraint in the female. While each is alike prohibited from partaking of these enjoyments but on the terms of marriage by the fluctuating and inefficacious influence of religion, the censure of the world denies it [to] the female part of the species under the severest penalties while the male sex is left free. No sooner is a woman known to have infringed this prohibition than either she is secluded from all means of repeating the offence, or upon her escaping from that vigilance she throws herself into that degraded class whom the want of company of their own sex render unhappy, and the abundance of it on the part of the male sex unprolific. This being the case, it appears the contribution which the male part of the species are willing as well as able to bestow is beyond all comparison greater than what the female part are permitted to receive. If a woman has a husband she is permitted to receive it only from her husband; if she has no husband she is not permitted to receive it from any man without being degraded into the class of prostitutes. When she is in that unhappy class she has not indeed less than she would wish, but what is often as bad to her—she has more.

It appears then that if the female sex are losers by the prevalence of this practise it can only be on this supposition—that the force with which it tends to divert men from entering into connection with the other sex is greater than the force with which the censure of the world tends to prevent those connections by its operation on the women. [196]

As long as things are upon that footing there are many cases in which the women can be no sufferers for the want of solicitation on the part of the men. If the institution of the marriage contract be a beneficial one, and if it be expedient that the observance of it should be maintained inviolate, we must in the first place deduct it from the number of the women who would be sufferers by the prevalence of this taste all married women whose husbands were not infected with it. In the next place, upon the supposition that a state of prostitution is not a happier state than a state of virginity, we must deduct all those women who by means of this prevalence would have escaped being debauched. The women who would be sufferers by it ab initio are those only who, were it not for the prevalence of it, would have got husbands.

The question then is reduced to this. What are the number of women who by the prevalence of this taste would, it is probable, be prevented from getting husbands? These and these only are they who would be sufferers by it. Upon the following considerations it does not seem likely that the prejudice sustained by the sex in this way could ever rise to any considerable amount. Were the prevalence of this taste to rise to ever so great a heighth the most considerable part of the motives to marriage would remain entire. In the first place, the desire of having children, in the next place the desire of forming alliances between families, thirdly the convenience of having a domestic companion whose company will continue to be agreeable throughout life, fourthly the convenience of gratifying the appetite in question at any time when the want occurs and without the expence and trouble of concealing it or the danger of a discovery

Were a man's taste even so far corrupted as to make him prefer the embraces of a person of his own sex to those of a female, a connection of that preposterous kind would therefore be far enough from answering to him the purposes of a marriage. A connection with a woman may by accident be followed with disgust, but a connection of the other kind, a man must know, will for certain come in time to be followed by disgust. All the documents we have from the ancients relative to this matter, and we have a great abundance, agree in this, that it is only for a very few years of his life that a male continues an object of desire even to those in whom the infection of this taste is at the strongest. The very name it went by among the Greeks may stand instead of all other proofs, of which the works of Lucian and Martial alone will furnish any abundance that can be required. Among the Greeks it was called *Paederastia*, the love of boys, not *Andrerastia*, the love of men. Among the Romans the act was called *Paedicare* because the object of it was a boy. There was a particular name for those who had passed the short period beyond which no man hoped to be an object of desire to his own sex. They were called *exoleti*. No male therefore who was passed this short period of life could expect to find in this way any reciprocity of affection; he must be as odious to the boy from the beginning as in a short time the boy would be to him. The objects of this kind of sensuality would therefore come only in the place of common prostitutes; they could never even to a person of this depraved taste answer the purposes of a virtuous woman.

WHAT SAYS HISTORY?

Upon this footing stands the question when considered a priori: the evidence of facts seems to be still more conclusive on the same side. There seems no reason to doubt, as I have already observed but that population went on altogether as fast and that the men were altogether as well inclined to marriage among the Grecians in whom this vitious propensity was most prevalent as in any modern people in whom it is least prevalent. In Rome, indeed, about the time of the extinction of liberty we find great complaints of the decline of population: but the state of it does not appear to have been at all dependent on or at all influenced by the measures that were taken from time to time to restrain the love of boys: it was with the Romans, as with us, what kept a man from marriage was not the preferring boys to women but the preferring the convenience of a transient connection to the expense and hazard of a lasting one.

IF IT WERE MORE FREQUENT THAN THE REGULAR CONNECTION IN WHAT SENSE COULD IT BE TERMED UNNATURAL?

The nature of the question admits of great latitude of opinion: for my own part I must confess I cannot bring myself to entertain so high a notion of the alluringness of this preposterous propensity as some men appear to entertain. I cannot suppose it to [be] possible it should ever get to such a heighth as that the interests of the female part of the species should be materially affected by it: or that it could ever happen that were they to contend upon equal ground the eccentric and unnatural propensity should ever get the better of the regular and natural one. Could we for a moment suppose this to be the case, I would wish it to be considered what meaning a man would have to annex to the expression, when he bestows on the propensity under consideration the epithet of unnatural. If contrary to all appearance the case really were that if all men were left perfectly free to choose, as many men would make choice of their own sex as of the opposite one, I see not what reason there would be for applying the word natural to the one rather than to the other. All the difference would be that the one was both natural and necessary whereas the other was natural but not necessary. If the mere circumstance of its not being necessary were sufficient to warrant the terming it unnatural it might as well be said that the taste a man has for music is unnatural.

My wonder is how any man who is at all acquainted with the most amiable part of the species should ever entertain any serious apprehensions of their yielding the ascendent to such unworthy rivals.

AMONG THE ANCIENTS— WHETHER IT EXCLUDED NOT THE REGULAR TASTE

A circumstance that contributes considerably to the alarms entertained by some people on this score is the common prejudice which supposes that the one propensity is exclusive of the other. This notion is for the most part founded on prejudice as may be seen in the works of a multitude of ancient authors in which we continually see the same person at one time stepping aside in pursuit of this eccentric kind of pleasure but at other times diverting his inclination to the proper object. Horace, in speaking of the means of satisfying the venereal appetite, proposes to himself as a matter of indifference a prostitute of either sex: and the same poet, who forgetting himself now and then says a little here and there about boys, says a great deal everywhere about women. The same observation will hold good with respect to every other personage of antiquity who either by his own account or that of another is represented to us as being infected with this taste. It is so in all the poets who in any of their works have occasion to say anything about themselves. Some few appear to have had no appetite for boys, as is the case for instance with Ovid, who takes express notice of it and gives a reason for it. But it is a never failing rule wherever you see any thing about boys, you see a great deal more about women. Virgil has one Alexis, but he has Galateas [blank] in abundance. Let us be unjust to no man: not even to a paederast. In all antiquity there is not a single instance of an author nor scarce an explicit account of any other man who was addicted exclusively to this taste. Even in modern times the real women-haters are to be found not so much among paederasts, as among monks and Catholic priests, such of them, be they more or fewer, who think and act in consistency with their profession.

REASON WHY IT MIGHT BE EXPECTED SO TO DO

I say even in modern times; for there is one circumstance which should make this taste where it does prevail much more likely to be exclusive at present than it was formerly. I mean the severity with which it is now treated by the laws and the contempt and abhorrence with which it is regarded by the generality of the people. If we may so call it, the persecution they meet with from all quarters, whether deservedly or not, has the effect in this instance which persecution has and must have more or less in all instances, the effect of rendering those persons who are the objects of it more attached than they would otherwise be to the practise it proscribes. It renders them the more attached to one another, sympathy of itself having a powerful tendency, independent of all other motives, to attach a man to his own companions in misfortune. This sympathy has at the same time a powerful tendency to beget a proportionable antipathy even towards all such persons as appear to be involuntary, much more to such as appear to be the voluntary, authors of such misfortune. When a man is made to suffer it is enough on all other occasions to beget in him a prejudice against those by whose means or even for whose sake he is made to suffer. When the hand of every man is against a person, his hand, or his heart at least, will naturally be against every man. It would therefore be rather singular if under the present system of manners these outcasts of society should be altogether so well disposed towards women as in ancient times when they were left unmolested.

WHETHER, IF IT ROBBED WOMEN, IT OUGHT AT ALL EVENTS TO BE PUNISHED?

The result of the whole is that there appears not any great reason to conclude that, by the utmost increase of which this vice is susceptible, the female part of the species could be sufferers to any very material amount. If however there was any danger of their being sufferers to any amount at all this would of itself be ample reason for wishing to restrain the practise. It would not however follow absolutely that it were right to make use of punishment for that purpose, much less that it were right to employ any of those very severe punishments which are commonly in use. It will not be right to employ any punishment, 1. if the mischief resulting from the punishment be equal or superior to the mischief of the offence, nor 2. if there be any means of compassing the same end without the expense of punishment. Punishment, says M. Beccaria, is never just so long as any means remain untried by which the end of punishment may be accomplished at a cheaper rate. [200c and 200d are blank] / [201]

INDUCEMENTS FOR PUNISHING IT NOT JUSTIFIED ON THE GROUND OF MISCHIEVOUSNESS

When the punishment [is] so severe, while the mischief of the offence is so remote and even so problematical, one cannot but suspect that the inducements which govern are not the same with those which are avowed. When the idea of the mischievousness of an offence is the ground of punishing it, those of which the mischief is most immediate and obvious are punished first: afterwards little by little the legislator becomes sensible of the necessity of punishing those of which the mischief is less and less obvious. But in England this offence was punished with death before ever the malicious destruction or fraudulent obtainment or embezzlement of property was punished at all, unless the obligation of making pecuniary amends is to be called a punishment; before even the mutilation of or the perpetual disablement of a man was made punishable otherwise than by simple imprisonment and fine. (It was the custom to punish it with death so early as the reign of Ed. 1st.)

BUT ON THE GROUND OF ANTIPATHY

In this case, in short, as in so many other cases the disposition to punish seems to have had no other ground than the antipathy with which persons who had punishment at their disposal regarded the offender. The circumstances from which this antipathy may have taken its rise may be worth enquiring to. 1. One is the physical antipathy to the offence. This circumstance indeed, were we to think and act consistently, would of itself be nothing to the purpose. The act is to the highest degree odious and disgusting, that is, not to the man who does it, for he does it only because it gives him pleasure, but to one who thinks [?] of it. Be it so, but what is that to him? He has the same reason for doing it that I have for avoiding it. A man loves carrion—this is very extraordinary—much good may it do him. But what is this to me so long as I can indulge myself with fresh meat? But such reasoning, however just, few persons have calmness to attend to. This propensity is much stronger than it is to be wished it were to confound physical impurity with moral. From a man's possessing a thorough aversion to a practise himself, the transition is but too natural to his wishing to see all others punished who give into it. Any pretense, however slight, which promises to warrant him in giving way to this intolerant propensity is eagerly embraced. Look the world over, we shall find that differences in point of taste and opinion are grounds of animosity as frequent and as violent as any opposition in point of interest. To disagree with our taste [and] to oppose our opinions is to wound our sympathetic feelings and to affront our pride. James the 1st of England, a man [more] remarkable for weakness than for cruelty, conceived a violent antipathy against certain persons who were called Anabaptists on account of their differing from him in regard to certain speculative points of religion. As the circumstances of the times were favorable to [the] gratification of antipathy arising from such causes, he found means to give himself the satisfaction of committing one of them to the flames. The same king happened to have an antipathy to the use of tobacco. But as the circumstances of the times did not afford the same pretenses nor the same facility for burning tobacco-smokers as for burning Anabaptists, he was forced to content himself with writing a flaming book against it. The same king, if he be the author of that first article of the works which bear his name, and which indeed were owned by him, reckons this practise among the few offences which no Sovereign ever ought to pardon. This must needs seems rather extraordinary to those who have a notion that a pardon in this case is what he himself, had he been a subject, might have stood in need of.

This transition from the idea of physical to that of moral antipathy is the more ready when the idea of pleasure, especially of intense pleasure, is connected with that of the act by which the antipathy is excited. Philosophical pride, to say nothing at present of superstition, has hitherto employed itself with effect in setting people a-quarreling with whatever is pleasurable even to themselves, and envy will always be disposing them to quarrel with what appears to be pleasurable to others. In the notions of a certain class of moralists we ought, not for any reason they are disposed to give for it, but merely because we ought, to set ourselves against every thing that recommends itself to us under the form of pleasure. Objects, it is true, the nature of which it is to afford us the highest pleasures we are susceptible of are apt in certain circumstances to occasion us still greater pains. But that is not the grievance: for if it were, the censure which is bestowed on the use of any such object would be proportioned to the probability that could be shewn in each case of its producing such greater pains. But that is not the case: it is not the pain that angers them but the pleasure.

How Far the Antipathy is a Just Ground

Meanwhile the antipathy, whatever it may arise from, produces in persons how many soever they be in whom it manifests itself, a particular kind of pain as often as the object by which the antipathy is excited presents itself to their thoughts. This pain, whenever it appears, is unquestionably to be placed to the account of the mischief of the offence, and this is one reason for the punishing of it. More than this—upon the view of any pain which these obnoxious persons are made to suffer, a pleasure results to those by whom the antipathy is entertained, and this pleasure affords an additional reason for the punishing of it. There remain however two reasons against punishing it. The antipathy in question (and the appetite of malevolence that results from it) as far as it is not warranted by the essential mischievousness of the offence is grounded only in prejudice. It may therefore be assuaged and reduced to such a measure as to be no longer painful only in bringing to view the considerations which shew it to be ill-grounded. The case is that of the accidental existence of an antipathy which [would have] no foundation [if] the principle of utility were to be admitted as a sufficient reason for gratifying it by the punishment of the object; in a word, if the propensity to punish were admitted in this or any case as a sufficient ground for punishing, one should never know where to stop. Upon monarchical principles, the Sovereign would be in the right to punish any man he did not like; upon popular principles, every man, or at least the majority of each community, would be in the right to punish every man upon no better reason.

If It Were, So Would Heresy

If this were admitted we should be forced to admit the propriety of applying punishment, and that to any amount, to any offence for instance which the government should find a pleasure in comprising under the name of heresy. I see not, I must confess, how a Protestant, or any person who should be for looking upon this ground as a sufficient ground for burning paederasts, could with consistency condemn the Spaniards for burning Moors or the Portuguese for burning Jews: for no paederast can be more odious to a person of unpolluted taste than a Moor is to a Spaniard or a Jew to an orthodox Portuguese.

Note

1. Louis Compton, "Gay Genocide," in L. Crewe, *The Gay Academic* (Palm Springs, CA: ETC Publications, 1978).

24.

THE BIOMEDICAL GAZE

How Medical Models Affect
Social Concepts of the Life Cycle

Robert B. Baker

In his watershed work, *Naissance de la Clinique* (Birth of the Clinic), French philosopher Michel Foucault (1926–1984) observed that the medical perception of the world, *the medical gaze*, as he called it, anatomizes persons, stripping away personhood, replacing it with a perception of biophysiological processes (Foucault [1963] 1973). The biomedical gaze strips the life cycle of its social meanings, perceiving only biophysiological events, blinded to the nested social relationships that surround them. Yet even as the medical gaze seeks to eschew social and religious meanings in the name of science, it is never free from their influence.

Consider the case of the ancient Greek philosopher Socrates (469–399 BCE). By the standards of Athenian society, Socrates had abnormal sexual predilections: he was a monogamous heterosexual. Normally, the sexual life cycle of upper-class Athenian males commenced with same-sex relationships with older males, moving on to heterosexual relationships in adulthood, when they were expected to marry and to have reproductive relationships with females. As males aged, however, they were expected to revert to same-sex relationships with younger males, completing their sexual life cycle. The typical sexual life cycle of

"The Biomedical Gaze" is drawn from R. Baker and L. McCullough, "Medical Ethics Through the Life Cycle in Europe and the Americas," *The Cambridge World History of Medical Ethics* (New York: Cambridge University Press), 2008, pp. 137–39, and is reprinted by permission of the author.

upper-class Athenian males thus involved bisexual maturation, evolving from same-sex to heterosexual to same-sex relationships (Dover 1989).

Unlike his contemporaries, Socrates was, abnormally, a committed heterosexual who became a faithfully monogamous married male. As an adult he had many relations with attractive young men (his students), yet, again abnormally, these relationships were consistently asexual. His fellow Athenians found Socrates' sex life odd. Nonetheless, the medical gaze was not particularly powerful in ancient Greece, and Socrates' "abnormal" heterosexual predilections were never medicalized.

In later eras, as the medical model came to dominate ever-larger swaths of the life cycle, sexuality became increasingly medicalized. In pre-Christian Europe, sexual intercourse was guiltless, reflecting the pro-erotic views of pagan culture. Medical authorities believed that regular ejaculations (spending one's seed) and intercourse were conducive to health; correlatively, that the retention of seed was unhealthy, causing headaches, lethargy, fainting, and bizarre behavior. Because the male sexual paradigm applied to females as well—as Aristotle (384–322 BCE) famously remarked, "a woman is as it were an impotent male, for it is through a certain incapacity that the female is female" (Aristotle, *On the Generation of Animals*, I, 20, 728a)—medical writers believed that females had seed or sexual fluid that needed to be expressed through orgasm. The general consensus was that retention of male seed in the testes or female seed or sexual fluids in the womb—a condition known as hysteria, from *hysterikos*, the Greek term for disturbances of the uterus—would manifest itself as fainting, fits, and other physical symptoms.

The most famous Greek physician of the Roman era, Galen (Claudius Galenus of Pergamum, 131–201) recommended either regular sexual intercourse or masturbation as a form of preventive medicine. Masturbation was also recommended as the appropriate treatment for hysteria. As evidence of its therapeutic efficacy, Galen cites the case of a widow afflicted with nervous tension. Diagnosing the problem as hysteria, a midwife manipulated the widow's sexual organs until she reached orgasm. As a result, Galen reported, the woman secreted a large quantity of fluid and was cured (Galen 1976, Book 6, Chapter 5, 185).

Judeo-Christian culture offered a radically different view of sexuality, eroticism, and masturbation. It perceived masturbation through the lens of Genesis 38:8–10—a short passage, in which God condemns and slays a man, Onan, for refusing to consummate a levirate marriage by having intercourse with his deceased brother's childless widow (so that the deceased brother will have offspring to carry on the line). Onan's nonconsummation involved "spilling his seed on the ground." No guidance is offered about whether the act for which God condemned and slew Onan was intentional defiance, refusal to consummate a levirate marriage, or spilling his seed, as either *coitus interruptus* or masturbation.

By the Renaissance, however, Christianity and Judaism interpreted Onan's sin as masturbation (Laquer 2003). Renaissance physicians thus felt the need to discard Galen's recommendations for the treatment of hysteria because "the spiritual harm outweigh[ed] any temporal gain" (Schleiner 1995, 123). By the eighteenth century, physicians began to project the Judeo-Christian moral critique of masturbation onto the act itself and masturbation came to be viewed as *unhealthy* as well as immoral. The transformation was initiated in 1710 when an anonymous medical tract, *Onania; or, The Heinous Sin of Self-Pollution*, was published in London (Anonymous [1723] 1986). Inverting the characteristics traditionally associated with retained seed or hysteria, the author claimed that the sin of masturbation carried with it such deleterious medical consequences as loss of appetite, weakness, sleeplessness, exhaustion, and fainting fits.

Circa 1760 a Swiss physician, Simon-Auguste-Andre-David Tissot (1728–1787), defended much the same thesis in *Onanism: Or a Treatise Upon the Disorders produced by Masturbation* (Tissot [1760] 1767), claiming that masturbation caused memory loss, clouded sight, and led to gout, rheumatism, weakness of the back, and consumption. Tissot had again inverted Galen's account of hysteria and its treatments, attributing to masturbation the very symptoms previously assigned to hysteria. Masturbation was thus instantly transformed from cure to cause, from therapy to pathology—not as a function of new scientific discoveries, but as an infusion of religious and social values into the seemingly objective medical gaze or model.

Conceived in the Victorian era (1819–1901), modern psychiatry assimilated Tissot's pathologizing of masturbation, taking the further step of transforming the act from a precipitating cause of various somatic or physical maladies into a psychiatric illness (Porter 1997, 203). In 1893 no less a figure than Sigmund Freud classified masturbation, not as a form of insanity per se, but rather as a leading cause of a condition known as neurasthenic neurosis (Freud 1971, I: 50).

Throughout the nineteenth and early twentieth centuries, treatments for masturbatory insanity, onanism, and neurasthenia were often extreme, ranging from electroshock to sexual surgery—including clitorectomy (removal of the clitoris for female masturbators), desensitizing scarification, and castration (typically for male masturbators), and institutionalization in an asylum (Barker-Benfield 1976; Engelhardt 1981). Under one name or another, masturbation remained an active psychiatric diagnosis through the 1930s. Its epitaph was written in the Kinsey reports of 1948 and 1953, which reported that 92 percent of males and 62 percent of females practiced masturbation (Kinsey 1948, 1953). Believing that something so common could not be unnatural, the pathologization of masturbation ceased. By the 1960s, the gynecologist-psychologist team of

William Masters (1915–2001) and Virginia Johnson completed the circle, returning the medical conception of masturbation to its classic roots, as a requisite of normality. In their studies on human sexuality they treat the capacity for masturbation as the litmus test for sexual health (Masters and Johnson 1966, 1970). Medical views of masturbation had thus come full circle: from a requisite of health, to a therapy, to a cause of disease, to a disease, and finally, once again, to a prerequisite of health—a normal part of puberty and integral aspect of maturation in the sexual life cycle.

The remarkable transformation in the medical understanding of masturbation in the sexual life cycle provides a striking example of the extent to which the seemingly objective medical gaze is prone to mirror social values. Pagan Greece and Rome celebrated sensuality and its medicine reflected these values, endorsing masturbation as both healthy and therapeutic. Judeo-Christianity, loathing eroticism and relegating sexuality to the realm of dutiful reproduction, saw masturbation as sinful. As medicine and psychiatry flourished in the eighteenth and nineteenth centuries, this sin was transformed into a sickness. When the influence of religion waned in twentieth-century Europe and North America, society became less puritanical and its medicine could accept normality of masturbation, once again treating it as a sign of healthy sexuality. At every turn, including its present incarnation, social values inform the medical gaze not only with respect to masturbation and homosexuality but also with respect to the life cycle generally. Any historical account of the relationships between biomedicine and the life cycle must thus address two countervailing tendencies: the tendency of the medical model to strip social and religious meaning from its account of the life cycle, and the countervailing tendency for society to reinfuse medicine's seemingly objective, non-value-laden accounts with the very social and religious meanings that the ideology of medicine ostensibly rejects.

BIBLIOGRAPHY

Anonymous. [1723] 1986. *Onania, or, The Heinous sin of self-pollution. A supplement to the Onania.* New York: Garland Publishing.

Aristotle, 1979. *Generation of Animals*, A. L. Peck, Trans. Cambridge, MA: Harvard University Press.

Barker-Benfield, G. J. 1976. *The Horrors of the Half-Known Life: Male Attitudes Toward Women and Sexuality in Nineteenth-Century America.* New York: Harper & Row Publishers.

Dover, K. J. 1989. *Greek Homosexuality.* Cambridge, MA: Harvard University Press.

Engelhardt, H. Tristram, Jr. 1974. "The Disease of Masturbation: Values and the Concept of Disease." *Bulletin of the History of Medicine* 48: 234–48.

————. [1974] 1981. "The Disease of Masturbation: Values and the Concept of Disease." In *Concepts of Health and Disease: Interdisciplinary Perspectives*, ed. Arthur L. Caplan, H. Tristram Engelhardt Jr., and James J. McCartney; foreword by Denton Cooley, pp. 267–80. Reprint. Reading, MA: Addison-Wesley, Advanced Book Program (World Science Division).

Foucault, Michel. [1963] 1973. *Naissance de la clinique: Une archèologie du règard medical*, translated as *The Birth of the Clinic: An Archaeology of Medical Perception*, by A. M. Sheridan Smith. New York: Pantheon.

Freud, Sigmund. 1971. *Heredity and the Aetiology of the Neuroses*. In *The Standard Edition of the Complete Psychological Works of Sigmund Freud*. London: Hogarth Press.

Galen. 1976. *On the Affected Parts*, trans. R. E. Siegel. Basle, Switzerland: Krager Publishers.

Kinsey, Alfred. 1953. *Sexual Behavior in the Human Female*. Philadelphia: W. B. Saunders.

————. 1948. *Sexual Behavior in the Human Male*. Philadelphia: W. B. Saunders.

Laqueur, Thomas W. 2003. *Solitary Sex: A Cultural History of Masturbation*. New York: Zone Books.

Masters, W. H., and V. E. Johnson. 1970. *Human Sexual Inadequacy*. Boston: Little, Brown.

————. 1966. *Human Sexual Response*. Philadelphia: Lippincott Williams & Wilkins Publishers.

Porter, Roy. 1997. *The Greatest Benefit to Mankind: A Medical History of Humanity from Antiquity to the Present*. London: HarperCollins.

Schleiner, Winfried. 1995. *Medical Ethics in the Renaissance*. Washington, DC: Georgetown University Press.

Tissot, Samuel Auguste. 1761. *Avis au peuple sur sa santé*. Lausanne: J. Zimmerli.

Tissot, Simon-Auguste-Andre-David. 1767. *Onanism: Or, a Treatise upon the Disorders produced by Masturbation*, 3rd ed., trans. A. Hume. London: W. Wilkinson.

25.

TAKING RESPONSIBILITY
FOR SEXUALITY*

Joyce Trebilcot

It is fundamental to feminism that women should take responsibility for ourselves, collectively and individually. In this essay I explore a central aspect of this project: taking responsibility for sexuality. I am particularly concerned here with women taking responsibility for our sexual identities as lesbian or heterosexual.

I write in part out of the struggle within feminism over whether feminism precludes women having affectional-sexual ties with men. As those familiar with feminist theory know, feminists advocate lesbianism on a variety of grounds. Some emphasize, for instance, that because virtually everyone's first erotic relationship is with a woman (mother), lesbianism is "natural" for women, as heterosexuality is for men. Another argument is based on the claim that, in patriarchy, equality in a heterosexual relationship is impossible; even if a man undertakes to renounce male privileges, he cannot do so entirely. A third argument holds that women who are committed to feminism should give *all* their energies to women. I am not concerned here to explore these arguments. Rather,

---

*This paper was originally prepared as a talk for a conference on women and mental health at the University of Oklahoma in the spring of 1982. That version appears in *Women and Mental Health: Conference Proceedings*, edited by Elaine Barton, Kristen Watts-Penny, and Barbara Hillyer Davis (Norman, OK: Women's Studies Program, University of Oklahoma, 1982). The paper was also presented at Union College, Schenectady, New York, in the spring of 1983.

I especially appreciate conversations about the topic of this essay with Sandra Lee Bartky.

I want to develop the idea of women taking responsibility for our own sexuality, whatever it may be. Feminism requires at least this of us.

Notice first that to take responsibility for a state of affairs is not to claim responsibility for having caused it. So, for example, if I take responsibility for cleaning up the kitchen I am not thereby admitting to any role in creating the mess; the state of the kitchen may be the consequence of actions quite independent of me. Similarly, in taking responsibility for her sexuality, a woman is not thereby claiming responsibility for what her sexuality has been, but only for what it is now and what it will be in the future.

In taking responsibility, a woman chooses to make a commitment about a specific state of affairs. The role of choice here constitutes an important link between the idea of taking responsibility and feminist values, for in feminist value schemes choice often has a central place.[1] Indeed, a feminist theory of responsibility might well involve the thesis that one is not to be held responsible for anything one has not agreed ahead of time to be responsible for.[2]

To take responsibility for one's sexuality, broadly conceived, is to take responsibility for the whole range of erotic/sexual/gender phenomena that are aspects of one's actions, attitudes, thoughts, wishes, style, and so on. In particular, it includes taking responsibility for oneself as lesbian or heterosexual or bisexual, or the celibate version of any of these: celibate lesbian, celibate heterosexual, celibate bisexual. It is to be expected that many women find these male-created labels and perhaps even their feminist redefinitions unsatisfactory.[3] Nevertheless, taking responsibility for one's sexuality does include locating oneself in terms of some such categories—categories that are already available or that one may invent.[4]

A paradigm case of taking responsibility for one's sexuality is coming out as a lesbian.[5] It is characteristic of first coming out, of coming out to oneself, that a woman does not know whether to say that she has *discovered* that she is a lesbian, or that she has *decided* to be a lesbian. The experience is one of acknowledging, of realizing what is already there, and at the same time of creating something new, a new sense of oneself, a new identity. In coming out, one connects up an already existing reality—one's feelings, one's sensations, one's identification with women—with one's values, i.e., with one's understanding or concept of who one is. This is the sort of process I mean to refer to here when I speak of taking responsibility for sexuality.

The process, then, is one of *discovery/creation*. Notice that there is no simple term for this process in patriarchal language, at least not in English. It might be suggested, for example, that coming out is a matter of interpretation, of interpreting or reinterpreting one's experiences and feelings in a certain way, as evidence of or elements in one's lesbianism. But this way of understanding coming out is incomplete because it captures only part of the process, the discovery part. To discover that one has been a lesbian all along is certainly to interpret past experiences in a new way, as experiences of a closeted lesbian. But coming out involves also deciding to be a lesbian, for now and in the future, which is to say, deciding not to participate in the institution of heterosexuality and to go on loving women. Coming out then is not merely a matter of reinterpreting one's past; it involves taking responsibility for being a lesbian both in the past and in the future.

Another received term that might be thought to apply to coming out is "conversion experience." There is certainly ample patriarchal literature about people undergoing conversions, mostly religious ones. But the idea of conversion doesn't capture coming out either. The patriarchal convert becomes what he was not. The lesbian becomes what she is.

But, it might be suggested, what about the expression "coming out" itself? Doesn't that convey the experience? This expression has been adopted by lesbians from gay male culture and by gay males presumably from the custom of debutantes coming out into society. It emphasizes not the creation of the self, but the presentation of the self to others. It omits, I think, the inwardness of lesbian experience, the fact that coming out is not merely (or at all) a social exercise but a subjective one, a kind of growth.

It is no accident, of course, that there is no term in patriarchy for the experience I am concerned with here, that there is no brief and clear way of accurately referring to it. Taking responsibility for one's own sexuality is not in the interest of patriarchy, which insists, for its own protection, that sexuality is only a given, that we have no role in creating it. The power of men over women in patriarchy, and of some men over others, is maintained in large part through the institution of heterosexuality, which requires not that women take responsibility for our own sexuality but, rather, that women act on rules that are given to us.[6]

Now, before I go on to discuss the meaning of taking responsibility for one's sexuality for heterosexual women, I want to trace briefly how patriarchy insists that sexuality is wholly given, even through changing ways of thinking about sexuality, through changing sexual values.

Consider first the traditional view that establishes heterosexuality as the norm, and lesbianism as a deviation or disease. On this view, one's sexuality is clearly a given only; it is inherited, or acquired in childhood; it is something that happens *to* an individual. This way of thinking about sexuality tends to keep one docile: one is passive, submissive, with respect to it; it is something received entire, not something one contributes to or creates. On this model, the lesbian, who is described as deviant or as suffering some illness or pathology, is supposed to require treatment by an expert: her sexuality, her "deviance," is not something she can take care of herself. On this traditional model, the question of taking responsibility for one's sexuality does not arise for either lesbian or heterosexual. Sexual identity for everyone is something one "gets," something that happens to one; and if it is not okay, then an expert is called in, but the woman herself remains passive.

In some circles this traditional way of conceiving sexuality has been replaced by pluralism. Pluralism rejects the view that only heterosexuality is normal and holds instead, in the spirit of liberalism, that there are alternative "sexual preferences"—lesbianism, bisexuality, heterosexuality—which are equally acceptable and which can all be equally "healthy." According to pluralism, sexual identity alone does not determine whether one is healthy or ill, normal or deviant. Such determinations are made in terms of how one "adjusts" to one's sexual identity, how well it satisfies one's needs, whatever they may be.

This way of thinking about sexual identity is equivalent to the more traditional view in terms of keeping women docile. Pluralism's message is: "Look, whatever you are, it's okay—don't worry about it. There are differences among us, but we can all live together happily." This message, of course, seeks to drown out the voice of the lesbian who understands lesbianism as part of the struggle against patriarchy. *Her* message is: "Pay attention to what each form of sexuality means for women. They are *not* all the same in terms of equality, in terms of power, in terms of domination." But this thinking is forbidden by an ethic that insists that all the alternatives are equally okay. So laissez-faire pluralism works against women thinking seriously about our sexuality as we must do if we are to take responsibility for it.

A third way of thinking about sexuality is to hold that everyone ought to be pansexual or at least bisexual, and so open to sexual encounters with persons of both sexes. This position is connected with the ideology, if not the practice (which was mainly heterosexual), of the "sexual revolution" of the sixties, and with leftist theories that advocate the release of sexuality from repression. On this view, the theoretical ideal is that everyone should be the same, bisexual. The theory itself tells us what to be. But if we don't have to decide for ourselves, we don't have to compare the different kinds of sexuality and consider reasons for and against them. We are simply to be obedient, to be bisexual, to be open to anything. This position, of course, has special potential for the exploitation of women. And, like the traditional and pluralistic models, it provides no support for individuals' taking responsibility for and defining their own sexuality.

None of these male-created value systems allows room for the idea that one might discover/create one's own sexuality on the basis of one's feelings and one's politics, on the basis of reasons, on the rational-emotional weighing of all one deems relevant. The same is true, of course, of patriarchal science. The scientific study of sexuality seeks to discover causes of lesbianism, and sometimes also of heterosexuality, and there is no space in these causal accounts for women to participate in the creating of our own sexual identities. A feminist theory of sexuality will not be a causal theory in any familiar sense, and will surely include an account of the role a woman herself may play in the development of her sexuality.[7]

It is, I believe, in the interest of all women to take responsibility for our sexuality. "Coming out," as I have suggested, provides a model for this process. But what could it possibly mean to "come out" as a heterosexual? Most heterosexual women accept the identities their conditioning provides for them, and so, it would seem, there is little or nothing for them to discover or create.

But to think in this way is again to fall into the trap of taking sexuality as merely given. Virtually all women can take responsibility for our sexuality. For a heterosexual woman to take responsibility for herself as heterosexual involves acknowledging the experiences and feelings she has that are parts of her heterosexuality, and also making the decision to participate or not in the institution of heterosexuality. Notice that the institution has many facets. It consists not just of sexual activity, but of a myriad of values and practices, including, for example, concepts of love, of couples, of faithfulness; meanings given to various fashions in clothes and personal appearance; ways of behaving with men and with women; and so on. A heterosexual woman taking responsibility decides which of the aspects of the institution she wishes to participate in (if any), and why. She may participate wholly, but if she is responsible, she does so not without thinking, but for reasons that she takes to be good ones.

Some women object to the idea that they should take responsibility for their own sexual identity on the ground that they have no choice, that they are what they are—lesbian, heterosexual—and cannot change. For example, it is not unusual for a feminist to claim that although the weight of *reason*, for her, is on the side of lesbianism, her *feelings* (perhaps as expressed in her fantasies), are irredeemably heterosexual, for she is sexually aroused by men but not by women. If such women sometimes identify as heterosexuals, they may claim that they cannot change the fact that they are sexually attracted to men, which they experience as a given, and so that they cannot take responsibility for their sexuality— that they are caught in a conflict between reason and feeling.

The peculiarity of this position is the assumption that one's feelings must determine one's sexual identity, that is, that one's genital twinges must determine whether one is lesbian, or heterosexual, or both. Granting that some women are sexually aroused only by men, they are not therefore locked into any of the familiar identities or excluded from any. Such women may, in the first place, choose for or against heterosexual *activity*. We know that there are many sexual impulses that ought to be suppressed rather than acted on, and women for whom the weight of reason is on the side of lesbianism have reason not to participate in heterosexual intercourse. It is also true that a woman may choose to make love to or with women, even though she is not sexually aroused. A woman's claim that she is not erotically responsive to women but only to men does not in itself limit her choices as between lesbianism, heterosexuality, or bisexuality, or celibacy of whatever variety. Sexuality is socially constructed; in reconstructing it we need not assume either that erotic feelings should lead to lovemaking or that lovemaking ought to occur only where there are erotic feelings.

Genital *sensations*, then, are not definitive of sexual identity; but clearly genital *activity* has a central role. Although there are, for example, lesbians who regularly engage in sexual intercourse with men (particularly, married lesbians and lesbian prostitutes), lesbian identity in these cases depends on there being special reasons (often economic) for continued heterosexual behavior. In the absence of such special reasons, regular heterosexual activity defeats the claim that one is a lesbian; such a woman would have instead to be identified as heterosexual or bisexual. Similarly, women who believe themselves to be heterosexual or bisexual, but who regularly engage in sexual activity with women but not with men, cannot, in the absence of special circumstances, sustain the claim of heterosexuality.

But what about the heterosexual feminist whose purported reason for engaging in heterosexual activity is just that she takes physical pleasure in it, physical pleasure she can experience in no other way? It would be too great a sacrifice, she says, to give up this pleasure, even for the political and personal benefits she thinks would come from an identification other than heterosexual. In exploring this issue, it often turns out that the physical pleasure is not after all separable from the economic, emotional, social, and other advantages that she gains from heterosexual relationships. For such a woman, identification as heterosexual is frequently based not primarily on some genital pleasure, but on a complex understanding of the role of heterosexual activity in her life.

A woman who has such an understanding can correctly be said to be taking responsibility for her own sexuality, even though the inconsistency between her reason (lesbian) and her genital feelings and behavior (heterosexual) remains. For she has come to understand her heterosexual identity not as a fate irrevocably determined by genital sensations, but as a choice she has made on the basis of a variety of factors, a choice pushed upon her, to be sure, by the power of the institution of heterosexuality, but also one that she might not have made and might yet revoke. Indeed, as she comes to understand her sexuality in the process of taking responsibility for it, her sexual identity may itself change, for the process of discovery/creation dialectically transforms preexisting reality.

It seems then that it does make sense to speak of all women—whatever our sexuality is and whatever it may become—as capable of taking responsibility for our sexuality, for discovering/creating our sexuality. I believe that we should take responsibility, for a variety of reasons I can only touch on here. First, if we define our own sexuality, if we are in control, we are more likely to be strong, self-creating, and independent, not merely about sexuality but generally, than if we simply do what is expected of us, that is, conform without question to the norms of heterosexuality. But also, to take responsibility for sexuality requires study and thought about the meanings of the different sexualities, and this consciousness-raising has important political implications. It means that there will be greater understanding among women of how patriarchy operates. It also means that there will be fewer heterosexuals, insofar as serious thought about heterosexuality leads women to withdraw from that institution. It not only contributes to a greater closeness in the women's community but also to a greater solidarity among all women through a lessening of heterosexism, lesbophobia, and lesbian-hating.

Let me focus briefly on this last idea, the connection between taking responsibility and overcoming these forms of lesbian oppression. Heterosexism is the conviction that heterosexuality is superior to other sexual identities; it includes heterosexist solipsism, that is, ignoring the existence of identities other than heterosexual. Heterosexism is commonly manifested in the assumption that everyone is heterosexual, or that lesbians are distant and rare, not one's friends and associates. Taking responsibility for sexual identity raises consciousness about lesbians and so makes women more aware of the presence of lesbians among their families, their friends, and in their workplaces. Heterosexism is expressed also, of course, by overt or subtle denigration of lesbians and lesbian culture. But a woman who takes seriously the project of defining her own sexuality has to consider the possibility that she herself could be a lesbian; having done this, I think, she is less likely to put down lesbians and things lesbian. If she rejects lesbianism, it is a reasoned rejection, not a prejudice (that is, not a judgment made prior to conscientious consideration of the issue). Heterosexism also takes the form of insensitivity, in heterosexual women, to the fact that the special privileges they enjoy as heterosexuals—privileges in jobs, housing, travel, and the like—are not privileges they *deserve* and lesbians do not, but rather, are privileges unfairly awarded to them by the heterosexual/patriarchal system and unfairly denied to their lesbian sisters. Again, women who take seriously their own sexual autonomy are likely to be more aware than others of the injustice of this system of privilege.

Lesbophobia, like heterosexism, may be lessened as one becomes conscious of one's sexual identity as something one has control over. Lesbophobia has a variety of forms. One is simply fear of the unknown: lesbians seem alien and threatening because one does not know what to expect from them. But part of taking responsibility for one's sexuality is finding out about lesbians and lesbianism.

Another form of lesbophobia is fear that I might be or become one too. But a woman who has a sense of responsibility about her sexuality, while she might find the idea of becoming a lesbian scary, knows that if she does identify as lesbian she does so because of her own discovery/decision; she knows that she herself is in control of her sexual identity, and whatever fear she has will be within her control as well.

Finally, lesbophobia may be a fear of being rejected by lesbians, of not being acceptable to them, or to some specific group of them, in terms of their values or standards or styles. This sort of lesbophobia is common among lesbians. But again, for lesbians and nonlesbians, the consciousness of creating one's own values and style mitigates the fear: the question is not after all whether one is acceptable to them, but, perhaps, whether one wants to expand one's own value system so as to include at least parts of theirs, so that one can be part of their group. This is something one can decide for oneself.

Hatred of lesbians, which frequently accompanies both heterosexism and lesbophobia, is, like misogyny, especially sad among women, for it is hatred of oneself, or of parts of oneself. Both lesbian and nonlesbian women can get into hating parts of ourselves and projecting those parts and that hatred onto lesbians. But taking responsibility involves getting in touch with dissonant, unacceptable, threatening, puzzling aspects of ourselves; if we acknowledge those aspects we are less likely both to project them and to hate them. Also, taking responsibility tends to increase self-esteem, and so to squeeze out self-hatred.

There are, then, excellent reasons why women, all women, should take responsibility for our own sexuality. We all *can* do so. For taking responsibility does not require a woman to be in a position to change the material conditions of her life; it requires only that she be able to understand her sexual identity as discovered and created by her in response to the pressures of patriarchy and the promise of the realization of feminism.

NOTES

1. This is so even though choice is associated with hierarchy and dualism, which most feminist theorists understand to be inconsistent with feminist values.

2. In feminist discourse, the concept of responsibility tends to drop out and is partially replaced by the notion of accountability. Accepting accountability is like taking responsibility in that one chooses what one is accountable for (one is not accountable if one did not make the commitment). Accepting accountability differs from taking responsibility in emphasizing relationships, in emphasizing those to whom one is accountable—one's community, friends, and lover. To urge that women should accept accountability for their sexuality, is to urge them to accept membership in a community or to make a com-

mitment to some relationship. In this essay I use the more patriarchal concept of responsibility because my focus is not so much on a woman's relationship to other women as on her giving reasons, perhaps only to herself, for the forms in which she expresses her sexual feelings.

3. For a discussion of feminist definitions of lesbianism, see Ann Ferguson, "Patriarchy, Sexual Identity, and the Sexual Revolution," *Signs* 7 (Autumn 1981): 158–72.

4. Some rebellious women may resist avowing an identity in these terms on the ground that they do not want to be labeled. But compare rejecting all labels to adopting a deviant's label with respect to their potential for expressing rebelliousness.

5. For accounts of coming out see *The Coming Out Stories*, edited by Julia Penelope Stanley and Susan J. Wolfe (Watertown, MA: Persephone Press, 1980).

6. In patriarchy, women may be expected to take some responsibility for aspects of their sexuality, for example, for allowing sexual access only to certain males or for birth control. But the idea that a woman can take responsibility for herself as lesbian or as heterosexual is foreign to patriarchy.

7. Heterosexuality is compulsory (Adrienne Rich, "Compulsory Heterosexuality and Lesbian Existence," *Signs* 5 [Summer 1980]: 631–60) and chosen (Marilyn Frye, Assignment: NWSA—Bloomington—1980: Speak on "Lesbian Perspectives on Women's Studies," *Sinister Wisdom* 14 [1980]: 3–7).

Notice, too, that it may be politically advantageous for gay men to interpret homosexuality as caused, as something they did not choose, in order to protect themselves from being perceived by straight men as breaking the bonds of fraternity.

26.

CULTURE AND WOMEN'S SEXUALITIES

Evelyn Blackwood*

Anthropological studies of women's same-sex relations in non-Western societies provide an important source for theorizing women's sexuality because they allow us to go beyond a narrow focus on Western cultures and concepts. Looking at studies from groups other than the dominant societies of Europe and America, I explore the diversity of women's sexualities and the sociocultural factors that produce sexual beliefs and practices. This article argues that sexual practices take their meaning from particular cultures and their beliefs about the self and the world. Cultural systems of gender, in particular, construct different sexual beliefs and practices for men and women. I conclude the article by suggesting some broad patterns at work in the production of women's sexualities across cultures.

Reprinted by permission from *Journal of Social Issues* 56, no. 2 (2000), pp. 223–38. © 2000 The Society for the Psychological Study of Social Issues.

*Correspondence concerning this article should be addressed to Evelyn Blackwood, Department of Sociology and Anthropology, Stone Hall, Purdue University, West Lafayette, IN 47907 [e-mail: blackwood@sri.soc.purdue.edu]. I would like to thank several wonderful colleagues who have provided ongoing support and stimulating discussions of these ideas: Deborah Elliston, Jeff Dickemann, and Saskia Wieringa. I also appreciate the thoughtful comments of the editors, Anne Peplau and Linda Garnets, as well as the anonymous reviewers.

This article explores women's sexuality from a cultural anthropology perspective. Anthropological evidence constitutes an important source for theorizing women's sexuality because it allows us to go beyond a sometimes narrow focus on the sexual categories of the dominant White societies of Europe and America (these groups will be glossed as "Western"). From a Western viewpoint, sexuality constitutes an essential or core attribute of identity; individuals are said to have fixed sexual identifies or orientations. Sexuality as it is understood in the United States and Europe, however, often bears little resemblance to sexual relationships and practices across cultures. By looking at cultural evidence from ethnic groups and countries other than the dominant White societies of Europe and America, I will explore the richness and diversity of women's sexualities and the sociocultural factors that constitute those sexualities.

The perspective I take in this article follows social construction theory, which argues that sexuality depends on the cultural context for its meaning. Although Freud saw human sexuality as a precultural given that must be controlled or regulated by society, social construction theorists argue that sexuality itself is a social product (Caplan, 1987; Foucault, 1978; Padgug, 1979; Rubin, 1975). There are a variety of strands of social construction theory; the differences lie mainly in the extent to which culture is thought to produce sexuality (Vance, 1989). The strong constructionist view holds that a general sexual potential is constructed into particular desires, meanings, and behaviors by culture. A weaker view states that culture shapes or constrains the form sexuality takes but "natural" desires set the baseline of sexuality. In my view social processes do not act as constraints to a "natural" sexuality but actually produce sexualities through discourses of desire, religion, gender, and so on. This view argues that sexual acts, or what appears to be sexual, take their meaning from particular cultures and their beliefs about the self and the world. It is these beliefs or ideologies that anthropologists investigate to understand the meaning of sexuality. Sexual meanings are produced through any number of factors, including ideologies of religion, ethnicity, class, gender, family, and reproduction, as well as the material and social conditions of everyday life. These factors provide the context for the production of sexual relationships, desires, and longings.

In this article I first take a number of case studies of women's same-sex relations in ethnic groups and countries other than the dominant White societies of Europe and America to illustrate the sociocultural factors that produce sexual beliefs and practices. Then I explore how cultural systems of gender construct different sexual beliefs and practices for men and women. In the third section I use two detailed examples of female sexualities, one from Suriname and one from West Sumatra, to argue that sexuality is neither a static category nor a fixed identity. I conclude by exploring some broad patterns at work in the production of women's sexualities across cultures.

Although many of the examples presented in this article involve women whom Americans might identify as "lesbians," I do not use that term generally. The term "lesbian" in the United States commonly refers to a woman whose primary sexual object choice is other women. When applied cross-culturally, "lesbian" invokes an essential linkage among practices whose connections may be tenuous at best (for further discussion of this point, see Wieringa & Blackwood, 1999). Since the term does not work in all cases across cultures, I use the term "same-sex relations" to refer to erotic relations or practices between women.

CULTURAL CONTEXTS OF SEXUALITY

Female same-sex sexuality has been noted in a number of colonized groups, postcolonial states, and sovereign countries since the beginning of European imperialism (Blackwood, 1986b; Blackwood & Wieringa, 1999). Case studies of women's same-sex relations illuminate the particular sociocultural processes that construct sexuality. I consider three different types of relations—intimate friendship, erotic ritual practice, and adolescent sex play—that represent both the varieties of sexualities as well as the complexities of the social processes involved.

Intimate Friendships

A study done in Lesotho, a small country surrounded by the nation of South Africa, documents intimate friendships between schoolgirls called "mummy-baby" relationships (Gay, 1986). Mummy-baby relations are institutionalized friendships between younger and older girls and women that became popular throughout much of Black southern Africa starting in the 1950s (Blacking, 1978). Prior to this time in rural communities, young women were educated at puberty in initiation schools run by women. Each initiate was appointed a "mother," an older girl who helped her "child" through initiation. This practice established strong networks between two age sets of women, ties that were maintained through visits and exchanges of gifts for many years (Blacking, 1978). Because of missionary efforts to stop this form of education, the schools are now virtually abandoned. Young women now attend public or boarding schools in neighboring towns or urban areas. Yet the bonds between initiates serve as a cultural model for the mummy-baby relations of contemporary schoolgirls and young women.

In the mummy-baby relationship, two young women start a relationship by arranging private encounters and exchanging love letters and gifts. The older girl, who becomes the mummy, might already have a boyfriend or other babies, while the younger one, the baby, is allowed to have only one mummy. The mummies are sources of guidance and "advice on sex and protection from aggressively courting young men" (Gay, 1986, p. 104) and appropriate partners in one's first romantic or sexual encounters. For girls who become mummies and babies to each other, their relationship is part of the romantic drama of growing up and learning the pleasures and responsibilities of relationships. They view their relationship as an affair or romance; hugging, kissing, and sexual relations are part of it. As they become older, they may in turn become mummies to their own babies or start to have their own boyfriends. For Lesotho women, the intensity of mummy-baby relations usually ends with marriage, when their attention is turned toward domestic responsibilities, but many women maintain the bonds of friendship with other women after marriage. Consequently, these relationships provide important emotional and economic ties for women within rural communities (Gay, 1986).

Mummy-baby relationships are constructed from a number of received cultural sources. The first source is the initiation school, where young girls received training for adult sexual practices and learned the importance of older girls and women as sources of friendship and social connection. In a culture where it is taboo for a mother to talk about sexuality with a daughter, older girls in initiation schools and now "mummies" are the culturally sanctioned source for this information. The second source comes from ideologies of sexuality. Although the Roman Catholic Church insists on virginity for Lesotho girls, within indigenous beliefs "female sensuality is both encouraged and restrained, but it is never denied" (Gay, 1986, p. 101). Young women's practice of lengthening the labia is seen as a way to make themselves "hotter." Their experiences with other girls teach them to develop and manage their own sexual feelings.

A third factor in the construction of mummy-baby relationships is the *motsoalle* (special friend), a special affective and gift exchange partnership practiced by women of an earlier generation in rural Lesotho (Kendall, 1999). In the past both married women and men had sexual partners other than their spouses (Nthunya, 1997). These cultural practices reflected an ideology of sexuality that sees women as agents of their own sexuality. These special friendships were long-term, loving, and erotic relationships that coexisted with heterosexual marriage. One woman, Nthunya (1997), who had a *motsoalle* relationship, was a poor, rural farmer most of her life. When she married her husband, she moved to his family home. She worked on their farm, raising sheep and growing maize. Her husband was often away on road construction or other wage labor jobs. Together they had six children. She describes her relationship with her female *motsoalle*:

> It's like when a man chooses you for a wife, it's because he wants to share the blankets with you. The woman chooses you the same way, but she doesn't want to share the blankets. She wants love only. When a woman loves another woman, you see, she can love her with a whole heart (Nthunya, 1997, p. 69).

Such relationships were publicly celebrated by gift-giving and feasting that involved the whole community. For the feast, a sheep was slaughtered, gifts were exchanged, and neighbors and kin from throughout the village came to eat, drink, and dance. The ritual feast was a public validation of the commitment the two women made to each other. A relationship with a *motsoalle* was neither an alternative nor a threat to marriage. According to Nthunya, her husband and her *motsoalle's* husband were both supportive of their relationship. Nthunya (1997, p. 72) said, "In the old days friendship was very beautiful—men friends and women friends. Friendship was as important as marriage. Now this custom is gone; everything is changing."

The poverty of Lesotho and the migration of husbands have often been used as explanations for women's intimate friendships. Such explanations assume that women love each other only when they are deprived of heterosexual outlets. The above case, however, shows the importance of other sociocultural factors in women's same-sex desires. Sexuality for women of Lesotho is constructed through the institution of women's friendships, the cultural tradition of age mates, and the cultural ideology of sexuality in which women have sexual agency. Consequently, close emotional and intimate bonds between women are seen as a natural part of growing up and an important source of social ties in adulthood.

Intimate friendships for both sexes are quite common in cultures of sub-Saharan Africa. The institution of bond friendships among Azande women of central Africa (located in the countries of Sudan and the Republic of Zaire), for example, relied on cultural patterns similar to those of the south. At the time that this institution was first noted in the 1930s (Evans-Pritchard, 1970), Azande society was composed of several kingdoms with noble and commoner classes. As in Lesotho, descent was traced through men, and children belonged to the husband's lineage. Men were allowed to marry several wives; each wife had her own dwelling in her husband's compound. The marital relationship was organized around economics, with the wife providing labor on her husband's land and receiving her own land to cultivate as well. Women maintained important trade relations to sell the produce that they grew. Exchange relations established across the village improved not only their economic resources but also their social connections and the numbers of people they could count on. Within this context Azande women looked to bond friendship as an important means to develop and broaden their networks (Blackwood, 1986a).

Bond friendships were formal relationships of exchange and service between two women. The relationship was established by holding a formal ceremony called *bagburu*, in which the two women exchanged small gifts, then divided a corn cob in half, each one taking a half to plant in her own garden. Bond friendships were not only exchange relationships; they established close emotional and sometimes erotic relationships between women. Unfortunately, most of what is known about *bagburu* relationships comes from Azande men and reflects their own fears and fantasies about their wives (Evans-Pritchard, 1970). Azande wives had to ask permission from their husbands to begin a *bagburu* relationship. The men believed that some women who were bond friends had sexual relations together. Husbands tried to discourage their wives from developing sexual attachments, although they rarely refused to give permission for the relationship itself. Evans-Pritchard reports little information about sexual practices between bond friends, but a story of two women's lovemaking after performing *bagburu* suggests that such behavior was not considered unusual (Evans-Pritchard, 1970, p. 1431). In this case the importance of social and trade networks with other women supports a construction of women's sexuality as something for them to explore and enjoy within and outside of marriage.

Erotic Ritual Practices

The homoerotic ritual practices of aboriginal Australian women constitute another case that resists a Western framework of sexual identities. Prior to colonization, Australian aborigines were seminomadic, egalitarian hunter-gatherers who lived in small camps. Their complex kinship system defined potential marriage partners as well as extramarital relations for both women and men (Roheim, 1933).

Young girls were initiated into their adult roles at first menstruation through a process of training and ritual that produced a girl's social identity. Adult women taught adolescent girls about sexuality and sexual magic through initiation ceremonies. These ceremonies conveyed messages about the configuration of tribal land, kinship categories, and proper social action; they also included homoerotic movements or performances between the women and the initiates. Earlier anthropologists, who seemed reluctant to discuss this aspect of ritual performances, described the movements of the women dancers as sexually suggestive, leading to so-called simulated intercourse. According to Kaberry (1939), the intent of this action was to ensure heterosexual success (getting or keeping a husband or male lover). More recent interpretations (Povinelli, 1992) suggest that these ceremonies include homoerotic "digging" (*yedabetj*). For the performers, "digging" constitutes erotic play that initiates young women into the complex social and kin categories of their adult lives (Povinelli, 1992). For Australian aboriginal groups, the social processes that produce erotic ritual play include both a cultural ideology in which women have sexual agency and a belief in the power of ritual to influence and control human action.

Adolescent Sex Play

Adolescent heterosexual play is well documented for many cultures. Its practice is closely tied to ideas about childhood, sexuality, and virginity. In societies such as the !Kung San of the Kalahari Desert of southern Africa, children and adolescents engage in both heterosexual and homosexual play. Due to colonization, few !Kung now live their nomadic hunter-gatherer lifestyle, but one !Kung woman, Nisa, has recounted a life history that sheds light on these adolescent sexual practices (Shostak, 1983).

The egalitarian !Kung lived in small communities of kin that moved with the rains and availability of food. Families had few possessions. The adult couple shared a small grass dwelling with their children. In such close quarters they waited until their children fell asleep before they engaged in sex. Adults insisted that they disapproved of childhood sex play (to disapproving missionaries, perhaps), but when children played at the things their parents did, it included sexual experimentation. Nisa recounted how she watched older girls play sexually with each other and then did the same with her girlfriends as she approached adolescence. As girls got older, they played sexually with the boys, although Nisa describes herself as initially reluctant to do so. All the young girls Nisa knew later married men. In this case marriage does not become the only adult locus of sexuality, since, according to Nisa, both men and women have sexual relations with partners other than their spouses.

The !Kung have constructed an adolescent phase of sexual experimentation that includes both same-sex and other-sex partners. This construction of sexuality is related to several sociocultural factors, including ideologies of gender, family, and childhood. Lacking any significant property or inheritance concerns vested in marriage, !Kung gender ideology is egalitarian. For !Kung families, neither marriage partner has exclusive sexual rights over the other. !Kung view adolescence as a time to learn sexual feelings and desires. All these factors combine to produce adolescence as a sexual "learning" period that precedes heterosexual marriage. In this case sexuality between young women is constructed as a part of sexual exploration.

The preceding section has described both the variety and complexity of sexuality in ethnic groups and countries other than the dominant White societies of Europe and America. As the cases show, a number of sociocultural processes construct sexuality, including initiation practices, institutions of women's friendships, the importance of social networks, and cultural traditions of age mates, as well as ideologies of gender, religion, marriage, and family. These processes give sexuality its meaning and provide the context through which it is constructed.

CONSTRUCTING MEN'S AND WOMEN'S SEXUALITIES

In this section I consider how gender ideologies, the cultural set of practices and beliefs about men and women and their relations to each other, construct men's and women's sexualities differently. Because gender includes beliefs about sexual behavior, it is one of the primary crucibles within which sexuality is produced. Sexualities are informed by and embedded in conceptions of gender; that is, they are embedded in gender ideologies that enable and structure differential practices for women and men. In the following examples I examine the way gender ideologies produce very different constructions of men's and women's sexualities. I use examples from the Sambia of Papua New Guinea and from patriarchal China to show the ways in which sexual ideologies for women in these cultures are quite distinct from those for men. The differences in sexual ideologies produce very different sexual practices for women and men.

Among the Sambia of Papua New Guinea, femininity is seen as inherent, an attribute that girls are born with. In contrast, masculinity is understood as something that boys lack and must acquire as they grow up. While ritual practices ensure that young boys acquire masculinity, no rituals are necessary for girls to acquire femininity. This gender ideology encodes very different ideas about the sexuality of men and women. Boys must acquire masculinity ritually by ingesting the semen of adult men (Herdt, 1981). According to Western categories, such practices would be considered "homosexual." In this Papuan New Guinea culture, however, insemination rituals are not seen as homosexual behavior but rather as ritual measures to ensure the proper development of masculine traits and reproductive competence. Once properly inseminated and achieving their full masculinity, these young men are ready for heterosexual marriage. This ritual practice is explicitly linked to notions of the efficacy of fluids for human development (Elliston, 1995). From all accounts, young girls do not engage in ritual "homosexual" practices because they already possess the necessary substances for femininity. But although girls' sexual development is unmarked, their bodily fluids are seen as sexually dangerous and polluting to men, resulting in a negative view of women's sexuality, which must be strictly circumscribed by ritual taboos. In this case, ideas about men's and women's attributes lead to very different conceptualizations of their sexuality, men needing "homosexual" insemination and women seen as polluting and dangerous.

Another example of cultural differences in men's and women's sexualities comes from patriarchal China. In nineteenth-century China, women were quickly married off to a husband and were expected to be subservient and sexually faithful. In contrast, men were entitled to control wives and family property and were allowed a number of wives as well as other sexual partners. Marriage for many women in patriarchal China was an oppressive institution. Because of the importance of reproducing the patrilineage and maintaining ancestor worship, arranged marriages were the norm; oftentimes the young couple did not meet before they were married. The new wife went to live in the household of her husband and was at first considered little more than a servant under the strict supervision of her mother-in-law. In the province of Guangdon, marriage presented an especially frightening prospect, since women not only married out of their village but in many cases into enemy territory (Sankar, 1986).

Following the development of silk production in Guangdon province in south China, the practice of marriage resistance and the creation of sisterhoods arose (Sankar, 1986; Topley, 1975). With the development of the silk factories in Guangdon in the mid-1800s, many young unmarried women went to work in the silk factories, earning money for themselves as well as their families. Because they were able to earn their own income, some of these women postponed marriage indefinitely. Women who refused to marry took a public vow to remain unwed and not to engage in sexual relations with men. This vow established their adult status, freeing their parents from any obligation to arrange a marriage and securing their rights to ancestor worship in their natal houses (Sankar, 1986). Sisterhoods of six to eight women each were formed, with such names as "Golden Orchid Association" or "Association for Mutual Admiration." The sisters lived in cooperative houses called "vegetarian halls" or "spinsters' halls," where they established joint funds to be used for holidays, emergencies, and their future retirement or death (Honig, 1985; Sankar, 1986). Sisters also formed sexual relationships with each other. "Larger sisterhoods may have contained several couples or ménage à trois" (Sankar, 1986). After the victory of the Red Army in 1949, the sisterhoods were banned as "feudal remnants" and many sisters fled to Malaysia, Singapore, Hong Kong, and Taiwan.

These sisterhoods were not simply a reaction to oppressive marriage conditions. Several other sociocultural factors were important in the development of the sisterhoods, including the institution of girls' houses, beliefs about ancestors, and sibling marriage order. First, it was the custom in this region for the kin group to build girls' houses for their adolescent daughters (Topley, 1975). Sleeping and eating in these houses, girls became close friends and confidants. Second, in patrilineal China, one's deceased parents must be given offerings regularly. Deceased wives are honored by their husband's family; unmarried or spinster women would have no one to honor them after they died. Women past the age of marriage were given a spinster ceremony through which they attained adult status and the right to have a house built for them where their kin could remember them after they died. Third, since younger sisters and brothers must wait until their elder siblings are married, the spinster ceremony allowed these siblings the right to marry. In addition to unique economic conditions, these factors contributed to the development of marriage resistance and sisterhoods in Guangdon China.

In the cases of the Chinese sisterhoods and the Papua New Guinea Sambia, cultural gender ideologies constructed different sexual practices for men and women. In the Sambia case a cultural practice rooted in an ideology of gender antagonism and the efficacy of bodily fluids legitimated particular insemination practices between men and boys, while creating women as inherently gendered and without need of adolescent homosexuality. In China patriarchal institutions created women's sexuality as subordinate to men's desires, while constructing men's sexuality more broadly to include the practice of taking male consorts, particularly among upper-class men and royalty (Ng, 1989). In China, the control of women's sexuality produced public resistance by women to oppressive marital and economic conditions, leading to the establishment of separatist sisterhoods.

In these cases, gender ideologies create different sexual roles, behaviors, meanings, and desires for women and men. Consequently, men and women in these cultures see themselves differently as sexual actors. For Sambian men, their sexuality must be developed in adolescence through insemination practices and sustained in adult life by strict ritual taboos. In contrast, Sambian women are constantly reminded that contact with their sexual organs and fluids is debilitating and even dangerous to men, resulting in limited heterosexual contacts. Historically in patriarchal China, men's desires were constructed broadly, whereas women's sexual experiences were strictly limited to their roles as wives or concubines to men.

From these cases it is clear that gender ideologies are critical to the production of men's and women's sexualities. Such ideologies work to produce very different sets of ideas about what men and women desire. By establishing certain ideas about who and what men and women are, gender ideologies create different possibilities for men's or women's understanding of their desires and their access to other sexual partners.

DECONSTRUCTING SEXUAL IDENTITIES

Studies of sexuality in Europe and America tend to take for granted the fixity of sexual object choice and sexual identity. Categories of homosexual, heterosexual, and bisexual, which are routinely used to define study populations, however, turn out to have little cross-cultural reliability. I now discuss two cases of female same-sex relations to highlight the problems with these Western sexual and gender categories. I explore cases from Suriname and West Sumatra in which women appear to be "lesbian" or "bisexual," but in fact their own understanding of their sexuality is quite different from the way it is constructed in the West.

The Mati Work

Erotic attachments between Creole women in the postcolonial state of Suriname, South America, pose a number of problems for Western categories of sexuality. The *mati* work is a widespread institution among Creole working-class women in the city of Paramaribo, Suriname (Wekker, 1999). Creoles, the second largest population group in Suriname, are the descendants of slaves brought from Africa, living mostly in urban areas. *Mati*, although by no means a monolithic category, are women who have sexual relationships with men and with women; they may have a relationship with a man and a woman occurring at the same time or one at a time. While some *mati*, especially older women who have borne and raised their children, do not have sex with men anymore, younger *mati* have a variety of arrangements with men, such as marriage, concubinage, or a visiting relationship. Women's relationships with women mostly take the form of visiting relationships, although a minority of female couples and their children live together in one household. These varied arrangements are made possible by the circumstance that most working-class Creole women own or rent their own houses and are single heads of households (Wekker, 1999).

The Creole concepts of self and sexuality are found in the framework of the Afro-Surinamese folk religion, called *Winti*. Unlike the Western version of the self as "unitary, authentic, bounded, static, trans-situational," the self in an Afro-Surinamese working-class universe is conceptualized as "multiplicitous, malleable, dynamic, and contextually salient" (Wekker, 1999, p. 125). *Winti* religion pervades virtually all aspects of life, from before birth to beyond death.

Within this framework both men and women are thought to be composed of male and female *winti*, gods. Both men and women are deemed full sexual beings with their own desires and possibilities of acting on these desires. Sexual fulfillment is important, but the gender of one's object choice is considered less important. According to one 84-year-old *mati*, who had relationships with men and bore a number of children, the "apples of her eye" throughout her long life were women:

> I never wanted to marry or "be in association with a man." My "soul"/"I" did not want to be under a man. Some women are like that. I am somebody who was not greedy on a man, my "soul," "I," wanted to be with women. It is your "soul" that makes you so. (Wekker, 1999, p. 125)

A *mati* is conceptualized as a woman, part of whose "I" desires and is sexually active with other women. Since the "I" is multiply and openly conceived, it is not necessary to claim a "truest, most authentic kernel of the self," a fixed "identity" that is attracted to other women. Rather, *mati* work is seen as a particularly pleasing and joyous activity, not as an identity (Wekker, 1999).

Surinamese *mati* (and Lesotho *motsoalle*) do not see themselves as lesbians or bisexuals; they have sex with each other, but their relations with men, including husbands and boyfriends, are also part of their sexuality. This case reflects the multiple sociocultural factors that produce the *mati* work. According to Wekker (1999), sexuality in this postcolonial working-class cultural nexus is multiply constructed through colonial discourses and Afro-Surinamese ideas about the self, sexuality, gender, and religion. But *mati* work is neither a sexual identity nor a distinct category of persons. It is encompassed by an ideology of sexuality in which men and women are seen as sexual beings whose sexuality is fluid and multiple.

Tombois in West Sumatra

One final example that complicates the Western categories of gender and sexuality comes from my own work on *tombois* among the Minangkabau in West Sumatra, Indonesia (Blackwood, 1998). The term *tomboi* (derived from the English word "tomboy") is used for a female acting in the manner of men (female here refers to physical sex of body, not gender). Although *tombois* are female, they see themselves as men who are attracted to normatively gendered women. In this overview I briefly explain the cultural factors that produce the *tomboi* identity and how this identity complicates any simple understandings of gender or sexuality.

Tombois pride themselves on doing things like Minangkabau men. They play *koa*, a card game like poker, which is perceived as a men's game. They smoke as men do; rural women rarely take up smoking. They go out alone, especially at night, which is men's prerogative. Like men, they drive motorcycles; women ride behind (women do drive motorcycles, but in a mixed couple the man always drives).

Tombois construct their desire for and relationships with women on a model of Minangkabau masculinity. The statement they often make is that their lovers are all feminine women. These women adhere to the codes of femininity assigned to female bodies. Female couples call each other *mami* and *papi*, and refer to other couples as *cowok* and *cewek*, Indonesian words that have the connotation of "guy" and "girl." Their use of gendered terms reflects *tombois'* understanding of themselves as situated within the category "man" (*laki-laki*).

Certain key social processes (cultural ideologies) in West Sumatra are involved in the production of the *tomboi* identity. The first of these is a gender ideology that constructs two genders as mutually exclusive; the second is a kinship ideology that situates women as producers and reproducers of their lineages. The Minangkabau have a matrilineal form of kinship in which inheritance and property pass from mothers to daughters. They are also devoutly Islamic. Typical of many Islamic cultures, the Minangkabau believe that men and women have different natures. Men are said to be more aggressive and brave than women are. Boys are admonished not to cry: Crying is what girls do. Women are expected to be modest and respectful, especially young, unmarried women. This gender ideology constructs differences in rights and privileges between men and women without, however, constituting men as superior (see Blackwood, 2000).

In the context of a rural kin-based society, heterosexual marriages are the key to the maintenance of a vital network of kin and in-laws. For Minangkabau women the continuation of this kinship network through marriage and children is critical to their own standing and influence both in their kin groups and in the community. Because daughters are essential to the continuation of the lineage, elders carefully monitor young women to ensure that they marry and marry well. Daughters are not just reproducers, however; they are also the leaders of the next generation of kin. Consequently, there are no acceptable fantasies of femininity or female bodies in rural villages that do not include marriage and motherhood.

The restrictive definitions and expectations of masculinity and femininity attached to male and female bodies help produce gender transgressions in the form of the *tombois*. One *tomboi* played too rough and enjoyed boys' activities when little, and was called *bujang gadis*, a term that meant "boy-girl." Identified as masculine by others, *tombois* make sense of their own gender behavior as being that of a man. Because their behavior falls outside the bounds of proper femininity, *tomboys* deny their female bodies and produce the only other gender recognized in this two-gender system, the masculine gender. The persuasiveness of the dominant gender ideology circulating in West Sumatra means that other expressions of womanhood are unimaginable if they blur the prescribed lines between women and men. Consequently, some masculine females appropriate the masculine gender because it is the most persuasive model available.

But a transnational lesbian and gay discourse circulating in Indonesia primarily through national gay organizations and newsletters complicates *tomboi* identity. First organized in the early 1980s, these predominantly urban groups have nurtured a small but growing nationwide community of gays and lesbians (Boellstorff, 2000). In the process they have fostered development of a new gay identity for Indonesians, which, although not the same as that of gay Europeans and Americans, shares with them the idea of a sexual identity distinct from gender identity.

The infusion of transnational gay discourse into the lives of *tombois* and their partners presents new cultural models of sexuality. Moving between urban and rural areas, these individuals confront urban gay and lesbian identities that they negotiate and claim in hybrid ways. Identity for *tombois* in West Sumatra at this point is a mix of local, national, and transnational identities. If their identity growing up was produced by local cultural processes that emphasized mutually exclusive genders and a gender-based model of sexuality, their movement between cities and rural areas means *tombois* are exposed to other models of sexuality and gender identity. They have used these identities to construct a new sense of themselves as *tombois* and *lesbis*.

These cases illustrate the way gender as well as sexuality is culturally produced. Rather than occupying a fixed category of gender or sexuality, *tombois* do not fit into any single Western category, being neither clearly lesbian, butch (a masculine lesbian), transgender, woman, or man. For their part, *mati* women do not claim an unchanging identity as lesbians, but rather an unchanging, joyous sexuality which includes both men and women partners. The different experiences and transformations over time substantiate a view of sexuality as the product of complex social processes.

THE SOCIAL PRODUCTION OF SEXUALITIES

My discussion of the cultural processes that construct sexualities is based on a small but growing number of case studies of women's same-sex relations cross-culturally. The lack of availability of adequate information makes systematic comparison difficult. One survey found reports of female same-sex practices in 95 indigenous cultures (Blackwood, 1984), but no comprehensive world survey has been conducted to date. The difficulties of coding the various types of behavior documented even in this short article raise other problems for statistical analyses. Despite the problems of formulating comparative analyses, some consistencies appear among the cases that allow for generalization about the social processes at work.

Anthropological and historical records suggest that in indigenous cultures it is rare to find a segregated community of women involved in affective or erotic relationships with each other. Rather what appears in different times and conditions is a range of sexualities that do not fall easily into Western binaries of heterosexual or homosexual. These diverse sexualities, which include intimate friendships between adult married women, adolescent sex play, and ritual same-sex practices, change over time in response to a broad range of cultural factors.

The broader patterns that appear in the cultural construction of sexuality can be connected to different types of gender ideologies, kinship systems, and class societies. Earlier attempts at comparative theories suggested that where men have greater control over women, or in societies stratified by class and gender, women's same-sex practices are subject to more oppression than men's (Rubin, 1975) or limited to clandestine relations or marginalized groups (Blackwood, 1986a). Both these suggestions rely on the "constraint" theory of sexuality by implying that without serious controls over them, women's same-sex relations would appear much more often.

In an effort to rework these earlier theories with a stronger constructionist approach, I want to emphasize the way culture produces ideas about sexuality. For instance, in strict patrilineal class societies the importance of inheritance and property rights for men requires that women be sexually active only with their husbands. This requirement is forcefully articulated in a discourse that aligns women's sexuality with reproduction and men's desires. Thus, good women save themselves for and desire only their husbands. Other options may be imaginable, since men are known to have other heterosexual and even homosexual contacts, but the harsh consequences for women in most cases foreclose any thought of going beyond the permissible. I do not mean that women's "natural" same-sex desire is thereby repressed, but rather that the experience and understanding of such an expression of sexuality as desirable or significant is foreclosed.

In contrast to the constraints placed on women's sexuality in patrilineal societies, women in gender-egalitarian, nonclass societies, such as the !Kung and Australian aborigines, participate in a range of adolescent and ritual same-sex practices. These societies have marriage requirements and prohibitions on certain forms of sexual relations. Yet lacking property relations or expectations about rights of access found in strict patrilineal societies and dovetailing with the importance of women's social bonds and their agency within the community, these cultures produce an ideology of sexuality as something powerful, diverse, enjoyable, and explorable. This is not to say that all nonclass societies will produce multiple sexualities. In some societies same-sex relations are said to be culturally unintelligible. The important point is that many sociocultural factors work together to produce sexual meanings; it is nearly impossible to predict which ones will produce particular forms of sexuality.

The way sexuality is constructed, the ideology of what is "natural"—for instance, who is considered more sexually aggressive or in need of more sex—has everything to do with concepts of gender, selfhood, kinship (inheritance and property rights), and marriage, among others. The cases presented here challenge the common assumption in Europe and the United States that sexuality and sexual identity comprise stable, coherent categories. The case studies show the importance of the cultural context in constructing sexuality; what needs to be investigated more fully is the way sexuality is constructed in particular contexts, historical eras, and cultural domains. Careful ethnographic analysis of sexual practices will continue to be important in efforts to deepen our understanding of women's sexualities.

REFERENCES

Blacking, J. (1978). Uses of the kinship idiom in friendships at some Venda and Zulu schools. In J. Argyle & E. Preston-Whyte (Eds.), *Social system and tradition in Southern Africa* (Cape Town, South Africa: Oxford University Press, pp. 101–17).

Blackwood, E. (1984). *Cross-cultural dimensions of lesbian relations*. Unpublished master's thesis, San Francisco State University, San Francisco, CA.

———. (1986a). "Breaking the mirror: The construction of lesbianism and the anthropological discourse in homosexuality." In E. Blackwood (Ed.), *The many faces of homosexuality: Anthropological approaches to homosexual behavior* (New York: Harrington Park Press, pp. 1–17).

——— (Ed.). (1986b). *The many faces of homosexuality: Anthropological approaches to homosexual behavior.* (New York: Haworth.)

———. 1998. "Tombois in West Sumatra: Constructing masculinity and erotic desire." *Cultural Anthropology* 13, no. 4:491–521.

———. 2000). *Webs of power: Women, kin and community in a Sumatran village* (Lanham, MD: Rowman and Littlefield).

Blackwood, E., & Wieringa, S. E. (Eds.). (1999). *Female desires: Same-sex relations and transgender practices across cultures* (New York: Columbia University Press).

Boellstorff, T. (2000). *The gay archipelago: Postcolonial sexual subjectivities in Indonesia.* Unpublished doctoral dissertation, Stanford University, Stanford, CA.

Caplan, P. (Ed.). (1987). *The cultural construction of sexuality* (London: Tavistock).

Elliston, D. (1995). "Erotic anthropology: 'Ritualized homosexuality' in Melanesia and beyond." *American Ethnologist* 22, no. 4:848–67.

Evans-Pritchard, E. E. 1970). "Sexual inversion among the Azande." *American Anthropologist* 72:1428–34.

Foucault, M. 1978). *History of sexuality. Vol. 1: An introduction* (New York: Pantheon).

Gay, J. 1986). "'Mummies and babies' and friends and lovers in Lesotho." In E. Blackwood (Ed.), *The many faces of homosexuality: Anthropological approaches to homosexual behavior* (New York: Harrington Park Press, pp. 97–116).

Herdt, G. 1981). *Guardians of the flute* (New York: McGraw-Hill).

Honig, E. 1985). "Burning incense, pledging sisterhood: Communities of women workers in the Shanghai cotton mills, 1919–1949." *Signs: Journal of Women in Culture and Society* 10, no. 4:700–14.

Kaberry, P. 1939). *Aboriginal woman, sacred and profane* (London: Routledge).

Kendall. 1999). "Women in Lesotho and the (Western) construction of homophobia." In E. Blackwood & S. E. Wieringa (Eds.), *Female desires: Same-sex relations and transgender practices across cultures* (New York: Columbia University Press, pp. 157–78).

Ng, V. W. 1989). "Homosexuality and the state in late Imperial China." In M. Duberman, M. Vicinus, & G. J. Chauncey (Eds.), *Hidden from history: Reclaiming the gay and lesbian past* (New York: Meridian Books, pp. 76–89).

Nthunya, M. M. 1997). *Singing away the hunger: The autobiography of an African woman* (Bloomington: Indiana University Press).

Padgug, R. A. 1979). "Sexual matters: On conceptualizing sexuality in history." *Radical History Review* 20:3–23.

Povinelli, B. (1992, November). *Blood, sex, and power: "Pitjawagaitj" / menstruation ceremonies and land politics in Aboriginal Northern Australia.* Paper presented at the 91st Annual Meeting of the American Anthropological Association, San Francisco.

Roheim, G. (1933). "Women and their life in Central Australia." *Journal of the Royal Anthropological Institute of Great Britain and Ireland,* 63:207–65.

Rubin, G. (1975). "The traffic in women: Notes on the political economy of sex." In R. Rapp (Ed.), *Towards an anthropology of women* (New York: Monthly Review Press, pp. 157–211).

Sankar, A. (1986). "Sisters and brothers, lovers and enemies: Marriage resistance in Southern Kwangtung." In E. Blackwood (Ed.), *The many faces of homosexuality: Anthropological approaches to homosexual behavior* (New York: Harrington Park Press, pp. 69–83).

Shostak, M. (1983). *Nisa: The life and words of a !Kung woman* (New York: Vintage Books).

Topley, M. (1975). "Marriage resistance in rural Kwangtung." In M. Wolf & R. Witke (Eds.), *Women in Chinese society* (Stanford, CA: Stanford University Press, pp. 57–88).

Vance, C. S. (1989). "Social construction theory: Problems in the history of sexuality." In *Homosexuality, which homosexuality?* (London: GMP), pp. 13–35.

Wekker, G. (1999). "'What's identity got to do with it?' Rethinking identity in light of the mati work in Suriname." In E. Blackwood & S. E. Wieringa (Eds.), *Female desires: Same-sex relations and transgender practices across cultures* (New York: Columbia University Press, pp. 119–38).

Wieringa, S. E., & E. Blackwood. (1999). "Introduction." In E. Blackwood & S. E. Wieringa (Eds.), *Female desires: Same-sex relations and transgender practices across cultures* (New York: Columbia University Press, pp. 1–38).

27.

THE FIVE SEXES

Why Male and Female Are Not Enough

Anne Fausto-Sterling

I n 1843 Levi Suydam, a twenty-three-year-old resident of Salisbury, Connecticut, asked the town board of selectmen to validate his right to vote as a Whig in a hotly contested local election. The request raised a flurry of objections from the opposition party, for reasons that must be rare in the annals of American democracy: it was said that Suydam was more female than male and thus (some eighty years before suffrage was extended to women) could not be allowed to cast a ballot. To settle the dispute a physician, one William James Barry, was brought in to examine Suydam. And, presumably upon encountering a phallus, the good doctor declared the prospective voter male. With Suydam safely in their column the Whigs won the election: by a majority of one.

Barry's diagnosis, however, turned out to be somewhat premature. Within a few days he discovered that, phallus notwithstanding, Suydam menstruated regularly and had a vaginal opening. Both his/her physique and his/her mental predispositions were more complex than was first suspected. S/he had narrow

Taken from *The Sciences* (March/April 1993). Reprinted with the permission of the New York Academy of Sciences, 7 World Trade Center, 250 Greenwich St, 40th Fl, New York, NY 10007-2157.

Anne Fausto-Sterling is Professor of Biology and Gender Studies in the Department of Molecular and Cell Biology and Biochemistry at Brown University. She is Chair of the Faculty Committee on Science & Technology Studies.

shoulders and broad hips and felt occasional sexual yearnings for women.
Suydam's "feminine propensities, such as a fondness for gay colors, for pieces of
calico, comparing and placing them together, and an aversion for bodily labor,
and an inability to perform the same, were remarked by many," Barry later wrote.
It is not clear whether Suydam lost or retained the vote, or whether the election
results were reversed.

Western culture is deeply committed to the idea that there are only two
sexes. Even language refuses other possibilities; thus to write about Levi Suydam
I have had to invent convention—*s/he* and *his/her*—to denote someone who is
clearly neither male nor female or who is perhaps both sexes at once. Legally, too,
every adult is either man *or* woman, and the difference, of course, is not trivial.
For Suydam it meant the franchise; today it means being available for, or exempt
from, draft registration, as well as being subject, in various ways, to a number of
laws governing marriage, the family and human intimacy. In many parts of the
United States, for instance, two people legally registered as men cannot have
sexual relations without violating anti-sodomy statutes.

But if the state and the legal system have an interest in maintaining a two-
party sexual system, they are in defiance of nature. For biologically speaking,
there are many gradations running from female to male; and depending on how
one calls the shots, one can argue that along that spectrum lie at least five sexes—
and perhaps even more.

For some time medical investigators have recognized the concept of the
intersexual body. But the standard medical literature uses the term *intersex* as a
catch-all for three major subgroups with some mixture of male and female characteristics: the so-called true hermaphrodites, whom I call herms, who possess
one testis and one ovary (the sperm- and egg-producing vessels, or gonads); the
male pseudohermaphrodites (the "merms"), who have testes and some aspects of
the female genitalia but no ovaries; and the female pseudohermaphrodites (the
"ferms"), who have ovaries and some aspects of the male genitalia but lack testes.
Each of those categories is in itself complex: the percentage of male and female
characteristics, for instance, can vary enormously among members of the same
subgroup. Moreover, the inner lives of the people in each subgroup—their special needs and their problems, attractions, and repulsions—have gone unexplored by science. But on the basis of what is known about them I suggest that
the three intersexes, herm, merm, and ferm, deserve to be considered additional
sexes each in its own right. Indeed, I would argue further that sex is a vast, infinitely malleable continuum that defies the constraints of even five categories.

Not surprisingly, it is extremely difficult to estimate the frequency of intersexuality, much less the frequency of each of the three additional sexes: it is not the

sort of information one volunteers on a job application. The psychologist John Money of Johns Hopkins University, a specialist in the study of congenital sexual-organ defects, suggests intersexuals may constitute as many as 4 percent of births. As I point out to my students at Brown University, in a student body of about 6,000 that fraction, if correct, implies there may be as many as 240 intersexuals on campus—surely enough to form a minority caucus of some kind.

In reality though, few such students would make it as far as Brown in sexually diverse form. Recent advances in physiology and surgical technology now enable physicians to catch most intersexuals at the moment of birth. Almost at once such infants are entered into a program of hormonal and surgical management so that they can slip quietly into society as "normal" heterosexual males or females. I emphasize that the motive is in no way conspiratorial. The aims of the policy are genuinely humanitarian, reflecting the wish that people be able to "fit in" both physically and psychologically. In the medical community, however, the assumptions behind that wish—that there be only two sexes, that heterosexuality alone is normal, that there is one true model of psychological health—have gone virtually unexamined.

The word *hermaphrodite* comes from the Greek names Hermes, variously known as the messenger of the gods, the patron of music, the controller of dreams, or the protector of livestock, and Aphrodite, the goddess of sexual love and beauty. According to Greek mythology, those two gods parented Hermaphroditus, who at age fifteen became half male and half female when his body fused with the body of a nymph he fell in love with. In some true hermaphrodites the testis and the ovary grow separately but bilaterally; in others they grow together within the same organ, forming an ovo-testis. Not infrequently, at least one of the gonads functions quite well, producing either sperm cells or eggs, as well as functional levels of the sex hormones—androgens or estrogens. Although in theory it might be possible for a true hermaphrodite to become both father and mother to a child, in practice the appropriate ducts and tubes are not configured so that egg and sperm can meet.

In contrast with the true hermaphrodites, the pseudohermaphrodites possess two gonads of the same kind along with the usual male (XY) or female (XX) chromosomal makeup. But their external genitalia and secondary sex characteristics do not match their chromosomes. Thus merms have testes and XY chromosomes, yet they also have a vagina and a clitoris, and at puberty they often develop breasts. They do not menstruate, however. Ferms have ovaries, two X chromosomes and sometimes a uterus, but they also have at least partly masculine external genitalia. Without medical intervention they can develop beards, deep voices and adult-size penises.

No classification scheme could more than suggest the variety of sexual anatomy encountered in clinical practice. In 1969, for example, two French investigators, Paul Guinet of the Endocrine Clinic in Lyons and Jacques Decourt of the Endocrine Clinic in Paris, described ninety-eight cases of true hermaphroditism—again, signifying people with both ovarian and testicular tissue—solely according to the appearance of the external genitalia and the accompanying ducts. In some cases the people exhibited strongly feminine development. They had separate openings for the vagina and the urethra, a cleft vulva defined by both the large and the small labia, or vaginal lips, and at puberty they developed breasts and usually began to menstruate. It was the oversize and sexually alert clitoris, which threatened sometimes at puberty to grow into a penis, that usually impelled them to seek medical attention. Members of another group also had breasts and a feminine body type, and they menstruated. But their labia were at least partly fused, forming an incomplete scrotum. The phallus (here an embryological term for a structure that during usual development goes on to form either a clitoris or a penis) was between 1.5 and 2.8 inches long; nevertheless, they urinated through a urethra that opened into or near the vagina.

By far the most frequent form of true hermaphrodite encountered by Guinet and Decourt—55 percent—appeared to have a more masculine physique. In such people the urethra runs either through or near the phallus, which looks more like a penis than a clitoris. Any menstrual blood exits periodically during urination. But in spite of the relatively male appearance of the genitalia, breasts appear at puberty. It is possible that a sample larger than ninety-eight so-called true hermaphrodites would yield even more contrasts and subtleties. Suffice it to say that the varieties are so diverse that it is possible to know which parts are present and what is attached to what only after exploratory surgery.

The embryological origins of human hermaphrodites clearly fit what is known about male and female sexual development. The embryonic gonad generally chooses early in development to follow either a male or a female sexual pathway; for the ovo-testis, however, that choice is fudged. Similarly, the embryonic phallus most often ends up as a clitoris or a penis, but the existence of intermediate states comes as no surprise to the embryologist. There are also urogenital swellings in the embryo that usually either stay open and become the vaginal labia or fuse and become a scrotum. In some hermaphrodites, though, the choice of opening or closing is ambivalent. Finally, all mammalian embryos have structures that can become the female uterus and the fallopian tubes, as well as structures that can become part of the male sperm-transport system. Typically either the male or the female set of those primordial genital organs degenerates, and the remaining structures achieve their sex-appropriate future. In hermaphrodites both sets of organs develop to varying degrees.

*   *   *

Intersexuality itself is old news. Hermaphrodites, for instance, are often featured in stories about human origins. Early biblical scholars believed Adam began life as a hermaphrodite and later divided into two people—a male and a female—after falling from grace. According to Plato there once were three sexes—male, female, and hermaphrodite—but the third sex was lost with time.

Both the Talmud and the Tosefta, the Jewish books of law, list extensive regulations for people of mixed sex. The Tosefta expressly forbids hermaphrodites to inherit their fathers' estates (like daughters), to seclude themselves with women (like sons), or to shave (like men). When hermaphrodites menstruate they must be isolated from men (like women); they are disqualified from serving as witnesses or as priests (like women), but the laws of pederasty apply to them.

In Europe a pattern emerged by the end of the Middle Ages that, in a sense, has lasted to the present day: hermaphrodites were compelled to choose an established gender role and stick with it. The penalty for transgression was often death. Thus in the 1600s a Scottish hermaphrodite living as a woman was buried alive after impregnating his/her master's daughter.

For questions of inheritance, legitimacy, paternity, succession to title, and eligibility for certain professions to be determined, modern Anglo-Saxon legal systems require that newborns be registered as either male or female. In the United States today sex determination is governed by state laws. Illinois permits adults to change the sex recorded on their birth certificates should a physician attest to having performed the appropriate surgery. The New York Academy of Medicine, on the other hand, has taken an opposite view. In spite of surgical alterations of the external genitalia, the academy argued in 1966, the chromosomal sex remains the same. By that measure, a person's wish to conceal his or her original sex cannot outweigh the public interest in protection against fraud.

During this century the medical community has completed what the legal world began—the complete erasure of any form of embodied sex that does not conform to a male-female, heterosexual pattern. Ironically, a more sophisticated knowledge of the complexity of sexual systems has led to the repression of such intricacy.

In 1937 the urologist Hugh H. Young of Johns Hopkins University published a volume titled *Genital Abnormalities, Hermaphroditism and Related Adrenal Diseases*. The book is remarkable for its erudition, scientific insight, and open-mindedness. In it Young drew together a wealth of carefully documented case histories to demonstrate and study the medical treatment of such "accidents of birth." Young did not pass judgment on the people he studied, nor did he attempt to coerce into treatment those intersexuals who rejected that option. And he showed unusual even-handedness in referring to those people who had had sexual experiences as both men and women as "practicing hermaphrodites."

example of non-conformity to male or female —→One of Young's more interesting cases was a hermaphrodite named Emma who had grown up as a female. Emma had both a penis-size clitoris and a vagina, which made it possible for him/her to have "normal" heterosexual sex with both men and women. As a teenager Emma had had sex with a number of girls to whom s/he was deeply attracted; but at the age of nineteen s/he had married a man. Unfortunately, he had given Emma little sexual pleasure (though *he* had had no complaints), and so throughout that marriage and subsequent ones Emma had kept girlfriends on the side. With some frequency s/he had pleasurable sex with them. Young describes his subject as appearing "to be quite content and even happy." In conversation Emma occasionally told him of his/her wish to be a man, a circumstance Young said would be relatively easy to bring about. But Emma's reply strikes a heroic blow for self-interest:

> Would you have to remove that vagina? I don't know about that because that's my meal ticket. If you did that, I would have to quit my husband and go to work, so I think I'll keep it and stay as I am. My husband supports me well, and even though I don't have any sexual pleasure with him, I do have lots with my girl-friends.

Yet even as Young was illuminating intersexuality with the light of scientific reason, he was beginning its suppression. For his hook is also an extended treatise on the most modern surgical and hormonal methods of changing intersexuals into either males or females. Young may have differed from his successors in being less judgmental and controlling of the patients and their families, but he nonetheless supplied the foundation on which current intervention practices were built.

By 1969, when the English physicians Christopher J. Dewhurst and Ronald R. Gordon wrote *The Intersexual Disorders*, medical and surgical approaches to intersexuality had neared a state of rigid uniformity. It is hardly surprising that such a hardening of opinion took place in the era of the feminine mystique—of the post–Second World War flight to the suburbs and the strict division of family roles according to sex. That the medical consensus was not quite universal (or perhaps that it seemed poised to break apart again) can be gleaned from the near-hysterical tone of Dewhurst and Gordon's book, which contrasts markedly with the calm reason of Young's founding work. Consider their opening description of an intersexual newborn:

> One can only attempt to imagine the anguish of the parents. That a newborn should have a deformity . . . [affecting] so fundamental an issue as the very sex

of the child . . . is a tragic event which immediately conjures up visions of a hopeless psychological misfit doomed to live always as a sexual freak in loneliness and frustration.

Dewhurst and Gordon warned that such a miserable fate would, indeed, be a baby's lot should the case be improperly managed; "but fortunately," they wrote, "with correct management the outlook is infinitely better than the poor parents—emotionally stunned by the event—or indeed anyone without special knowledge could ever imagine."

Scientific dogma has held fast to the assumption that without medical care hermaphrodites are doomed to a life of misery. Yet there are few empirical studies to back up that assumption, and some of the same research gathered to build a case for medical treatment contradicts it. Francies Benton, another of Young's practicing hermaphrodites, "had not worried over his condition, did not wish to be changed, and was enjoying life." The same could be said of Emma, the opportunistic hausfrau. Even Dewhurst and Gordon, adamant about the psychological importance of treating intersexuals at the infant stage, acknowledged great success in "changing the sex" of older patients. They reported on twenty cases of children reclassified into a different sex after the supposedly critical age of eighteen months. They asserted that all the reclassifications were "successful," and they wondered then whether reregistration could be "recommended more readily than [had] been suggested so far."

The treatment of intersexuality in this century provides a clear example of what the French historian Michel Foucault has called biopower. The knowledge developed in biochemistry, embryology, endocrinology, psychology, and surgery has enabled physicians to control the very sex of the human body. The multiple contradictions in that kind of power call for some scrutiny. On the one hand, the medical "management" of intersexuality certainly developed as part of an attempt to free people from perceived psychological pain (though whether the pain was the patient's, the parents', or the physician's is unclear). And if one accepts the assumption that in a sex-divided culture people can realize their greatest potential for happiness and productivity only if they are sure they belong to one of only two acknowledged sexes, modern medicine has been extremely successful.

On the other hand, the same medical accomplishments can be read not as progress but as a mode of discipline. Hermaphrodites have unruly bodies. They do not fall naturally into a binary classification: only a surgical shoehorn can put them there. But why should we care if a "woman"—defined as one who has breasts, a vagina, a uterus, ovaries, and who menstruates—also has a clitoris large enough to penetrate the vagina of another woman? Why should we care if there

Cultural need to define

are people whose biological equipment enables them to have sex "naturally" with both men and women? The answers seem to lie in a cultural need to maintain clear distinctions between the sexes. Society mandates the control of intersexual bodies because they blur and bridge the great divide. Inasmuch as hermaphrodites literally embody both sexes, they challenge traditional beliefs about sexual difference: they possess the irritating ability to live sometimes as one sex and sometimes the other, and they raise the specter of homosexuality.

But what if things were altogether different? Imagine a world in which the same knowledge that has enabled medicine to intervene in the management of intersexual patients has been placed at the service of multiple sexualities. Imagine that the sexes have multiplied beyond currently imaginable limits. It would have to be a world of shared powers. Patient and physician, parent and child, male and female, heterosexual and homosexual—all those oppositions and others would have to be dissolved as sources of division. A new ethic of medical treatment would arise, one that would permit ambiguity in a culture that had overcome sexual division. The central mission of medical treatment would be to preserve life. Thus hermaphrodites would be concerned primarily not about whether they can conform to society but about whether they might develop potentially life-threatening conditions—hernias, gonadal tumors, salt imbalance caused by adrenal malfunction—that sometimes accompany hermaphroditic development. In my ideal world medical intervention for intersexuals would take place only rarely before the age of reason; subsequent treatment would be a cooperative venture between physician, patient, and other advisers trained in issues of gender multiplicity.

I do not pretend that the transition to my utopia would be smooth. Sex, even the supposedly "normal," heterosexual kind, continues to cause untold anxieties in Western society. And certainly a culture that has yet to come to grips—religiously and, in some states, legally—with the ancient and relatively uncomplicated reality of homosexual love will not readily embrace intersexuality. No doubt the most troublesome arena by far would be the rearing of children. Parents, at least since the Victorian era, have fretted, sometimes to the point of outright denial, over the fact that their children are sexual beings.

All that and more amply explains why intersexual children are generally squeezed into one of the two prevailing sexual categories. But what would be the psychological consequences of taking the alternative road—raising children as unabashed intersexuals? On the surface that tack seems fraught with peril. What, for example, would happen to the intersexual child amid the unrelenting cruelty of the schoolyard? When the time came to shower in gym class, what horrors and humiliations would await the intersexual as his/her anatomy was displayed in all its nontraditional glory? In whose gym class would s/he register to begin with? What bathroom would s/he use? And how on earth would Mom and Dad help shepherd him/her through the minefield of puberty?

In the past thirty years those questions have been ignored, as the scientific community has, with remarkable unanimity, avoided contemplating the alternative route of unimpeded intersexuality. But modern investigators tend to overlook a substantial body of case histories, most of them compiled between 1930 and 1960, before surgical intervention became rampant. Almost without exception, those reports describe children who grew up knowing they were intersexual (though they did not advertise it) and adjusted to their unusual status. Some of the studies are richly detailed—described at the level of gym-class showering (which most intersexuals avoided without incident); in any event, there is not a psychotic or a suicide in the lot.

Still, the nuances of socialization among intersexuals cry out for more sophisticated analysis. Clearly, before my vision of sexual multiplicity can be realized, the first openly intersexual children and their parents will have to be brave pioneers who will bear the brunt of society's growing pains. But in the long view—though it could take generations to achieve—the prize might be a society in which sexuality is something to be celebrated for its subtleties and not something to be feared or ridiculed.

28.

A HISTORY OF INTERSEX

From the Age of Gonads to the Age of Consent

Alice Domurat Dreger

This marks the first time an entire volume has been dedicated to the exploration of the ethics of intersex treatment. It could not be more timely; professional conferences, gender clinics, and the popular media are abuzz with the controversy over how medicine and society should handle intersex and intersexuals. The volume will provide some much-needed perspective.

The chapters that follow explain the phenomena known collectively as intersexuality in some depth. For the uninitiated, I will simply note here that "hermaphroditism" and "intersex" are blanket terms used to denote a variety of congenital conditions in which a person has neither the standard male nor the standard female anatomy. Of course, what counts as "standard" male or female is open to interpretation. How big does a "clitoris" have to be before it is "non-standard"—and is size all you should count? Should facial hair be considered "standard" in men and not in women and children, even though some men have little facial hair and some women much? Should our "standards" of sex be based on hidden parts like gonads or chromosomes even though most of us don't know with certainty the nature of our gonads and chromosomes?

["set" normality standards — handwritten margin note]

Questions such as these become more numerous and more difficult as one investigates the myriad of human sex variations. In fact, because of ever-more discoveries of sexual variation and ever-more developments in sexual politics, medical and lay definitions of "male" and "female" have changed repeatedly and continue to change. These definitional shifts have been driven by technological and theoretical advances in biomedical fields (for example, genetics), but they have also been driven by anxious responses to hermaphroditism. As I've learned from nearly nine years of study, intersexuality messes up just about every rule you have been led to believe about sex and gender. Anxiety ensues, and often in reaction to this anxiety, non-intersexuals have demanded order out of intersexuals.

THE AGE OF GONADS

Consider what happened in France and Britain in the late 19th century. At that time, medical doctors were already feeling rather worried about the instability of political-sexual identities. The recently named "homosexual" was showing up in alarming numbers, and a vocal minority of women agitated for equal rights under the law, in the professions, and in the universities. During this already anxious time, doctors started to discover an astonishing number of physically hermaphroditic subjects. As I argue in *Hermaphrodites and the Medical Invention of Sex*,[1] this was due in part to the rise of gynecology and the fact that more people were seeing doctors. But anxiety about sex roles probably also contributed to the rapid rise in medical reports of hermaphrodites by making physicians sensitive to their patients' sexual identities, anatomies, and practices.

In an effort to forestall physical sexual confusion (hermaphroditism) lest it amplify social sexual confusion, biomedical experts in the late 19th century groped around looking for stable and non-overlapping definitions of "male," "female," and "true hermaphrodite." Only if non-overlapping categories could be found would the two-sex social system truly be safe. Apparent salvation came in the form of what I call the Gonadal Definition of Sex.

In 1896, led by two British experts, George F. Blacker (1865–1948) and T. W. P. Lawrence (1858–1936), American and European medical men rallied around the idea that the anatomical nature of the gonads (as ovarian or testicular) alone should determine a subject's "true sex," no matter how confusing or mixed her or his other parts. Henceforth, no matter how manly a patient looked, even if he had a full-sized penis, no vagina, a full beard, and a reputation for bedding down (and satisfying) young maidens, if he had ovaries, he would be labeled a female—in this case a "female pseudo-hermaphrodite." No matter how womanly a patient looked, no matter if she had a vagina, fine and rounded breasts, a smooth face, and a husband she loved, if she had testes, she would be labeled a male—in this case a "male pseudo-hermaphrodite."

So strong was doctors' belief in the Gonadal Definition of Sex and the primacy of the gonads that in Britain the "problem" of "women" with testes was sometimes "solved" by removing the testes from these women, and in France by imploring these patients to stop their "homosexual" alliances with men.[2] (As you might guess, incredulous hermaphroditic patients sometimes thought their doctors daft or cruel.) Commenting on the case of L. S., a testes-laden woman labeled by her doctors "frankly homosexual" because she passionately loved only men, a pair of French experts observed, "The possession of a [single] sex [as male or female] is a necessity of our social order, for hermaphrodites as well as for normal subjects."[3] And so nearly everyone would be labeled male or female, even if pseudo (falsely) hermaphroditic.

During this Age of Gonads, the only "true hermaphrodite" was that subject whose gonads—upon *microscopic* verification by *teams* of experts—were confirmed to contain both ovarian and testicular tissue. Non-emergency exploratory surgeries were quite rare, and biopsies basically unheard of; and so, conveniently, the only true hermaphrodite was a dead hermaphrodite, or at least a castrated (and therefore non?) hermaphrodite. With this intellectual set-up, most sexually challenging patients could be labeled "truly" male or female, and only in the most unlikely and extraordinary cases would a patient be labeled "truly hermaphroditic."

Surely this Gonadal Definition came about in 1896 in part because of recent discoveries in endocrinological and embryological research. The gonads looked to be pretty important physiologically and developmentally, and certainly they are. But allegiance to science alone cannot explain the fierce adherence to the Gonadal Definition. For doctors did not care if the ovarian or testicular tissue in any given patient *functioned*, nor did they ever give up on believing that sex signs showed up all over the body—on the face, the chest, in the tastes, desires, and behaviors, even (in some professional minds) in the color of the fingernails and the bend of the knee. Doctors liked the Gonadal Definition because it kept almost every living body to only one "true" sex, male or female.[4]

Again, note that *only* claims of *true* hermaphroditism required microscopes and teams of experts. The identity of "male" or "female" (even if "pseudo-hermaphroditic") was seen as largely unproblematic; labeling patients truly male or female kept the sexes down to the safe number of two, and so it was pretty easy for a doctor to label a patient "male" or "female" without his colleagues giving him grief. But try to label a patient truly hermaphroditic, and the wrath of the high-powered and numerous defenders of the Gonadal Definition would rain down. One living body, one sex. That was the rule. Sex stabilized. Problem solved.

Well, not quite. Advancing technologies soon made it possible to discover and verify living true hermaphrodites via tissue-sparing biopsies, and doctors started to question what it would mean for social order to label a living person a "true hermaphrodite" or an astoundingly womanly patient (like L. S.) "male" just because she had testes. Thanks to the new diagnostic technologies, the old Gonadal Definition of Sex was failing.

By 1915, one physician harkened the end of the Age of Gonads by raising the question of whether doctors shouldn't abandon the Gonadal Definition. William Blair Bell (1871–1939), then staff surgeon to the Royal Infirmary at Liverpool, considered the latest findings of endocrinology and the trouble caused by the new diagnostic technologies, and wrote, "Since it is now possible to demonstrate the fact that the psychical and physical attributes of sex are not necessarily dependent on the gonads, I think that each case should be considered as a whole; that is to say, the sex should be determined by the obvious predominance of characteristics, especially the secondary, and not by the non-functional sex-glands alone, for this is neither scientific nor just."[5]

In spite of his revolutionary prescription for sex diagnosis, one that moved overtly and consciously away from the Gonadal Definition, Blair Bell's position was conservative in two fundamental ways. First, Blair Bell was, like his predecessors, motivated in theory and practice by an interest in maintaining clear, medically sanctioned divisions between the two sexes in each individual case and in society as a whole. Indeed, this was largely the reason Blair Bell suggested the abandonment of the gonad-as-exclusive-marker rule. It didn't work anymore. Like his colleagues, Blair Bell wanted to quiet sex anomalies, not accentuate them as the Gonadal Definition now threatened to do.

Second, Blair Bell maintained the idea that every body did indeed have *a single true sex*, even if "neither the sex-gland nor the genital ducts necessarily influence or give any indication of the true sex of the individual, as shown by the secondary characteristics."[6] Blair Bell recommended that medical doctors not only diagnose a single sex for anomalous bodies, but that they then *help it along*, by eliminating any sexually "anomalous" characteristics and accenting those that matched the so-diagnosed sex. Blair Bell concluded, "our opinion of the gender [of a given patient] should be adapted to the peculiar circumstances and to our modern knowledge of the complexity of sex, and surgical procedures should in these special cases be carried out to establish more completely the obvious sex of the individual."[7]

So, "true sex" would, perhaps, no longer be dictated exclusively by the anatomical nature of the gonads, but only two true sexes would still exist, with a limit of one to each body, and the medical expert would still be the interpreter—and now, when necessary and possible, the amplifier—of true sex.

To the Age of Surgery

This—the assignment to and the surgical construction of a single, believable sex for each ambiguous body—was indeed the wave of the future. Blair Bell's work sounded the end of the Age of Gonads, and it harkened in a successor era that we could call the Age of Surgery. In this period—still going on today—each body would be allowed only a single true sex, and the medical doctor would be the determiner or even the creator of it. Sex would now be consciously and literally constructed by the surgeon.

So we now flash forward. Since the work of John Money and his colleagues at Johns Hopkins in the 1950s, expert clinicians' understanding has been that, if children are to develop stable gender identities (and by consequence be happy and mentally healthy), they must have "correct" looking genitalia. Money's theory holds that (1) all children, intersexed and non-intersexed, are psychosexually neutral at birth, and (2) you can therefore make virtually any child either gender as long as you make the sexual anatomy reasonably believable.[8]

In one way this is the extreme opposite of the Victorian philosophy, which could be thought of as understanding sexual identity purely as a matter of "nature" (flesh and bones). Money's approach assumes nurture is the way you get to sexual identity, or what he would call gender identity. But in other ways this approach is still rather like the Victorian philosophy: it assumes doctors should be the determiners of sexual identity; it still takes the body as key; it cannot conceive of allowing a hermaphroditic identity.

Following the wide dispersal of Money's theory of gender identity development, people born intersexed are now typically subject as children to "normalizing" surgeries and hormone treatments. The general rule is this: If a child is born intersexed and has a Y chromosome, his phallus will be carefully examined. If it looks like a believable penis to the doctors, or if they think they can make it look like what they think a penis should look like, the child will be assigned the boy gender. Doctors will examine this child at regular intervals and work—using surgical and endocrinological technologies—to make him look like a "true" boy. If his phallus is less than 2.5 centimeters (1 inch) stretched at birth, however, most specialist clinicians will assign this child the girl gender, and use surgery and hormone treatments to make the patient look like what the doctors think girls should look like.

If a child is born intersexed and without a Y chromosome, doctors will assign that child the girl gender. If her clitoris is longer than 1 centimeter stretched at birth, surgeons will seek to surgically reduce it because they think it will bother the child's parents and interfere with bonding and gender identity formation. If she does not have a vagina that is, in the doctors' opinion, big enough for penetration with a penis, she will have surgery for that. Hormone treatments will eventually be used, if necessary, to get her breasts to grow, and so on.

Since the overarching rule of this system is "avoid psychological confusion about the patient's gender identity," doctors often do not tell intersexuals and their parents all that the doctors know, lest information about intersexuality confuse or complicate the family's understanding of gender. All of the professional energy is aimed at producing a physically "right" girl or boy who, presumably, the parents will then be able to raise in an unambiguous way. At the end of it all, the process is supposed to result in a well-adjusted (happy and behaviorally unambiguous) heterosexual (sleeping with people assigned the other gender) adult who complies with ongoing medical treatments (like hormone therapy), who has a fine relationship with her family, and who doesn't know she was born intersexed.

[handwritten margin note: deception]

[handwritten margin note: supposed results]

Until very recently, this practice was apparently considered—by those who knew of it—beneficent and not worth questioning. Of course, few did know of it, because intersexuality was considered rare and touchy, perhaps even taboo. Lately, however, ethicists, clinicians, and intersexuals themselves have begun to doubt the dominant clinical paradigm.

A RAPID SHIFT

Indeed, Bruce Wilson and William Reiner argue that there is now taking place a paradigm shift in intersex management—from the older techno-centric treatment paradigm to a newer, ethically informed, patient-centered paradigm. Wilson and Reiner, both clinicians who work with intersexed children, argue that the older treatment model is fundamentally unsound—that it lacks empirical support and that it contradicts fundamental medical ethical principles, including "first, do no harm."

Without a doubt, the speed with which the intersex scene has been changing during this decade seems to indicate a major paradigm shift. I will add to this volume's contributors' stories my own anecdotal "postcard from the paradigm shift": A few months ago, as I was in the midst of working on this volume, I gave a talk about intersexuality at a university. My audience was diverse and included many people from outside the university system, and so I kept my presentation pretty basic. About halfway through, I showed a three-minute clip from the activist video *Hermaphrodites Speak!*[9] and contrasted this with a three-minute introductory segment from a surgery training film entitled *Surgical Reconstruction of Ambiguous Genitalia in Female Children.*[10] ("Female children" means children assigned the female gender.)

A few days after my talk, a woman in her early twenties who had been in attendance contacted me to ask me more questions about intersexuality. I'll call her Sarah. Over the course of our conversation, Sarah volunteered the information that she has a very large clitoris. She said that, though she had never been diagnosed as intersexed, she had always had a feeling that she had better hide her unusual anatomy from doctors, and had managed to do so remarkably successfully—and, after seeing the surgery video, she was glad she had. She told me she never really thought about how odd it might be that she uses her clitoris to penetrate her partner's vagina. I had mentioned in my presentation that while a large clitoris is not a medical problem—it just looks and feels different—it might indicate an underlying metabolic danger. Sarah wanted to know if she should be concerned for her health. She remembered vaguely a "hernia" operation from childhood, and now wondered if that had really been exploratory surgery to see if she had testicles.

Four years ago, in 1995, had I given this talk I would have used only pathologized images of intersexuals. No non-pathologizing images of living intersexuals (like those in this book and in *Hermaphrodites Speak!*) were available to me. As a consequence, Sarah might have been too ashamed to talk with me afterwards—indeed, I might have inadvertently made her feel positively freakish. (Heaven only knows what she or her partner would have concluded about her from my original "curiosity shop" talks on this subject.)

In 1995, had Sarah come and told me what she did, I would have actually been skeptical that she was telling me the truth. All evidence to the contrary, I still thought of intersexuality as quite rare, and frankly I had so bought into the medical textbook image of intersex that I would have had trouble believing that this articulate, three-dimensional woman could really be intersexed. (I realized recently that I had long been afraid to meet intersexuals because I figured subconsciously that when they walked up to me they would all be in black-and-white, nude, with their eyes blacked out, standing up next to a big measuring stick. What a shock it was when I realized that they look pretty much like the rest of us when you meet them at an airport, a coffee shop, or a university.)

Most significantly, in 1995 I would not have known where to refer Sarah for help. I did not know of any doctors I could trust not to cause her emotional and maybe physical pain. In spite of the fact that in 1990 Suzanne Kessler published an excellent critique of the medical management of intersex,[11] I had yet to find a physician who saw a problem with the dominant treatment system. I would have been afraid that what few support groups existed would be too nascent to really help her.

But in 1998, I could and did believe Sarah when she told me about her anatomy. Anne Fausto-Sterling has found that the frequency of intersex states is significantly higher than has generally been appreciated,[12] and I've finally come around to the data. I can now tell people with virtual certainty that we have all, in the course of our lives, met one intersexual (and probably many more). Naturally the frequency among my audiences must be even higher than the population at large; I expect to find intersexuals at about every other talk I give. Before Sarah, I had already met two other women who managed to go through life with big clitorises, so I knew that could happen. (Incidentally, all three have no interest in surgical reduction.) So I did not run away frightened from Sarah, and I did not tell her she was delusional or naive.

In 1998, I could and did refer Sarah to a select few physicians whom I could trust not to treat her with a pejorative attitude, bald voyeurism, minced words, or unwanted "corrections." I also could and did refer her to several vibrant support groups who could put her in touch with people who shared her experiences, people who could give her insight into her life history, her identity, and her future. I could send her to Suzanne Kessler's excellent new book, *Lessons from the Intersexed*.[13] A network of helpers was in place to catch Sarah as she fell into the realization of this new identity. So, as I worked on this volume, I helped guide her through the first stages of self-discovery and realized with amazement how much the world has changed for intersexuals in just four years.[14]

PROBLEMS WITH THE DOMINANT MODEL

In conversations I have had with them, some surgeons have argued that we ought not to hastily throw out the older Age of Surgery model of intersex management for a new model. They say we first need evidence that the older model has failed and that a different model would work better. Four responses come to mind.

First, there is no real evidence that the older model works. As several of the contributors in this volume note (and as I and others have noted previously),[15] what few outcome studies there have been of intersex management have basically focused on how good the specific surgical repair turned out. In other words, we know a little about which kind of vaginoplasty results in less stenosis (scarring up), but we know almost nothing about how the women who received those vaginoplasties as girls have fared psychologically or sexually. This in spite of the fact that the older approach is premised on an understanding of intersex as a psychosocial problem. Like Wilson and Reiner, in chapter 16, Justine Marut Schober, a pediatric urological surgeon who works with intersexed children, sounds a strong note of caution and expresses concern over the long-term use of a treatment model that lacks supporting data.

Kenneth Kipnis and Milton Diamond argue that this lack of follow-up studies is scandalously irresponsible; they call for cessation of unconsented surgeries until broad-based follow-up studies are done. Kipnis and Diamond also allude to evidence that the theoretical basis for the older model may well be fundamentally flawed; they cite cases and studies that suggest that children are *not* born psychosexually neutral and infinitely malleable in terms of gender formation.

Relatedly, the second response to the "keep the older model for awhile" argument is this: We do have some evidence that the older model has failed a large number of patients. Some of that is provided here, especially in parts 2 and 3. Kipnis and Diamond follow up on the famous Joan-John case. Sherri Groveman, a woman with androgen insensitivity syndrome (AIS) who leads a support group for AIS women, provides an eloquent essay explaining the dangers of doctors' withholding the whole truth from intersexed patients. She includes stories from AIS women to give us some sense of what it is like to have a key element of your identity shaped by medical professionals. In an essay premiering her original research, Sharon Preves, a sociologist, summarizes interviews she recently conducted with 40 adults born intersexed. She finds evidence that certain features of the older treatment paradigm—including unconsented surgeries and withholding information from patients—directly undermine the goal of producing a happy and healthy patient. Preves argues that intersex clinical treatment needs to be reworked to a point where it meets the clinicians' intentions of positive psychological outcomes.

Cheryl Chase quotes parents at wits' end with regard to failed "corrective" surgeries performed on their sons' penises. She questions surgeons' claims that most intersex surgeries leave patients with "normal" looking genitalia and good sexual sensation. Chase throws into doubt the efficacy and safety of current-day surgeries, and while Chase's critique is at the expert level, it doesn't take an expert to realize that most clitoral reduction surgeries will, by their very nature, reduce clitoral sensation.

Third, while it would be assuring to have long-term studies that show us that an alternative model works better than the older model, given enormous variation in nature and nurture, how could adequate controls ever be put into place for such a comparative study? As Wilson and Reiner also point out, even if we could design such a study, we would have to wait decades for the results, and in the meantime a large number of children would be subject to a medical model more and more people have concluded is unethical.

This then brings us to the fourth response to the "hold the older line for awhile" argument: Even if we had evidence that the older treatment paradigm works most of the time—which we certainly don't—we would still have to face the fact that it violates basic ethical principles now widely accepted in all realms except the treatment of children born intersexed.[16] Many of the following articles discuss this in depth, so I will just summarize the point here.

TRUTH-TELLING

[handwritten: basic ethical principles violated by older model of surgical correction]

The older model necessitates a basic deception. Parents are, at least in most cases, not told that the treatment model is not proven to work, is based on a peculiar theory of gender identity formation, and is increasingly widely criticized. Intersexed children, as they grow older, are kept in the dark about their conditions, even though they usually know something about them is different. (It is hard not to feel that way when doctors keep examining your genitals.) In no other realm in medicine do doctors regularly argue for active, nearly wholesale deception.

INFORMED CONSENT

The absence of full disclosure about the questionable theoretical basis of the practice and its lack of empirical support means that parents and later intersexuals themselves cannot be said to be giving informed consent. The fact that many intersexuals are not told (even when they ask) their diagnoses means they are not informed at the most basic level. Withholding of diagnoses also prevents them from researching their own condition and treatment and finding peer support.

BENEFICENCE

The older model, while designed to be beneficent, appears in many cases to actually harm intersexed children and their families by treating them as pathological and then failing to fully educate them, support them with psychological counseling by trained professionals, or refer them to peer support groups.

AUTONOMY *[handwritten: - what it is to be a human person]*

Intersexed people have their autonomy violated because their doctors and parents are allowed to make decisions about how their genitals should look. While intersex may signal an underlying metabolic danger, intersexed genitals are not diseased and do not have to be treated as pathological. Cosmetic surgeries are performed without the subject's consent because of adults' discomfort with intersexuality. Robert Crouch notes in his contribution that the treatment of intersex has been more about "us"—non-intersexuals—than them. These surgeries risk the subjects' sexual pleasure, health, and fertility. Several of the contributors to this volume argue that it is unethical to use such risky "cosmetic" genital surgeries on anyone who does not herself consent to them.

TOWARD THE AGE OF CONSENT

In his classic study of paradigm shifts, Thomas Kuhn showed that major theoretical shifts tend to occur not because the evidence for a newer theory outweighs the evidence for an older one, but rather because core beliefs change.[17] The shift in intersex management now taking place follows this model. Clinicians are beginning to abandon the older model of intersex management not because we have vast quantities of data to show that a newer model works better, but because medicine as a whole has moved toward patient-centered, ethically principled care. The fact that intersex management has taken so long to catch up can only be due to the fact that we treat "abnormality"—especially the sexual sort—as a special case.

While the following articles differ in some fine points, this general new model for intersex management arises from them:

° PROVIDE PSYCHOLOGICAL SUPPORT TO PARENTS

When a child is born intersexed (or diagnosed as intersexed prenatally), parents should immediately be offered psychological support. We know in part from Joan Ablon's research on families dealing with achondroplasia that parents of children born with unusual anatomies typically undergo a grieving process in which they grieve the loss of the anticipated "normal" child.[18] Parents of intersexuals therefore need to be referred to professional counselors who understand grief, parenting, and the complexities of gender. They also need to be referred to peer support groups so that they receive assurance from other parents that their feelings and concerns are normal and manageable.[19] From my conversations with intersexuals and their parents, it is clear that the role of counselor should not be left to an endocrinologist, urologist, geneticist, or surgeon.

° ASSIGN A GENDER

All children—no matter how intersexed—can and should be assigned a male or female gender. This consists of physicians helping parents understand which gender assignment makes the most sense (that is, which is likely to be the one the child will ultimately identify with). Will some intersexed children assigned, say, the boy gender decide later they are girls? Yes. And so will some non-intersexed boys. Hard as it is to accept, we have to recognize that *every* gender assignment is preliminary, whether the child being assigned a gender is intersexed or non-intersexed.

Provide Non-Pathologized Images

Intersexuals, their parents, medical students, residents, genetic counselors, and so on need to be provided with non-pathologized images of intersexuals, or they will inevitably see intersexuality as deeply pathological. These images should be of all types—textual, visual, face-to-face, and so on. This book provides a place to start. Support groups are the best sources for more of these resources.[20]

Delay Cosmetic Surgeries and Hormone Treatments

Medical problems of intersex children should obviously be addressed. Some of those problems will require surgery, for example when a child is born with a urinary tract that drains in such a way as to lead to repeated infections. But surgeries and hormone treatments designed simply to change the look of genitalia should not be done unless explicitly requested by the patient him/herself. At that time, the patient should be informed of the risks of the treatment options, and should be provided with long-term results of the options. How old should a child have to be before she or he can be said to be capable of informed consent? This is obviously a difficult and persistent question in medical ethics, but the fact that it is a difficult question does not mean that the question should be subverted by allowing risky and unnecessary surgeries on children before they can consent.

Limit Stressful Clinical Displays

Virtually all the of intersexed people who write in this volume stress the trauma caused by being repeatedly "put on display" for medical students, residents, and attending physicians. While medical professionals need to be educated about intersex by seeing real cases, they must also recognize the psychological harm done to intersexed patients—especially children—when they are repeatedly obligated to make their genitalia available for visual and physical examination by students and physicians. Clinicians will need to develop ways to educate without making intersexed patients feel freakish and violated.

Provide Psychological Support to the Child

Intersexed children face special psychosocial problems. Everyone agrees on this. Therefore intersexed children should be provided with pediatric counselors and peer support groups. Their concerns, fears, and questions should be answered honestly.

RECOGNIZE INTERSEXUALS AS EXPERTS

A major failure of the older model has arisen from the failure to recognize inter-sexed people as experts of their own experiences. A patient-centered model of intersex would take seriously intersexuals' opinions and critiques of various treatments. This would include long-term studies with all intersexed patients to determine which kinds of treatments helped or hurt them.

The reader will see that the following articles mostly agree on this overall strategy. I would like to note that I worked to find an author who would defend the older treatment model of intersex. My requests for contributions from pro-ponents of the older model were met with silence or the apology that potential contributors lacked the time to write for this volume.

BEYOND THE FIVE SEXES

When I speak about intersexuality, people often express to me the suspicion that science will eventually sort out this whole sex thing, and then we'll be able to say for sure what makes a male, what a female, and what a hermaphrodite. But such a hope is chasing after ghosts. In a groundbreaking article in 1993, Anne Fausto-Sterling argued that we need to recognize that there are five sexes in the human population: females, males, female pseudo-hermaphrodites, male pseudo-hermaphrodites, and true hermaphrodites.[21] But we know now that this very division into "five sexes" developed in 1896 as just one more cultural attempt to keep the threat of the hermaphrodite at bay. The fact that the term "true her-maphrodite" is still reserved for people born with both ovarian and testicular tissue is just a Victorian hangover.

So what is a true hermaphrodite? We can't really say. Anatomy is never going to tell us for sure what sex is all about or who is really an intersexual. As humans we decide that. We decide who gets to count as a male, what you have to have or do to count as a female, and what happens to you if you get labeled intersexed. Indeed, sociological and anthropological research indicates that we don't all even think of "man" and "woman" the same, no less intersex. In other times and other places, some people have even held up the hermaphrodite as an ideal, or as a sacred identity. (Robert Crouch discusses some of these alternative visions in his chapter.)

All theory aside, in real life sexual variation blends imperceptibly one kind into the next. The treatment of people born with notably unusual anatomies isn't going to be resolved by the discovery of some gene that reveals the ultimate nature of sexual identity. John Money was right in at least one way—we make it up as we go along, and yes, the body does matter—but in ways that continue to surprise and vary from person to person. In the end, all intersexuals are now asking is to be treated according to the same ethical principles as everybody else. This volume seeks to explore what that would mean.

NOTES

1. A. D. Dreger, *Hermaphrodites and the Medical Invention of Sex* (Cambridge, MA: Harvard University Press, 1998), pp. 25–26.

2. Ibid., pp. 119–26.

3. T. Tuffier and A. Lapointe, "L'Hermaphrodisme: Ses variétés et ses conséquences pour la pratique médicale (d'après un cas personnel)," *Revue de gynécologie et de chirurgie abdominale* 17 (1911): 209–68, at 256.

4. For more on the motivations for the Gonadal Definition, see Dreger, *Hermaphrodites and the Medical Invention of Sex,* note 1 above, pp. 150–54.

5. W. B. Bell, "Hermaphroditism," *Liverpool Medico-Chirurgical Journal* 35 (1915): 272–92, at 291.

6. Ibid., p. 277.

7. Ibid., p. 292. Incidentally, this is the first use I can find of the word "gender" in medical literature on hermaphroditism.

8. For a review and critique of Money's work, see C. Chase, "Hermaphrodites with Attitude: Mapping the Emergence of Intersex Political Activism," *GLQ: A Journal of Gay and Lesbian Studies* 4, no. 2 (1998): 189–211. Also see A. Fausto-Sterling, "How to Build a Man," in *Science and Homosexualities,* ed. V. A. Rosario (New York: Routledge, 1997), pp. 219–25.

9. *Hermaphrodites Speak!* Intersex Society of North America (ISNA), 26 minutes, 1997, videocassette. Copies may be obtained from ISNA, P.O. Box 31791, San Francisco, CA 94131; http://www.isna.org.

10. R. S. Hurwitz, H. Applebaum, and S. Muenchow, *Surgical Reconstruction of Ambiguous Genitalia in Female Children,* ACS/USSC Educational Library, no. ACS-1613, 21 minutes, 1990, videocassette. Copies may be obtained from Cine-Med, 127 Main St. North, P.O. Box 745, Woodbury, CT 06798; telephone (800) 633-0004.

11. S. J. Kessler, "The Medical Construction of Gender: Case Management of Intersexed Infants," *Signs* 16 (1990): 3–26.

12. M. Blackless et al., "How Sexually Dimorphic Are We?" *American Journal of Human Biology* (forthcoming). On the difficulty of calculating the frequency of intersexuality, see Dreger, *Hermaphrodites and the Medical Invention of Sex,* see note 1 above, pp. 40–43.

13. S. J. Kessler, *Lessons from the Intersexed* (Piscataway, NJ: Rutgers University Press, 1998).

14. For a summary of this recent history, see Chase, "Hermaphrodites with Attitude," see note 8 above.

15. See A. D. Dreger, "'Ambiguous Sex'—or Ambivalent Medicine? Ethical Issues in the Treatment of Intersexuality," *Hastings Center Report* 28, no. 3 (May/June 1998): 24–35; see also J. M. Schober, "Feminizing Genitoplasty for Intersex," in *Pediatric Surgery and Urology: Long Term Outcomes*, ed. M. D. Stringer et al. (London: W. B. Saunders, 1998), pp. 549–58.

16. For more on this argument, see Dreger, "'Ambiguous Sex'—or Ambivalent Medicine?" see note 15 above.

17. S. Kuhn, *The Structure of Scientific Revolutions* (Chicago: University of Chicago Press, 1996, 1962).

18. J. Ablon, "Ambiguity and Difference: Families with Dwarf Children," *Social Science and Medicine* 30, no. 8 (1990): 879–87.

19. The easiest way to locate intersex support groups is through the home page of the Intersex Society of North America, see note 10 above.

20. Ibid.

21. A. Fausto-Sterling, "The Five Sexes," *Sciences* 33 (1993): 20–25.

29.

PEDIATRIC ETHICS AND THE SURGICAL ASSIGNMENT OF SEX

Kenneth Kipnis and Milton Diamond

I t has been standard pediatric practice to recommend surgery for infants with ambiguous genitalia or loss of the penis. The parents of these patients are told to raise them without ambiguity and, in consequence, many adults who have had these operations in infancy have never been candidly informed of their medical histories. This management approach, which can involve a reassignment of sex, has its basis in research done on hermaphrodites and a single set of nonhermaphroditic identical twins originally tracked more than two decades ago. The current article reviews this practice and its epistemic foundations. It is argued that there should be a moratorium on such surgery; that the medical profession should complete comprehensive look-back studies to assess the outcomes of past interventions; and that efforts should be made to undo the effects of past deception.

This work was supported by the Eugene Garfield Foundation, Philadelphia, and the Queens Medical Center Research Fund, Honolulu.

This chapter first appeared in the *Journal of Clinical Ethics* 9, no. 4 (Winter 1998): © 1998 by the *Journal of Clinical Ethics*; used with permission.

CASE REPORT

In 1983, one of the authors of this study (KK) received a call from a pediatric sur-geon to do a clinical ethics consultation following the birth of a full-term baby boy with multiple congenital anomalies. While other deficits will be described below, the surgeon was immediately concerned about the child's abnormally small penis: technically, a micropenis. Apprehensive about the possibility of the child being shamed in the boys' locker room—psychosocial distress as he matured—the pediatric surgeon was counseling immediate surgical reassign-ment as a girl. According to the surgeon's plan, the testes would be removed and the genitalia fashioned into a cosmetic vulva before the baby left the hospital. The parents would be instructed to raise the infant as an unambiguous girl. At about the age of 12, estrogens would be administered to stimulate the develop-ment of female secondary sex characteristics. Eventually doctors would create an artificial vagina. Although the resulting woman would be unable to bear chil-dren, the surgeon anticipated that prompt surgical attention would allow the infant to enjoy a better and more normal life as a female than would be possible for a male with a very small penis.

The boy's mother was livid with rage and bitterness. Having given birth only days earlier, her dreams of a perfect child had disintegrated into a nightmarish reality. Pronouns were failing her and she did not know what to say to relatives. Communication had broken down with the surgeon and she was unable to dis-cuss reassignment with him much less consent to it. It fell to the ethics consultant to try to resolve the impasse by investigating the issues and making a recommen-dation. Research went in two directions: a survey of the literature on ambiguous genitalia and an inquiry into the medical condition of the infant. It was in the context of this case that the authors of the present article first began to work together: the philosopher-ethicist consulted with his colleague (MD) across the campus at the John A. Burns School of Medicine.

The literature review led immediately to the work of John Money, then a psychologist at the Gender Identity Clinic at the Johns Hopkins University. In a series of articles and a landmark 1972 book (*Man & Woman, Boy & Girl*),[1] Money and Anka Ehrardt described the case of a pair of identical male twins born in the 1960s. At the age of seven months, the boys were scheduled for cir-cumcision because of phimosis (a narrowing of the opening of the foreskin). An electrocautery knife used on one of the boys severely burned his penis, destroying it. A psychiatrist at the time expressed what one supposes was the conventional wisdom about the boy's probable future: "He will be unable to con-summate marriage or have normal heterosexual relations; he will have to recog-nize that he is incomplete, physically defective, and that he must live apart."[2]

Crushed by the loss, the parents learned of Money's work at Johns Hopkins and the early sex-change operations that were being done there. Following consultation, Money recommended to the parents that the boy be surgically reassigned and raised as a girl. Accordingly, at the age of 17 months, surgeons removed his testes and reshaped his scrotum to approximate a vulva. John, as he later became known in the literature, had become Joan, to be raised as a normal girl without any suspicion of early trauma.

Money's earlier research had convinced him that hermaphroditic children who appeared physiologically similar to each other could nonetheless develop into adults identifying and behaving either as men or as women.[3] Inferring from this work that all infants are sexually neutral at birth and malleable during a window period that remains open until about 18 to 24 months when gender becomes fixed, Money concluded that social imprinting and learning were the key factors in psychosexual development: an account that was consistent with research in language acquisition. Finally, echoing Freud,[4] Money surmised that the presence or absence of the penis was the critical anatomical factor. In a nutshell, the theory held that sexually neutral infants, both consciously and subconsciously, notice the presence or absence of a penis, observe the social distinctions between males and females, and characteristically comport with local standards of gender. Thus, given an unambiguous upbringing, normal behavior would follow perceived anatomy. While earlier reports had described the reassignment of infants with ambiguous genitalia, the appearance of unambiguously male identical twins, one needing attention, offered an unparalleled opportunity to confirm the theory of sexual neutrality at birth.

The twins were evaluated regularly at Hopkins and, in a series of celebrated publications,[5] Money described their psychosexual development to about the onset of puberty: the one surgically reassigned as a girl and the other identical twin, in effect, a control. Glowingly relating remarkable results, Money wrote in 1975: "No one . . . would . . . ever conjecture [that Joan was born a boy]. Her behavior is so normally that of an active little girl, and so clearly different by contrast from the boyish ways of her twin brother, that it offers nothing to stimulate one's conjectures."[6] Reported in professional publications and the national media,[7] Money's writings dramatically confirmed the plasticity of gender: an infant, born as an unambiguous male, had been surgically reassigned as female and successfully reared as a normal girl.

Drawing on Money's research and his theory of psychosexual development, pediatricians caring for infants with ambiguous genitalia inferred that genetic makeup and prenatal endocrinology could largely be ignored in the clinical assignment of sex. They reasoned that the penis had to be plainly absent or present from infancy on, and that these children had to be raised as girls or boys with no hint of abnormality. Accordingly, pediatric surgeons would strive to benefit these patients by "normalizing" ambiguous genitalia: reducing enlarged clitorides (eliminating visible penis-like structures in babies assigned as females) and, because of the technical difficulty of creating functional and cosmetically believable male genitals, refashioning anomalous male genitalia as female.

Well before the 1983 birth of the boy with micropenis, Money's published work had emerged as the epistemic foundation for the new pediatric standard of practice. Thus it was clear why the surgeon wanted to reassign the baby boy as a girl. Pediatric textbooks, then and now, characteristically recommend surgery when the size of the stretched penis is less than about 2.0 centimeters[8] or when the size of the clitoris is greater than about 1 centimeter.[9] If surgical disambiguation could succeed with an infant born unambiguously male, it would—it was thought—surely benefit other babies with ambiguous genitalia. These medical interventions, done with parental consent, as soon after birth as possible, were taken as beneficial, like the pediatric correction of cleft palate. The hermaphrodite and twin studies, it was thought, provided evidence that surgery benefited children with ambiguous genitalia and that, eventually, as one would suppose for infants with cleft palate, they too would have reason to thank their parents and doctors for medical ministrations received as infants.

In this case, while the literature supported the surgeon's 1983 recommendation, doubts arose following inquiry into other aspects of the boy's medical condition. There were other congenital anomalies. A second physician called attention to the boy's undeveloped eyes; the baby was blind. There was evidence of deafness and a probability of other central nervous system deficits, the nature and extent of which had not yet been determined. Accordingly, the child was unlikely to experience locker-room derision and might even go through life without being conscious of gender. The ethics consultant concluded that surgery could not be expected to benefit this particular patient and recommended that reassignment be delayed indefinitely. The surgeon and the parents concurred and the procedure was not done.

While more can be said about this case, here we want to observe both the narrowness of the clinical vision—the focus of attention initially did not extend above the pubis—and the mechanical application of a standard of practice calling for surgical reassignment on the basis of micropenis. We will revisit these themes below.

THE FURTHER HISTORY OF JOHN / JOAN

Notwithstanding that Money and Ehrardt's twin study had only a single experimental subject and a single control, such publications were nonetheless decisive in establishing what quickly became the standard of practice in pediatrics. As recently as April of 1996, the American Academy of Pediatrics (AAP) issued recommendations governing the "Timing of Elective Surgery on the Genitalia of Male Children . . .":

> Research on children with ambiguous genitalia has shown that sexual identity is a function of social learning through differential responses of multiple individuals in the environment. For example, children whose genetic sexes are not clearly reflected in external genitalia (i.e., hermaphroditism) can be raised successfully as members of either sex if the process begins before the age of 2 years. Therefore, a person's sexual body image is largely a function of socialization.[10]

The three works cited by the AAP in support of these findings list John Money as the lead author. No corroborating research is referenced. In fact, Money's theory and recommendations had been vigorously challenged in medical and scientific literature.[11] Suzanne Kessler has written: "Almost all of the published literature on intersexed infant case management has been written or co-written by one researcher, John Money. . . . Even though psychologists fiercely argue issues of gender identity and gender role development, doctors who treat intersexed infants seem untouched by those debates. . . . Why Money has been so single-handedly successful in promoting his ideas about gender is a question worthy of a separate substantial analysis."[12]

It is worthwhile to note that as early as 1966, medicine was coming to terms with transsexuals, individuals whose sexual self-identification is in opposition to their genital configuration and rearing.[13] Despite appropriate anatomy and socialization, the existence of these adults should have stimulated the AAP to question its acceptance that "sexual identity is a function of social learning."

It is conservatively estimated that one in 2,000 newborns are found to have ambiguous external genitalia,[14] that 100 to 200 pediatric surgical sex reassignments are performed in the United States annually, and that, globally, thousands of these procedures have been done since the initial publication of the twins case.[15] It is notable that, notwithstanding more than three decades of clinical experience with the surgical reassignment of infants, there have been no systematic, large-scale studies done to assess the outcome of these procedures. (Some small-scale reviews have been done by Kessler,[16] Schober,[17] and others noted below.) It is also notable that Money's narrative of the twins case ends before his subjects reach adolescence. In his last update, in 1978, Money writes: "Now prepubertal in age, the girl has . . . a feminine gender identity and role distinctly different from that of her brother. . . . The final and conclusive evidence awaits the appearance of romantic interest and erotic imagery."[18] This evidence never appears, and John/Joan, like many of these patients, is "lost to follow-up."

While several recent developments have called into question the venerable basis for the standard of pediatric practice, perhaps the most dramatic has been the reopening of the John/Joan case. In 1994, one of the authors of this study (MD) located and interviewed the former research subject. A richer and more comprehensive picture has emerged of the childhood that loomed so prominently in the literature of the 1970s.[19]

The child never was and never became a normal girl. Now in his thirties, having married a woman with three children, John lives as a man. He, his mother, and his brother now recall that Joan regularly rejected girls' toys, clothes, and activities. His mother says that, despite an attractive female appearance, Joan's movements and speech "gave him away and the awkwardness and incongruities became apparent."[20] John's twin brother has said: "When I say there was nothing feminine about Joan, I mean there was *nothing* feminine. She talked about guy things, didn't give a crap about cleaning house, getting married, wearing makeup" [emphasis in original]. At the age of six or seven, Joan told her brother she wanted to be a garbage man: "Easy job, good pay."[21] Despite the absence of a penis, Joan often stood to urinate. Other girls at school eventually barred her from their bathroom, threatening to kill her if she came in. Eventually she would use a back alley for urination.[22] Contrary to Money's earlier reports, Joan's behavior during childhood failed to be "so normally that of an active little girl."

Despite rearing as a girl, Joan dreamed of a future as a he-man type with a mustache and sports car. Although placed on estrogens at the age of 12, she often discarded the drugs, disliking how they made her feel. She was disturbed by her developing breasts. At one point she told her endocrinologist that she had suspected she was a boy since the second grade. She adamantly refused the surgery that would give her a vagina and complained to her psychiatrist how she dreaded the trips to Johns Hopkins where people looked at her and showed her pictures of nude bodies. At the conclusion of her final visit in 1978, Joan told her mother she would kill herself if she had to go again. By 1980 Joan's relationship with her clinicians at Hopkins had reached an impasse. "Do you want to be a girl or not?" her endocrinologist had demanded. "No!" replied Joan emphatically. At the age of 14, without knowing the history, she decided to cease living as a girl: Joan became John.[23]

Following the transition, John's father, on the advice of a psychiatrist, revealed what had happened during infancy. Until that moment her parents and clinicians had tried to conceal all that was problematic about her gender, to give her the unambiguous rearing as a girl they were told to provide. Listening intently to his father tell the story of the botched circumcision and surgery, John experienced relief. A puzzling past began to make sense. At John's request, male hormones were subsequently administered, a mastectomy was performed, and surgeons eventually created a penis. John now takes satisfaction as a husband, father, and breadwinner.

In retrospect, it seems clear that the surgical refashioning of infants' genitalia must be assessed during the adulthoods of those patients, after the sexual organs take on their distinctive importance in intimate and procreative relationships. To judge success by genital appearance and psychosexual development prior to puberty is to fall victim to narrowed vision.[24] When viewed comprehensively, the life of John/Joan undercuts both the standard of practice and the theory that children observe the distinction between male and female and comport with local standards of gender. Though Joan learned all she was supposed to, her behavior nonetheless exhibited quintessential male elements, and she failed to identify as female. Feminine social imprinting did not occur. In the end, the medical intervention had added the insults of infertility, emotional trauma, and ego loss to the injury of an accidental penectomy. Castration now necessitates a continuing regimen of male hormone replacement.

OTHER DEVELOPMENTS

The outcome of the John/Joan case has been observed with comparable patients. In a recent and ongoing study, Reiner tracked six boys who had lost their penises in infancy and were being reared as girls. These children behaved more like boys than girls and, in two cases, not knowing they were XY, the children autonomously changed gender and assumed male roles.[25] Reiner has stated: "it would be wrong to say that these two children wished to be boys or felt they were boys in girls' bodies: they believed they were boys."[26]

Another significant development has been the emergence of the Intersex Society of North America (ISNA) and related advocacy and support groups. The ISNA membership includes adults who were surgically "normalized" as children, generally without being told, and other intersexuals who have not had surgery. Having attempted unsuccessfully to dialogue with medical organizations in the United States, some intersexuals have taken to picketing hospitals and conferences.[27] Unlike those with surgically corrected cleft palates, intersex patients are condemning physicians for their surgeries and for withholding the truth about their medical condition and treatment. The John/Joan case, the Reiner study, the activist protests, and other cases reported in the literature[28] strongly suggest that pediatric reassignment may often be failing the "thank you test" for clinical beneficence,[29] and that these poor outcomes may not be isolated droplets of misfortune in a downpour of excellent results.

There is some research exploring what happens when infants do not receive surgery. One well-known outcome study has been done on adult males with micropenis who would have been reassigned in infancy as females under the present standard of practice. While six of these 12 postpubertal males admitted to having been teased about a small penis, all "felt male," were gynecophilic, and had erections and orgasms. Nine had sexual intercourse satisfactory to themselves and their partners; seven were married or cohabiting, and still others were sexually active. One had become a father.[30] Another study reported success in helping men with very small penises who presented at a clinic for counseling. All were sexually functional. They and their partners were able to come to terms with their differences.[31] Contrary to conventional wisdom, it is not inevitable that such a man must "recognize that he is incomplete, physically defective, and that he must live apart."

The locker-room argument—that an individual without a penis would be subject to ridicule by peers—has recently received attention. A preoperative female-to-male transsexual has related showering routines that allow one to manage without embarrassment.[32]

A review of the literature has failed to turn up a single article on the hazards, psychosocial or otherwise, of having a large clitoris.[33] Most individuals are not aware that a size standard exists and, indeed, in some cases the parents were unaware of the presence of their daughters' hypertrophied clitoris until clinicians pointed it out in the context of recommending surgery.[34] On the contrary, there are reports of such women and their sexual partners enjoying the configuration (personal cases of MD). For women who have had the surgery, some retain a capacity for orgasm[35] while others complain about pain and insensitivity.[36] Research has not shown that any of the reduction procedures in use reliably preserve full erotic sensitivity into adulthood.

Finally, Kessler has polled adult men and women on their attitudes toward surgery in infancy.[37] Women were asked if they would want surgical correction had they been born with a clitoris 1.0 to 2.5 centimeters; 93 percent said they would not have wanted treatment unless the condition was life threatening and the surgery would not reduce pleasurable sensitivity. Over half of the women would not have wanted the surgery even if the condition were unattractive and made them feel uncomfortable; 12 percent of the women would not have wanted the surgery under any circumstance. Men were likewise asked whether they would want reassignment as a female had they been born with micropenis. Over half would not have wanted the reassignment under any condition. Almost all would have refused surgery if it reduced pleasurable sensitivity or orgasmic capability. The responses of Kessler's subjects are consistent with the reasonable view that the roles that procreative capacity and sexual pleasure play in intimate adult relationships are far more important than the normality of genital appearance. Despite dissent,[38] the pediatric standard of practice makes precisely the opposite ranking.

SEX AND GENDER

The conceptual distinction between male and female persons (men/women, boys/girls, ladies/gentlemen, etc.) is standard cognitive equipment in culture, deeply implicated in self-identification and social ideology. Particularly in the West, it is taken for granted that humanity comes in two mutually exclusive sexes, and that these are readily distinguishable at birth by the presence or absence of a penis, which, in turn, signals a vast array of other permanent physiological and behavioral variations, both present and in the developmental future. Most of us check off the "M" or the "F" box and choose the corresponding clothing, hair removal routines, rest rooms, careers, urination positions, intimate partners, and underarm deodorants.

Intersexuality—biologically variant sexuality—disturbs the conventional: both our institutional practices and our ways of thinking and behaving. Though we are typically educated to think in binary terms, there are common medical conditions that move human beings away from the male and female norms. In this context it is useful to sketch and explain some of the principle dimensions of "normality," both at the biological level (that is, sexuality) and the psychosocial level (that is, gender). We now sketch some complexities of sexual variation in the light of everyday concerns.

LOCKER-ROOM APPEARANCE

At the biological surface is what we look like in the locker room: male or female? While typical male and female genitalia (and breast development) represent the familiar bimodal distribution, there is a full spectrum in between.

EXTERNAL GENITALIA

The roots of sexual difference are to be found in embryology. It is a useful over-simplification to see baby girls as the default outcome of gestation, the developmental route that is taken unless androgenic hormones are present. For XY (male) embryos, a region on the Y chromosome induces the development of testes from undifferentiated gonadal tissue. The testes in turn produce virilizing androgens in sequences and quantities that can cause that which would otherwise become the labia majora to fuse into a scrotum, and cause that which would otherwise become the labia minora and clitoris to elongate and enlarge into a penis: In the absence of male hormones, which also inhibit feminization, the gonads become ovaries and the vagina and uterus develop.[39]

Apart from differences in size and shape, common visible anatomical variations for XY males include hypospadias, where the penis is open at some location other than at the end; bifid (divided) scrotum; and undescended testicles. Conversely, an XX female may have an enlarged clitoris, an absent or shallow vagina, partially fused labia, and so on.[40] In sum, external genitalia can be typically male, typically female, or virtually anywhere in between. A very large clitoris and a very small penis may be indistinguishable except for the term used to describe them.

FUNCTIONALITY

There are three principle dimensions in which function can be assessed. The first takes into account the *individual's ability to have sexual intercourse.* Is there a functional penis or vagina? A second dimension takes into account *erotic potential.* It is common for genital surgery to compromise erotic sensitivity and, to that extent, the intimate relationships that depend upon it. The third dimension considers *reproductive potential.* Is it possible to become a genetic and/or gestational mother or a genetic father?

GONADS

It is possible to have both ovarian and testicular tissues: true hermaphrodites by definition have both. Gonadal tissue may also be undeveloped in an adult (neither testicular nor ovarian), or it may develop anomalously (mixed gonadal dysgenesis). And gonadal tissue may be completely absent.[41]

ENDOCRINOLOGY

This dimension calls attention to hormone levels, their timing, and the body's responsiveness to them. Among many variations, two common ones can serve as examples. A condition called congenital adrenal hyperplasia (CAH) causes some XX fetuses to develop male-like external genitalia. Their adrenal glands produce large amounts of androgens, virilizing the fetus.[42] These children will sometimes menstruate through the phallus after puberty. A second condition called androgen insensitivity syndrome (AIS) causes XY fetuses to develop female external genitalia. Their testes produce androgens, but, because of a cellular abnormality that partially or completely inhibits response to the hormone, gestational development proceeds toward a female external morphology.[43]

GENETICS

In addition to the most common XX and XY karyotypes, there are also, for example, XO (Turner's syndrome, a sex chromosome missing), XXY (Klinefelter's syndrome), XYY, XXXY, XXYY, and XXXYY. Embryos can also develop with XX cells in one part of the body and XY or other type cells in another part (mosaicism).[44]

CENTRAL NERVOUS SYSTEM

Hormones also organize the brain to bias an individual for future male-typical or female-typical behaviors. Laboratory experiments on mammals, for example, have elicited male behavior patterns in adult XX females after *in utero* exposure to androgens at critical stages of fetal development.[45] Likewise, female behavior patterns have been promoted in XY male mammals by prenatal exposure to anti-androgens.[46] Analogous phenomena have been observed with humans. This type of research supports the view that prenatal endocrinology biases psychosexual development by affecting the central nervous system. Rather than having been born neutral, the androgen-rich ambience in which John/Joan's brain developed probably accounts for her later masculine behavior and her suspicion, against the evidence, that she was really a boy.[47]

PSYCHOSOCIAL LIFE

While it remains to be seen how deeply our gendered behavior is neurologically hard-wired, there are at least three aspects of it that deserve consideration. The first calls attention to one's *sexual identity*. How does one see oneself at the deepest level? In addition to female and male, some now self-identify as intersexed. The second calls attention to one's *gender role*. How does one present publicly in dress, speech, gesture, and so on—as man or woman? And the third calls attention to *sexual orientation*. The condition of intersexuality precludes the application of terms like hetero- and homosexuality that conceive sexual desire, and its idealized object, in relation to the subject's sex. Instead, we reaffirm the recommendation to substitute the terms androphilic, gynecophilic, and ambiphilic.[48]

Because variation occurs independently at many of these levels, the total number of biological/psychosocial possibilities will be very large indeed. The study of intersexuality forces us far from the view that humanity comes in two mutually exclusive sexes, readily distinguishable at birth by the presence or absence of prominent external genitalia.

The discussion so far highlights four critical limitations in our capacity to manage intersexuality clinically. First, in the face of what to many is an astonishing variability, it appears impossible to draw any bright line that decisively and non-arbitrarily separates males and females. Second, even if there were such a procedure, parents lack the ability to engineer the psychosocial development of a target gender.[49] Third, we are unable to predict with confidence the gender that an intersexed newborn will settle into during adulthood. (Indeed, we are often enough mistaken even with anatomically typical infants.) And finally, given the deep and largely uncharted pervasiveness of the effects of being a typical male or female, it is unlikely that surgical reassignment will ever truly "normalize."

In the face of these four practical limitations, and the high probability that they will long endure, it may be time to accept that sex and gender have never been strictly binary; that, on the contrary, there have always been persons in between. In some cultures—various American Indian tribes and societies in Africa and New Guinea, for example—there are societal categories for persons who are neither men nor women as we understand these terms.[50] Intersexuality is common and understandable. Rather than an occasion for emergency surgery and concealment, the birth of a baby with ambiguous genitalia may be an occasion for medical, parental, and social humility and reflection, perhaps even for celebration.

But, as Alice Dreger suggests,[51] the standard of practice represents not humility at all, but a striking appropriation by doctors of the authority to use the arts of medicine to police the boundary between male and female in the defense of cultural norms. Whether this *hubris* is intentional or not, the surgical concealment of intersexuality lends support to those who take for granted that there are but two sexual configurations, each associated with a distinct gender and sexual preference. In making available routine procedures for reconciling deviant anatomy to cultural expectations, medicine vastly empowers the implementation of "normality" even, we would add, as it diminishes the value of difference.

Several commentators have observed the analogy between "normalizing" genital surgery and what has been called "female genital mutilation" as practiced on young girls in Islamic Africa. While both impose morbidity and loss of function in the course of conforming a child's genitalia to cultural expectations, medicine has been vocal in its condemnation of the latter, even as it continues to recommend the former. We question whether physicians should ever sacrifice the organic functionality of any nonconsenting child—Somali or American—on the altar of cultural expectation.

THREE RECOMMENDATIONS

First Recommendation

That there be a general moratorium on such surgery when it is done without the consent of the patient. In arriving at this first recommendation, we do not appeal to the premise that normalizing surgery in infancy does more harm than good. As noted earlier, the large-scale studies that could confirm this are yet to be done. While only a skeptical premise is warranted—that is, that we do not now know that surgery does more good than harm—it suffices nonetheless to justify a moratorium.

As a firm rule, doctors should never undertake surgery, especially without consent, unless there are disproportionate hazards associated with all of the other options: Above all, do no harm. The presumption has always to be against surgery unless two types of evidence are at hand. First, one needs to know that comparable patients generally do well after the surgery: such data are not at hand regarding the adult beneficiaries of these surgeries. And second, one needs to know that comparable patients generally do badly without the surgery. Since surgery is always harmful per se, it should never be done unless there is an expectation of ample compensating benefits. Because this evidence is lacking, the surgical assignment of sex remains an experimental procedure: one in which the results cannot be properly assessed until at least 20 years after the intervention.

Accordingly, it is not possible for a patient's parents to give informed consent to these procedures, precisely because the medical profession has not systematically assessed what happens to the adults these infant patients become. Doctors can't tell parents what the long-term risks and benefits are because they haven't done the studies and don't know.

With the publication of the rest of the John/Joan story, and the additional research sketched above, the standard of practice appears to have lost the epistemic foundation it was earlier thought to have. And yet for some reason these operations continue, despite the erosion of their justification. We recommend that all pediatric surgical assignments be suspended until these issues are resolved.

Two caveats: We are not arguing that medically justified surgical interventions be withheld. Many conditions—bladder exstrophy, certain types of CAH—are associated with risks of morbidity, mortality, and loss of function. Such conditions should always be treated appropriately. And second, we are not suggesting that intersexed children be raised without gender. The choice of gender assignment should take into account the infant's condition, including its causes, and whatever is known about the prognosis.[52] The aim must be to raise infants in a way that will most probably turn out to be comfortable for the maturing child. But gender assignment has to be provisional, subject to revision by the intersexed child as he or she matures. Our objection is to the *surgical* assignment of sex, not to gender assignment per se.

Second Recommendation

That this moratorium not be lifted unless and until the medical profession completes comprehensive look-back studies and finds that the outcomes of past interventions have been positive. In part, this recommendation emerges from sympathy with the view that early surgery may be medically indicated for some types of intersexuality. We need to know more, for example, about the high incidence of cancer in cases of mixed gonadal dysgenesis.

But a stronger justification flows from medical integrity: the profession's ethical commitment to learn as much as it can, even when it makes mistakes.[53] Luckily, a 20-year double-blind prospective study is unnecessary. There are now many thousands of grown intersexuals who have and who have not had surgical and hormonal treatment. Retrospective outcome studies can now be done on these adults, uncovering the comparative effects of treatment and nontreatment. The willingness to subject its practices to honest scrutiny is part of what any profession owes to the community it serves, part of what makes the profession worthy of its community's trust.[54] Pediatrics has an obligation to assess the mature products of its handiwork.

Finally, these studies may be of significant benefit to intersexuals themselves. If the studies find these patients to be at risk for certain medical conditions, this information should be passed along so they can plan and act accordingly.

Third Recommendation

That efforts be made to undo the effects of past deception by physicians. For years, pediatric surgeons have stressed the necessity of rearing postsurgical intersexed infants as unambiguous boys or girls. We do not question that. However, in implementing this approach, parents and clinicians have often concealed aspects of surgery and treatment from the child and excluded maturing children from medical management decisions. Joan Hampson, one of Money's early co-authors, has remarked: "Oddly, even in children old enough to have some opinion, in our experience it has been rare that they have been given any opportunity to express it."[55] This practice can take the form of a well-intentioned, albeit deceptive, conspiracy between family and clinicians and against the child.

Taking the long view, one might ask when, if ever, these former patients should be told of their medical histories. Should it be the intention, at infancy, that these patients never be told or, rather, is the mature or maturing patient entitled to know? There is no standard that the pediatrician advise parents to disclose when their child reaches puberty or adulthood or at any other time. Adults who have had these procedures in childhood are now presenting at clinics, quite ignorant of their histories. This secrecy does damage to the patient. For success in deception entails that the adult patient not understand his or her medical condition. Just to the extent that these adults are misled, they cannot act rationally out of a realistic appraisal of their situation.

But a second objection proceeds from the observation that these cultivated illusions cannot be nurtured reliably and indefinitely. Often patients will discover their condition from an inadvertent family slip, community gossip, or personal investigation into puzzling aspects of their lives. As these children mature into full adulthood and initiate independent clinical relationships, the web of deception will weaken, at least to the extent that the patient develops genuine relationships of trust and confidence with doctors. Unless the entire profession is complicit (thereby ruling out genuine relationships of trust and confidence), one must expect that the truth will emerge. And when it does, the patient will learn, anyway, what she or he was never supposed to have found out. If the patient is going to find out *anyway*, surely it is better for the physician to initiate disclosure.

But even more disturbing than discovering the secret, the former patient will also discover that his or her deformity is unspeakably shameful in the minds of parents and physicians. Moreover, the former patient will learn that she or he has since childhood been systematically deceived by the very people who should have been the most trustworthy. These patients will often avoid physicians and become estranged from their parents. All of this is damaging. Most of it is needless. On a broader scale, it will not be only those patients who learn that physicians are willing to participate in deception. It will be the general community who come to know that doctors choreograph familial mendacity.

We recommend that the medical profession find ways to own up to these adults, initiating disclosure of the medical histories doctors have helped to conceal from their former pediatric patients. In addition to the ethical obligation, clinicians may even have legal duties to warn their former patients when matters of importance are discovered.[56]

One final conjecture. It may well be that this lack of candor is at the root of the profession's failure to do the needed outcome studies, the reason why so many former patients are "lost to follow up." For researchers cannot easily question former patients on the effects of surgery done in infancy when those same patients have never been informed of the surgery, let alone the reasons for it. Although our recommendations are threefold, they speak to a single complex problem. Parents cannot be informed of the expected outcome of the pediatric surgery because the adult outcome studies have not been done. And the adult outcome studies have not been done because these adults have not been informed of the surgery. We may have here an epistemological "black hole" that entraps parents, patients, and physicians in lies, secrets, and avoidable ignorance. While it will take intellectual integrity and professional courage for these pediatric practitioners to extricate themselves, we expect the profession will rise to this occasion.

ACKNOWLEGMENT

This work was supported by the Eugene Garfield Foundation, Philadelphia, and the Queens Medical Center Research Fund, Honolulu.

This chapter first appeared in the *Journal of Clinical Ethics* 9, no. 4 (Winter 1998): © 1998 by the *Journal of Clinical Ethics*; used with permission.

NOTES

1. J. Money and A. A. Ehrhardt, *Man and Woman, Boy and Girl* (Baltimore, MD: Johns Hopkins University Press, 1972).

2. The psychiatrist is quoted in J. Colapinto, "The True Story of John/Joan," *Rolling Stone* (December 1997): 54–58, 60, 62, 64, 66, 68, 70, 72–73, 92, 94–97.

3. J. Money, J. G. Hampson, and J. L. Hampson, "An Examination of Some Basic Sexual Concepts: The Evidence of Human Hermaphroditism," *Bulletin of the Johns Hopkins Hospital* 97 (1955): 301–19; J. Money, J. G. Hampson, and J. L. Hampson, "Hermaphroditism: Recommendations Concerning Assignment of Sex, Change of Sex and Psychological Management," *Bulletin of the Johns Hopkins Hospital* 97 (1955): 284–300.

4. S. Freud, *Three Essays on the Theory of Sexuality*, standard ed. 7 (London: Hogarth Press, 1953, 1905); S. Freud, "Some Psychical Consequences of the Anatomical Distinction between the Sexes," in *Collected Papers by Sigmund Freud*, vol. 5, ed. J. Strachey (London: Hogarth Press, 1925).

5. Money and Ehrhardt, *Man and Woman*, see note 1 above; J. Money, "Prenatal

Hormones and Postnatal Socialization in Gender Identity Differentiation," *Nebraska Symposium on Motivation* 21 (1973): 221–95; J. Money, "Ablatio Penis: Normal Male Infant Sex-Reassignment as a Girl," *Archives of Sexual Behavior* 4 (1975): 65–71.

6. Money, "Ablatio Penis," see note 5 above.

7. "Biological Imperatives," *Time,* January 8, 1973, p. 34.

8. E. A. Catlin and J. D. Crawford, "Neonatal Endocrinology," in *Principles and Practice of Pediatrics,* 2nd ed., ed. F. A. Oski et al. (Philadelphia: Lippincott, 1994), 421–29; P. K. Donahoe and J. J. Schnitzer, "Evaluation of the Infant Who Has Ambiguous Genitalia, and Principles of Operative Management," *Seminars in Pediatric Surgery* 5 (1996): 30–40; M. Sifuentes, "Ambiguous Genitalia," in *Pediatrics: A Primary Care Approach,* ed. C. D. Berkowitz (Philadelphia: W. B. Saunders, 1996), pp. 261–65.

9. R. Azziz et al., "Congenital Adrenal Hyperplasia: Long-Term Results Following Vaginal Reconstruction," *Fertility & Sterility* 46 (1986): 1011–14; P. K. Donahoe, D. M. Powell, and M. M. Lee, "Clinical Management of Intersex Abnormalities," *Current Problems in Surgery* 28 (1991): 517–79.

10. American Academy of Pediatrics, "Timing of Elective Surgery on the Genitalia of Male Children with Particular Reference to the Risks, Benefits, and Psychological Effects of Surgery and Anesthesia," *Pediatrics* 97 (1996): 590–94.

11. D. Cappon, C. Ezrin, and P. Lynes, "Psychosexual Identification (Psychogender) in the Intersexed," *Canadian Psychiatric Association Journal* 4 (1959): 90–106; M. Diamond, "A Critical Evaluation of the Ontogeny of Human Sexual Behavior," *Quarterly Review of Biology* 40 (1965): 147–75; M. Diamond, "Sexual Identity, Monozygotic Twins Reared in Discordant Sex Roles and a BBC Follow-Up," *Archives of Sexual Behavior* 11 (1982): 181–85; B. Zuger, "Gender Role Determination: A Critical Review of the Evidence from Hermaphroditism," *Psychosomatic Medicine* 32 (1970): 449–63.

12. S. J. Kessler, *Lessons from the Intersexed* (Piscataway, NJ: Rutgers University Press, 1998).

13. H. Benjamin, *The Transsexual Phenomenon* (New York: Julian Press, 1966).

14. M. Blackless et al., "How Sexually Dimorphic Are We," *American Journal of Human Biology* (in press).

15. This estimate is by William Reiner, MD, quoted in Colapinto, "The True Story of John/Joan," see note 2 above.

16. Kessler, *Lessons from the Intersexed,* see note 12 above.

17. J. M. Schober, "Long-Term Outcome of Feminizing Genitoplasty for Intersex," in *Pediatric Surgery and Urology: Long-Term Outcomes,* ed. P. D. E. Mouriquand (Philadelphia: W. B. Saunders, in press).

18. J. Money and M. Schwartz, "Biosocial Determinants of Gender Identity Differentiation and Development," in *Biological Determinants of Sexual Behavior,* ed. J. B. Hutchison (New York: John Wiley & Sons, 1978).

19. M. Diamond and H. K. Sigmundson, "Sex Reassignment at Birth: Long-Term Review and Clinical Implications," *Archives of Pediatrics and Adolescent Medicine* 151 (1997): 298–304.

20. Diamond, "Sexual Identity," see note 11 above.

21. Colapinto, "The True Story of John/Joan," see note 2 above.

22. Diamond and Sigmundson, "Sex Reassignment," see note 19 above.

23. Colapinto, "The True Story of John/Joan," see note 2 above; Diamond and Sigmundson, "Sex Reassignment," see note 19 above.

24. M. A. Mureau et al., "Satisfaction with Penile Appearance after Hypospadias Surgery: The Patient and Surgeon View," *Journal of Urology* 155 (1996): 703–706.

25. W. G. Reiner, "To Be Male or Female—That is the Question," *Archives of Pediatric and Adolescent Medicine* 151 (1997): 224–25.

26. William Reiner, MD, quoted in Colapinto, "The True Story of John/Joan," see note 2 above.

27. C. Chase, "Hermaphrodites with Attitude: Mapping the Emergence of Intersex Political Activism," *Gay & Lesbian Quarterly* 4 (1998): 189–211.

28. C. J. Dewhurst and R. R. Gordan, "Change of Sex," *Lancet* 309 (1963): 1213–17; M. Diamond, "Sexual Identity and Sexual Orientation in Children with Traumatized or Ambiguous Genitalia," *Journal of Sex Research* 34 (1997): 199–222; V. Khupisco, "The Tragic Boy Who Refuses to Be Turned into a Girl," *Sunday Times of Johannesburg* (May 21, 1995): A-1.

29. K. Kipnis and G. Williamson, "Nontreatment Decisions for Severely Compromised Newborns," *Ethics* 95 (1984): 90–111.

30. J. M. Reilly and C. R. J. Woodhouse, "Small Penis and the Male Sexual Role," *Journal of Urology* 142 (1989): 569–72.

31. A. P. van Seters and A. K. Slob, "Mutually Gratifying Heterosexual Relationship with Micropenis of Husband," *Journal of Sex & Marital Therapy* 14 (1988): 98–107.

32. B. Craffey, "Showering 'Sans Penis,'" *Chrysalis: The Journal of Transgressive Gender Identities* 2, no. 5 (Fall 1997/Winter 1998): 55–56.

33. Schober, "Long-Term Outcome," see note 17 above.

34. Kessler, *Lessons from the Intersexed*, see note 12 above.

35. J. Randolph, W. Hung, and M. C. Rathlev, "Clitoroplasty for Females Born with Ambiguous Genitalia: A Long-Term Study of 37 Patients," *Journal of Pediatric Surgery* 16 (1981): 882–87; A. Sotiropoulos et al., "Long-Term Assessment of Genital Reconstruction in Female Pseudohermaphrodites," *Journal of Urology* 115 (1976): 599–601.

36. Randolph, Hung, and Rathlev, "Clitoroplasty for Females," see note 35 above; T. M. Barrett, E. T. Gonzales, "Reconstruction of the Female External Genitalia," *Urologic Clinics of North America* 7 (1980): 455–63.

37. Kessler, *Lessons from the Intersexed*, see note 12 above.

38. Ibid., K. I. Glassberg, "The Intersex Infant: Early Gender Assignment and Surgical Reconstruction," *Journal of Pediatric and Adolescent Gynecology* 11 (1998): 151–54; J. Schober, "Early Feminizing Genitoplasty," *Journal of Pediatric and Adolescent Gynecology* 11 (1998): 154–56.

39. M. Diamond, "Human Sexual Development: Biological Foundation for Social Development," in *Human Sexuality in Four Perspectives*, ed. F. A. Beach (Baltimore, MD: Johns Hopkins Press, 1976): 22–61.

40. M. M. Grumbach and F. A. Conte, "Disorders of Sex Differentiation," in *Williams Textbook of Endocrinology*, ed. J. D. Wilson et al. (Philadelphia: W. B. Saunders, 1998), 1303–1425.

41. Grumbach and Conte, "Disorders of Sex Differentiation," see note 40 above.

42. Ibid.

43. C. Quigley et al., "Androgen Receptor Defects: Historical, Clinical and Molecular Perspectives," *Endocrine Reviews* 16 (1995): 271–321.

44. C. Overzier; *Intersexuality* (New York: Academic Press, 1963).

45. C. H. Phoenix et al., "Organizing Action of Prenatally Administered Testosterone Propionate on the Tissues Mediating Mating Behavior in the Female Guinea Pig," *Endocrinology* 65 (1959): 369–82; R. W. Goy, J. E. Wolf, and S. G. Eisele, "Experimental Female Hermaphroditism in Rhesus Monkeys: Anatomical and Psychological Characteristics," in *Handbook of Sexology*, ed. J. Money and H. Musaph (Amsterdam, the Netherlands: Elsevier/North-Holland Biomedical Press, 1977), pp. 139–56.

46. J. Vega-Matuszczyk and K. Larsson, "Sexual Preference and Feminine and Masculine Sexual Behavior of Male Rats Prenatally Exposed to Antiandrogen or Antiestrogen," *Hormones and Behavior* 29 (1995): 191–206.

47. Diamond, "Human Sexual Development," see note 39 above; M. Diamond, "Sexual Identity and Sex Roles," in *The Frontiers of Sex Research*, ed. V. Bullough (Amherst, NY: Prometheus Books, 1979), pp. 33–56.

48. Diamond, "Sexual Identity," see note 28 above.

49. J. R. Harris, *The Nurture Assumption* (New York: Free Press, 1998).

50. R. B. Edgerton, "Poket Intersexuality: An East African Example of the Resolution of Sexual Incongruity," *American Anthropologist* 66 (1964): 1288–99; W. L. Williams, *The Spirit and the Flesh: Sexual Diversity in American Culture* (Boston: Beacon Press, 1986).

51. A. D. Dreger, *Hermaphrodites and the Medical Invention of Sex* (Cambridge, MA: Harvard University Press, 1998).

52. M. Diamond and H. K. Sigmundson, "Management of Intersexuality: Guidelines for Dealing with Persons with Ambiguous Genitalia," *Archives of Pediatrics and Adolescent Medicine* 151 (1997): 1046–50.

53. A. M. Schwitalla, "The Real Meaning of Research and Why it Should Be Encouraged," *Modern Hospital* 33 (1929): 77–80; B. Barber, "The Ethics of Experimentation with Human Subjects," *Scientific American* 234 (1976): 25–31.

54. K. Kipnis, "Professional Responsibility and the Responsibility of Professions," in *Profits and Professions*, ed. W. L. Robison, M. S. Pritchard, and J. Ellin (Clifton, NJ: Humana Press, 1983): 9–22.

55. J. G. Hampson, "Hermaphroditic Genital Appearance, Rearing and Eroticism in Hyperadrenocorticism," *Bulletin of the Johns Hopkins Hospital* 96 (1955): 265–73.

56. A. G. Nadel, "Duty of Medical Practitioner to Warn Patient of Subsequently Discovered Danger from Treatment Previously Given," *American Law Reports* 12, no. 4 (1981): 41.

30.

THE INTERNATIONAL BILL OF GENDER RIGHTS

As adopted June 17, 1995, Houston, Texas, USA.

Preface by Phyllis Randolph Frye

"The International Bill of Gender Rights (IBGR), strives to express human and civil rights from a gender perspective. However, the ten rights enunciated below are not to be viewed as special rights applicable to a particular interest group. Nor are these rights limited in application to persons for whom gender identity and gender role issues are of paramount concern. All ten sections of the IBGR are universal rights which can be claimed and exercised by every human being."

The International Bill of Gender Rights (IBGR) was first drafted in committee and adopted by the International Conference on Transgender Law and Employment Policy (ICTLEP) at that organization's second annual meeting, held in Houston, Texas, August 26–29, 1993.

June 17, 1995, http://inquirer.gn.apc.org/GDRights.html (August 14, 2007). **Source URL:** http://www.pfc .org.uk/node/275.

The IBGR has been reviewed and amended in committee and adopted with revisions at subsequent annual meetings of ICTLEP in 1994 and 1995.

The IBGR is a theoretical construction which has no force of law absent its adoption by legislative bodies and recognition of its principles by courts of law, administrative agencies, and international bodies such as the United Nations.

However, individuals are free to adopt the truths and principles expressed in the IBGR, and to lead their lives accordingly. In this fashion, the truths expressed in the IBGR will liberate and empower humankind in ways and to an extent beyond the reach of legislators, judges, officials, and diplomats.

When the truths expressed in the IBGR are embraced and given expression by humankind, the acts of legislatures and pronouncements of courts and other governing structures will necessarily follow. Thus, the paths of free expression trodden by millions of human beings, all seeking to define themselves and give meaning to their lives, will ultimately determine the course of governing bodies.

The IBGR is a transformative and revolutionary document but it is grounded in the bedrock of individual liberty and free expression. As our lives unfold, these kernels of truth are here for all who would claim and exercise them.

This document, though copyrighted, may be reproduced by any means and freely distributed by anyone supporting the principles and statements contained in the International Bill of Gender Rights.

THE INTERNATIONAL BILL OF GENDER RIGHTS

1. The Right to Define Gender Identity

All human beings carry within themselves an ever-unfolding idea of who they are and what they are capable of achieving. The individual's sense of self is not determined by chromosomal sex, genitalia, assigned birth sex, or initial gender role. Thus, the individual's identity and capabilities cannot be circumscribed by what society deems to be masculine or feminine behavior. It is fundamental that individuals have the right to define, and to redefine as their lives unfold, their own gender identities, without regard to chromosomal sex, genitalia, assigned birth sex, or initial gender role.

Therefore, all human beings have the right to define their own gender identity regardless of chromosomal sex, genitalia, assigned birth sex, or initial gender role; and further, no individual shall be denied Human or Civil Rights by virtue of a self-defined gender identity which is not in accord with chromosomal sex, genitalia, assigned birth sex, or initial gender role.

2. The Right to Free Expression of Gender Identity

Given the right to define one's own gender identity, all human beings have the corresponding right to free expression of their self-defined gender identity.

Therefore, all human beings have the right to free expression of their self-defined gender identity; and further, no individual shall be denied Human or Civil Rights by virtue of the expression of a self-defined gender identity.

3. The Right to Secure and Retain Employment and to Receive Just Compensation

Given the economic structure of modern society, all human beings have a right to train for and to pursue an occupation or profession as a means of providing shelter, sustenance, and the necessities and bounty of life, for themselves and for those dependent upon them, to secure and retain employment, and to receive just compensation for their labor regardless of gender identity, chromosomal sex, genitalia, assigned birth sex, or initial gender role.

Therefore, individuals shall not be denied the right to train for and to pursue an occupation or profession, nor be denied the right to secure and retain employment, nor be denied just compensation for their labor, by virtue of their chromosomal sex, genitalia, assigned birth sex, or initial gender role, or on the basis of a self-defined gender identity or the expression thereof.

4. The Right of Access to Gendered Space and Participation in Gendered Activity

Given the right to define one's own gender identity and the corresponding right to free expression of a self-defined gender identity, no individual should be denied access to a space or denied participation in an activity by virtue of a self-defined gender identity which is not in accord with chromosomal sex, genitalia, assigned birth sex, or initial gender role.

Therefore, no individual shall be denied access to a space or denied participation in an activity by virtue of a self-defined gender identity which is not in accord with chromosomal sex, genitalia, assigned birth sex, or initial gender role.

5. The Right to Control and Change One's Own Body

All human beings have the right to control their bodies, which includes the right to change their bodies cosmetically, chemically, or surgically, so as to express a self-defined gender identity.

Therefore, individuals shall not be denied the right to change their bodies as a means of expressing a self-defined gender identity; and further, individuals shall not be denied Human or Civil Rights on the basis that they have changed their bodies cosmetically, chemically, or surgically, or desire to do so as a means of expressing a self-defined gender identity.

6. The Right to Competent Medical and Professional Care

Given the individual's right to define one's own gender identity, and the right to change one's own body as a means of expressing a self-defined gender identity, no individual should be denied access to competent medical or other professional care on the basis of the individual's chromosomal sex, genitalia, assigned birth sex, or initial gender role.

Therefore, individuals shall not be denied the right to competent medical or other professional care when changing their bodies cosmetically, chemically, or surgically, on the basis of chromosomal sex, genitalia, assigned birth sex, or initial gender role.

7. The Right to Freedom from Psychiatric Diagnosis or Treatment

Given the right to define one's own gender identity, individuals should not be subject to psychiatric diagnosis or treatment solely on the basis of their gender identity or role.

Therefore, individuals shall not be subject to psychiatric diagnosis or treatment as mentally disordered or diseased solely on the basis of a self-defined gender identity or the expression thereof.

8. The Right to Sexual Expression

Given the right to a self-defined gender identity, every consenting adult has a corresponding right to free sexual expression.

Therefore, no individual's Human or Civil Rights shall be denied on the basis of sexual orientation; and further, no individual shall be denied Human or Civil Rights for expression of a self-defined gender identity through sexual acts between consenting adults.

9. The Right to Form Committed, Loving Relationships and Enter into Marital Contracts

Given that all human beings have the right to free expression of self-defined gender identities, and the right to sexual expression as a form of gender expression, all human beings have a corresponding right to form committed, loving relationships with one another, and to enter into marital contracts, regardless of their own or their partner's chromosomal sex, genitalia, assigned birth sex, or initial gender role.

Therefore, individuals shall not be denied the right to form committed, loving relationships with one another or to enter into marital contracts by virtue of their own or their partner's chromosomal sex, genitalia, assigned birth sex, or initial gender role, or on the basis of their expression of a self-defined gender identity.

10. The Right to Conceive, Bear, or Adopt Children; the Right to Nurture and Have Custody of Children and to Exercise Parental Capacity

Given the right to form a committed, loving relationship with another, and to enter into marital contracts, together with the right to express a self-defined gender identity and the right to sexual expression, individuals have a corresponding right to conceive and bear children, to adopt children, to nurture children, to have custody of children, and to exercise parental capacity with respect to children, natural or adopted, without regard to chromosomal sex, genitalia, assigned birth sex, or initial gender role, or by virtue of a self-defined gender identity or the expression thereof.

Therefore, individuals shall not be denied the right to conceive, bear, or adopt children, nor to nurture and have custody of children, nor to exercise parental capacity with respect to children, natural or adopted, on the basis of their own, their partner's, or their children's chromosomal sex, genitalia, assigned birth sex, initial gender role, or by virtue of a self-defined gender identity or the expression thereof.

Comments, suggestions, or questions regarding the IBGR should be forwarded to Sharon Stuart, IBGR Project, P.O. Box 930, Cooperstown, NY 1332B, USA. Telephone: (607) 547–4118. FAX: (607) 547–2198. E-Mail: StuComOne@aol.com.

Universities, libraries, academicians, attorneys, judges, government officials, social workers, and others may obtain bound proceedings from each of the annual ICTLEP conferences. Contact Phyllis Randolph Frye at PRFrye@aol.com.

For more information and an online version of The International Bill of Gender Rights, go to http://www.transgenderlegal.com/ibgr.htm.

Published on Press for Change (http://www.pfc.org.uk).

31.

TO CUT OR NOT TO CUT

Kathleen J. Wininger

". . . you are the incarnation of morality. . . . Your conscience is clear and your duty done when you have called everybody names."[1]

I n *Major Barbara*, the main character, armaments manufacturer Andrew Undershaft, rebukes his wife, Lady Britomat, for a moral piety; to have the correct view on things is more important than what is to be done. He suggests moral philosophy consists in naming and casting judgment on the problems of the world rather than doing something about them. Moral philosophy is dealing with more complex sexual and psychosexual issues every day. The issues of naming and passing judgment exist alongside the need to act or refrain from acting.

Dealing with most substantial philosophical issues takes one beyond philosophy in its narrowest parameters. In some ways the profession is recapturing its earliest breadth, taking back from sister disciplines a wide scope of informed thought. The writings of the late Sixties on sex and gender relied on fairly simple ideas of the relation between a binary biological distinction—male and female. Since much contemporary writing by biologists and philosophers, sociologists and anthropologists questions these binaries and suggests how they were constructed, it is not surprising to find that philosophers consider sex, gender, and sexual preference as problematic categories. The prevalence of the binary, and the need to affirm it, has led social practices to sometimes literally reconstruct the genitalia of sexually ambiguous people. This forces their "biology": genitalia and hormonal configurations to conform as nearly as possible to one of the two available sexual assignments. The prevalence of surgical solutions to the problem of intersexuals shows that not only is gender a matter of considerable complexity, even the assignment of sex is a matter which should be considered much more carefully. The implications for desire can also be profound since the surgery can deprive the individual of sensation, affecting sexuality regardless of gender role and sexual preference. The presence of debate around genital pleasure and its restriction or suppression involves us in issues challenging the epistemic authority of experts. For example, in the case of the intersex child, developmental psychologists and other experts argue against the delay of sex/gender assignments because they believe this delay is psychologically damaging from a developmental perspective. Controversies within transsexual and intersexed communities continue, and to give but one example, Alice Dreger's work is sometimes criticized because some believe[2] she has pathologized the intersex conditions. In calling them "disorders of sex development" and in her desire to have intersex recognized she has turned to diagnostic categories. In the broader social context sometimes "overpathologizing" is seen as necessary for justifications of medical interventions and insurance claims. The complexity of the issues and the heat of the debates arise from the different notions of identity, differing pragmatic strategies, and the legacy of intransigent models of sexuality and gender.

It is not only the existence of cases like the intersexed, but the decision to treat cases within a range of normality, rather than monstrous, that affects our theoretical constructions. Europeans have looked to practices of clitorectomy and infibulation in other cultures and found them to be barbaric, unhygienic, etc. Theorists have done this without interrogating their own practices of male circumcision or of the European practices of performing hysterectomies, clitorectomies (for "oversexed" females, for epilepsy), and transgender surgeries. If the areas of biological dimorphism are themselves complicated, then clearly the issues of gender assignment, gender changes, and sexual preferences provide places of variation as well.

The simple idea that gender is based on biology has been challenged by examining intra-cultural practices and by doing extra-cultural comparisons. Although this book concentrates upon debates within the contemporary United States, those debates are informed by the new information we have about a variety of complex cultures with varied social practices. Information regarding cultures, for example, the Mohave "berdache," who recognize between three and five gender assignments, or the practice of woman-to-woman marriage in many

African countries, has led to serious questions about gender categorizations in all cultures. There is a lively debate among African intellectuals about whether the European category of gender is ever applicable in the African context.[3]

When, a decade ago, anthropologist Deborah Elliston[4] wrote on this issue, she said:

> I find it problematic that female genital mutilation in Africa regularly reappears. . . . as a locus of feminist research interest, and that it more generally is treated as a legitimate topic of US-based feminist writing. US-feminist authored writings on the topic thus far demonstrate to me only that FGM [Female Genital Mutilation] cannot be analyzed or theorized from a US-based perspective. When US feminists write about FGM, their writings almost invariably become vehicles for placing non-Western women once more 'under Western eyes', to borrow a phrase from Chandra Mohanty: African women end up constructed, in these works, as thoroughly oppressed victims (of their men, their 'culture') while Western women are the free and enlightened thinkers who would rescue them, or at least draw back the 'veil' over these practices and 'expose' them to the enlightened light of US feminist criticism.

Yet her viewpoint on Female Genital Mutilation caused her to be accused of cultural relativism, of not having firm enough moral beliefs to transcend cultural mores. To this she countered:

> Rather than promoting the further exoticization of African women from those few societies within which some women undergo FGM, rather than adopting the colonial assumption that it is in 'other places' that one finds the more radical practices which "mutilate" female bodies and desires, US-based feminist scholars interested in FGM would stand on much firmer ground—methodologically, epistemologically, and ethically—if they looked to "female mutilation" in their own backyards: Breast implants, anyone? "Cosmetic" surgeries? Belly tucks? Liposuction?[5]

We can add to this list the mutilated body of the European woman, although self-inflicted, as being in the interest of sexual attractiveness and thus worthy of study.

The mixture of fascination and outrage of the European at adornment practices—genital cutting and manipulation—that is a part of so many cultures seems paradoxical when we consider, for example, that many Americans' default position on male circumcision is to lop off these children's penises without anesthetic, and often with the same justifications of other cultural practices' attractiveness of the member: cleanliness, tradition.[6] Note here that these are the precise justifications found in Africa and Asia and in addition to the women being less likely to seek auto-erotic fulfillment. Obioma Nnaemeka, the brilliant Nigerian theorist, wrote an article titled "If Female Circumcision Did Not Exist, Western Feminism Would Invent It."[7]

Nnaemeka wrote of the re-inscription on the African woman's body of colonial assumptions and practices, of a second attempt to display the African woman's body and expose her private parts in a way no European woman would experience outside of private medical treatment.

But perhaps Nnaemeka speaks too soon. In the United States, women's vaginas and labias are under the scrutiny of consumer capitalism—one more place to cut.

And what of American and European women's vaginas?

> Laser Vaginal Institute of Michigan offers elective female genital surgeries, the primary selling points being enhanced sexual gratification for the woman and aesthetically pleasing results.... Or a woman can become 'revirginized' and have an approximation of her hymen restored. (This is particularly popular among Middle Eastern women who need to 'fake' their virginity before marriage.) And if she wants to combine more than one surgery, she can end up paying more than $10,000 for newer, tighter, prettier genitals. This is the latest facet of cosmetic surgery—designer vaginas. Women have already nipped, tucked, implanted, and vacuumed every other part of their bodies, and are now turning their perfection-obsessed eyes to their own genitals."[8]

Where twenty years ago people were talking about homosexuality as an issue of social morality and justice, contemporary debates also consider the question of categorization. What is a man; a woman; a heterosexual; a homosexual? What is gender and its relation to the way sexuality is expressed? If a male chooses the vestments of a female, yet chooses a female partner, or a lesbian chooses to have a sex change operation, but keeps her sexual preference, what does that mean about what constitutes a lesbian, what constitutes a man, what constitutes femininity and masculinity?

There are apparently superficial yet often profound paradoxes in our discussions of surgical inventions on issues of gender. Arguments for bodily integrity, which rely on a biological and naturalized model of sexuality and gender, such as those mentioned above, exist side by side with interventionist models that advocate such practices as cultural genital cutting, male circumcision, elective sexual reassignment, infibulations, and clitorectomies. Ironically, we sometimes find ourselves in ideologically and theoretically peculiar positions when we advocate rights to surgical intervention for those with elective affinities for a gender assignment—which requires surgical and hormonal interventions—while simultaneously making arguments for allowing the "naturally" intersexed to find their way in a profoundly bivalent gender system. At the same time there are arguments for earlier interventions in transgender people that would allow them to make the switch before puberty and therefore before most ages of consent.

It is easy to see how many of these issues really come from a culturally enforced sex/gender division that requires on religious or other cultural grounds a simplistic female/male dichotomy. This, like other European categorizations, comes from a policing of sexuality, which, if it didn't begin with these theories, used sexology, psychoanalysis, and biologically based views to enforce these bivalent categories. The issue before us now, the challenge to us, is to have theories that allow us to discuss rather than pronounce on the very complex and varied issues involving the preservation and modifications of sexualized and gendered selves.

Notes

1. George Bernard Shaw, *Major Barbara* (Middlesex, England: Penguin Books, 1985), p. 146.

2. M. Diamond, "Variations of Sex Development Instead of Disorders of Sex Development," 2006, http://adc.bmjjournals.com/cgi/eletters/91/7/554#2460. Replying to I. A. Hughes et al., "Consensus Statement on Management of Intersex Disorders," *Archives of Disease in Childhood* 91 (2006): 554–63, http://adc.bmj.com/cgi/content/extract/91/7/554?rss=1, Copyright © 2006 BMJ Publishing Group Ltd. & Royal College of Paediatrics and Child Health.

3. April 3 and 4, 1997. Topic: Female Genital Mutilation, http://userpages.umbc.edu/~korenman/wmst/fgm2.html (accessed December 2, 2007). Oyewùmí, Oyèrónké, *African Women and Feminism: Reflecting on the Politics of Sisterhood* (Trenton, NJ: Africa World Press: 2003), *The Invention of Women: Making an African Sense of Western Gender Discourses* (Minneapolis: University of Minnesota Press, 1997); Ifi Amadiume, *Male Daughters, Female Husbands: Gender and Sex in an African Society* (Zed Press, 1987); *Africa After Gender?* ed. Catherine M. Cole, Takyiwaa Manuh, and Stephan F. Miescher (Indiana University Press, 2007).

4. April 3 and 4, 1997. Topic: Female Genital Mutilation, http://userpages.umbc.edu/~korenman/wmst/fgm2.html (accessed December 2, 2007).

5. Ibid.

6. The precise justifications found in Africa and Asia.

7. Obioma Nnaemeka, "If Female Circumcision Did Not Exist, Western Feminism Would Invent It," in *Eye to Eye: Women Practicing Development across Cultures,* ed. Celeste Schenck and Susan Perry (London: Zed Press, 2001), pp. 171–89.

8. Sara Klein, "Does This Make My Labia Look Fat? Medicine and Marketing Collide Below the Belt," originally published March 9, 2005, http://metrotimes.com/editorial/story.asp?id=7405 (accessed December 2, 2007).

Part 3.

DESIRE, PORNOGRAPHY, AND RAPE

32.

PATRIARCHAL SEX

Robert Jensen

Patriarchal sex (example 1): Four male undergraduates at Cornell University post on the Internet the "Top 75 reasons why women (bitches) should not have freedom of speech." Reason #20: "This is my dick. I'm gonna fuck you. No more stupid questions."[1]

Patriarchal sex (example 2): Rhonda was separated from her husband but was on generally friendly terms with him. One night he entered her home. For the next seven hours, he raped her. "It was like something just snapped in him. He grabbed me and said, "We gonna have sex, I need to fuck."[2]

I begin with a working definition of patriarchal sex: Sex is fucking.[3] In patriarchy, there is an imperative to fuck—in rape and in "normal" sex, with strangers and girlfriends and wives and estranged wives and children. What matters in patriarchal sex is the male need to fuck. When that need presents itself, sex occurs.

From that, a working definition of what it means to be a man in this culture: A man is a male human who fucks.[4]

First published in the *International Journal of Sociology and Social Policy* 17, nos. 1–2 (1987). Reprinted with the permission of the publisher.

What I'm Trying to Do and What I'm Not Trying to Do

In this essay I want to analyze patriarchal sex and theorize about strategies for moving away from it. In simple terms, I want to think about how we males might stop fucking and stop being men.

I draw on the work of radical feminist theorists and activists; my research on pornography and sexuality, and my experience as a man in US culture in the last half of the twentieth century. I move without apology between personal narrative and reflection, and more formal scholarly writing. I reject the conventional academic obsession with splitting off mind and body, reason and emotion, objective and subjective, scholarship and activism. One of the ways I know about the world is by living in it, and the knowledge I have gained has led me to a political position that makes certain actions on my part morally necessary. Decades of feminist and other critical work more than adequately justify this kind of engaged scholarship.[5]

What follows is part of my long-term project of trying to make sense of a system into which I was born, a system that privileges certain people with certain attributes (e.g., white, male, heterosexual, educated—all of which I have or have had at one point in my life) and works to maintain the concentration of power in the hands of a relatively small group of people.

This essay is not a "men's studies" or "gender studies" project. It is a feminist-inspired project.[6] I am a man working within feminist theory to try to understand the nature of oppression, specifically in this essay the nature of gender oppression and the role of sexuality in that oppression. My goal is to be a traitor to my gender, as well as to my race and my class. I routinely fail at this goal, though sometimes I get glimpses of what success looks like. I am fortunate to have the support of many feminist women[7] and a few like-minded male colleagues.[8] Integral to that support is their willingness to hold me accountable for my actions and words; the critique is a key part of the support.

Also, this essay is not an attempt to tell women what they should think or how they should behave. I am trying to talk primarily to other men about my struggle and what I have learned from it. I do this work both out of a yearning for justice for those oppressed in patriarchy (women, particularly lesbians, children, and to some extent gay men) and out of self-interest (the desire to live a more fulfilling life in a more just, humane, and compassionate world). I work both out of hope for the future and out of fear.

"What's your problem—are you afraid of sex?"

That question has been posed to me often as I have been involved in anti-pornography work. For a long time, my answer was, "No, of course not. Me, afraid? I'm no prude."

I am not a prude, but I have come to realize that I am very much afraid of sex. I am afraid of sex as sex is defined by the dominant culture, practiced all around me, and projected onto magazine pages, billboards, and movie screens. I am afraid of sex because I am afraid of domination, cruelty, violence, and death. I am afraid of sex because sex has hurt me and hurt lots of people I know, and because I have hurt others with sex in the past. I know that there are people out there who have been hurt by sex in ways that are beyond my words, who have experienced a depth of pain that I will never fully understand. And I know there are people who are dead because of sex.

Yes, I am afraid of sex. How could I not be?[9]

A common response from people when I say things like that is, "You're nuts." Sometimes, when I'm feeling shaky, a voice in the back of my head asks, "Am I nuts?"

I have been doing research and writing on pornography and sexuality for about eight years.[10] In the past few years, I have been trying to figure out how to talk to people who think I am crazy and how to deal with my own fear that they may be right. I have been trying to understand why the attack on the feminist critique of patriarchal sex has been so strong and so successful, and how it connects to the backlash against feminist work on sexual violence.

Here's one tentative explanation: It is too scary to be afraid of sex. To go too far down the road with the radical critique of sexuality means, inevitably, acknowledging a fear of patriarchal sex. And if all the sex around us is patriarchal, then we are going to live daily with that fear. And if patriarchal sex seems to be so overwhelmingly dominant that it sometimes is difficult to believe that any other sex is possible, then maybe we are always going to be afraid. Maybe it's easier to not be afraid, or at least to repress the fear. Maybe that's the only way to survive.

But maybe not. Maybe being afraid of sex is the first step toward something new. Maybe things that seem impossible now will be possible someday. Or maybe we will find that we won't need what we thought we needed.[11] Maybe being afraid is the first step out of the fear and into something else that we cannot yet name.

EXPANDING THE WORKING DEFINITION OF PATRIARCHAL SEX

I was born in 1958 in a small city in the upper Midwest to white parents who, after some years of struggle, settled into the middle class. I went to a Protestant church and public school. I had friends, mostly other boys. We talked about sex and we begged, borrowed, and stole pornography. I watched a lot of television and went to a lot of movies. I had a G. I. Joe doll and toy guns. I played sports. I was a quirky kid in some respects, physically smaller than most and a bit of an egghead from an early age. Maybe my family was a little more emotionally abusive than most, but maybe not. In many regards, I grew up "normal." And I got a normal education in sex.

Here is the curriculum for sex education for a normal American boy: Fuck women.

Here is the sexual grammar lesson I received. "Man fucks women; subject verb object."[12]

The specifics varied depending on the instructor.

Some people said, "Fuck as many women as often as you can for as long as you can get away with it." Others said, "Fuck a lot of women until you get tired of it, and then find one to marry and just fuck her." And some said, "Don't fuck any women until you find one to marry, and then fuck her for the rest of your life and never fuck anyone else."

Some said, "Women are special; put them on a pedestal before and after you fuck them." Others said, "Women are shit; do what you have to do to fuck them, and then get away from them."

Most said, "Only fuck women." A few said, "Fuck other men if you want to."

The basic concepts were clear: Sex is fucking. Fucking is penetration. The things you do before you penetrate are just warm-up exercises. If you don't penetrate, you haven't fucked, and if you haven't fucked, you haven't had sex. Frye defines this kind of heterosexual, and heterosexist, intercourse as, "male-dominant-female-subordinate-copulation-whose-completion-and-purpose-is-the-male's-ejaculation."[13] That is sex in patriarchy.

All the teachers (parents, friends, ministers, celebrities, pornographers, movie directors, etc.) tend to agree on the one primary rule about sex in patriarchy: You gotta get it. You have to fuck something at some point in your life. If you don't get it, there's something wrong with you. You aren't normal. You aren't really alive. You certainly aren't a man.

When I was a kid, I'm not sure I really wanted to fuck anyone. But eventually I figured out that if didn't learn to do it, I was going to be an outcast. So I learned, though later than most of my peers.

My first sex was with pornography. I was about six years old the first time I saw it. For the next two decades, it was part of my life on an irregular basis. I had sex with women in person, and I had sex with women in magazines and movies (masturbating to pornography is a way of having sex, of sexually using the women in it). As far as I can tell from research and conversations with men, I had a fairly typical sex life. I learned to like being in control. That was part of the appeal of sex with pornography: I had control over when I used it, and I was in control of the women in it.[14] That was part of the appeal of sex with women: I was the man, and I was in control because men "naturally" take control of sex. Once the details of access with a particular woman were negotiated, I was in control. Patriarchal sex practices vary from person to person, from attempts at more egalitarian interaction to the sadomasochistic. My preferred practices, on the surface, leaned more toward the egalitarian, but when I think about my sexual history I can connect every practice to a need for control, either of the woman or of the woman's pleasure.

When I started to realize that, I realized I was in trouble. When I realized that most everyone around me was in trouble, I started to get scared. When I got real scared, I stopped having patriarchal sex. That meant I stopped having sex with other people, including the people in pornography. At first, I didn't do this consciously. I just found it more and more difficult to have sex. At some point, I consciously made a decision to quit. As I began to understand more about how deeply I had been trained in the rules of patriarchal sex, it became more clear that I would have to stop participating in that system. I would have to stop fucking. I could no longer pretend that I was "working it out" by trying to put into practice new ideas about sex. Patriarchal sex was too deeply rooted in my body and my psyche. Before I could reconstruct my sexuality, I needed time to deconstruct, free of the pressure to have sex.

THE RADICAL FEMINIST CRITIQUE

By the time I came to understand that I wanted, and needed, to stop having patriarchal sex, I had a framework within which to understand what was happening to me. Radical feminist critiques of pornography and patriarchal sex gave me a vocabulary, a way to make coherent in words what was happening in my body and mind. That made it possible though by no means easy, to begin the process. Many feminist activists and theorists have contributed to this critique.[15] Here's my summary:

Men in contemporary American culture (I make no claim to cross-cultural or historical critique; I am writing about the world in which I live) are trained through a variety of cultural institutions to view sex as the acquisition of pleasure by the taking of women. Sex is a sphere in which men (by this I don't mean that every man believes this, but that many men believe this is true for all men) believe themselves to be naturally dominant and women naturally passive. Women are objectified and women's sexuality is commodified. Sex is sexy because men are dominant and women are subordinate; power is eroticized. In certain limited situations, those roles can be reversed (men can play at being sexually subordinate and women dominant), so long as power remains sexualized and power relations outside the bedroom are unchanged.

Summed up by Andrea Dworkin:

The normal fuck by a normal man is taken to be an act of invasion and ownership undertaken in a mode of predation; colonializing, forceful (manly) or nearly violent; the sexual that by its nature makes her his.[16]

One of the key sites in which these sexual values are reflected, reinforced, and normalized is pornography. Domination and subordination are sexualized, sometimes in explicit representations of rape and violence against women, but always in the objectification and commodification of women and their sexuality.[17] This results in several kinds of harms to women and children: (1) the harm caused in the production of pornography; (2) the harm in having pornography forced on them; (3) the harm in being sexually assaulted by men who use pornography; and (4) the harm in living in a culture which pornography reinforces and sexualizes women's subordinate status.

In a world in which men hold most of the social, economic, and political power, the result of the patriarchal sexual system is widespread violence, sexualized violence, and violence-by-sex against women and children. This includes physical assault, emotional abuse, and rape by family members and acquaintances as well as strangers. Along with the experience of violence, women and children live with the knowledge that they are always targets.

Attention to the meaning of the central male slang term for sexual intercourse —"fuck"—is instructive. To fuck a woman is to have sex with her. To fuck someone in another context ("he really fucked me over on that deal") means to hurt or cheat a person. And when hurled as a simple insult ("fuck you") the intent is denigration and the remark is often prelude to violence or the threat of violence. Sex in patriarchy is fucking. That we live in a world in which people continue to use the same word for sex and violence, and then resist the notion that sex is routinely violent and claim to be outraged when sex becomes overtly violent, is testament to the power of patriarchy. In this society, sex and violence are fused to the point of being indistinguishable. Yet to say this out loud is to risk being labeled crazy: "What's wrong with you—are you afraid of sex? Are you nuts?"

THE WRONG WAYS OUT OF THIS PROBLEM

1. All women and most men I've met are against rape. That is, they are against those acts the law defines as rape. But most aren't against fucking, because fucking is sex and how can you be against sex, which is seen as natural? This view is summed up in the phrase "Rape is a crime of violence, not of sex." But rape is a crime of sex; to de-sex rape is to turn away from the possibility of understanding rape. This is not to say that men don't seek power over women through rape and that the power isn't expressed violently; it is to acknowledge that men seek power over women through sex of all kinds, including rape.

I think people, men and women, want to believe that rape is violence—not sex—because to acknowledge that rape is sex requires that we ask how it is that so many men can decide that rape is an acceptable way to get sex. Rape is not the result of the aberrant behavior of a limited number of pathological men, but is "normal" within the logic of the system. When sex is about power and control, and men are socially, and typically physically, more powerful than women and children, then sexual violence is the inevitable outcome. As Dworkin argues, "Rape is no excess, no aberration, no accident, no mistake—it embodies sexuality as the culture defines it."[18]

This does not mean that every man is a rapist in legal terms. It means that we live in a society in which men, both legally designated rapists and nonrapists, are raised with rapist ethics.[19] Raping is a particularly brutal kind of fucking, but the difference between "deviant" rape and the "normal" fuck is often difficult to see.[20] Timothy Beneke, looking at how metaphors frame sex as an expression of male power and conquest, concludes:

> [E]very man who grows up in America and learns American English learns all too much to think like a rapist, to structure his experience of women and sex in terms of status, hostility, control, and dominance.[21]

So, the conventional view is that rape can't be about sex and has to be about violence, because if it's about sex then each one of us has to ask how deeply into our bodies the norms of patriarchal sex have settled. Men have to ask about how sexy dominance is to them, and women have to ask how sexy submission is to them. And if we think too long about that, we face the question of why we're still having patriarchal sex. And if we face that question, we may have to consider the possibility of stopping. And if we aren't having sex, then we have to face the dominant culture's assumption that we aren't really alive because we aren't having sex.

2. Women aren't victims, some say, and radical feminism has tried to turn women into victims by focusing on the harms of patriarchal sex.[22] This is a deceptively appealing rhetorical move. When members of one class (women) identify a way that members of another class (men) routinely hurt them, those who are hurt are told they are responsible for the injury because they identified it. If women would stop talking about these injuries, the logic seems to be, then the injuries would stop. This strategy seems popular with some women and lots of men lately. I understand why men take this stance; it relieves them of any obligation to evaluate their own behavior and be responsible. And I understand why women don't want to see themselves as always at risk of men's violence and sexual aggression. But saying you aren't at risk because you don't want to be at risk doesn't take the risk away.

What does the word "victim" mean? Dworkin writes:

It's a true word. If you were raped, you were victimized. You damned well were. You were a victim. It doesn't mean that you are a victim in the metaphysical sense, in your state of being, as an intrinsic part of your essence and existence. It means somebody hurt you. They injured you. . . . And if it happens to you systematically because you are born a woman, it means that you live in a political system that uses pain and humiliation to control and to hurt you.[23]

Understanding one's victimization is not the same as playing the victim. Acknowledging that women often are victimized is not an admission of weaknesses or a retreat from responsibility. Instead, it makes possible organized and sustained resistance to the power that causes the injuries. By clearly identifying the victimizers (most always men) and the system within which the injury is ignored or trivialized (patriarchy), political change becomes possible.

We live in a world in which some people exercise their power in a way that hurts others. It has become popular to pretend the injuries are the product of the overactive imaginations of whiners. White people routinely tell nonwhite people that racism is not a big problem and that if the nonwhites would stop complaining, all would be fine. Rich people tell poor and working people that there is no such thing as class in the United States and that if we all would just work hard together everything would be fine. Straight people tell lesbian and gay people that if they would just stop making such a public nuisance of themselves everyone would leave them alone and things would be fine. But things aren't fine. We live in racism. Poor and working people are being crushed by a cruel economic system. Heterosexism oppresses lesbians and gays. And men keep fucking women.

If patriarchy is this dominant and patriarchal sex this colonizing, one might ask what hope there is in resistance. Would it not make more sense to go along and get along?

No system, no matter how overwhelming and oppressive, is beyond challenge. Borrowing a metaphor from Naomi Scheman, we can think of patriarchy as being like concrete in the city. It covers almost everything. It is heavy and seemingly unmovable, and it paves the world. But the daily wear and tear produces cracks, and in those cracks, plants grow—weeds, grass, sometimes a flower. Living things have no business growing up out of concrete, but they do. They resist the totality of the concrete.

No system of power can obliterate all resistance. All systems yield space in which things can grow. I have seen resistance to patriarchal sex grow, even flourish, in the cracks. I have friends, the people who helped me sort these things out and move forward, who continue to survive and grow in resistance to patriarchal sex. In my life I have met few people interested in this project of resistance, but it doesn't take many people for me to feel as if resistance is worthwhile. But

I also seek more than just a few friends who are scattered around the country. I would like to be part of an epistemic community in which these questions can be explored.

EPISTEMIC COMMUNITIES

What kind of investigation is required for confronting patriarchal sex? I am not after THE solution to the problem. At times, I am not entirely sure about the questions. Lorraine Code suggests that when epistemology is construed as a quest for understanding, the appropriate question becomes not "What can I know?" but "What sort(s) of discourse does the situation really call for?"[24] It is from conversation and the sharing of richly detailed narratives that understanding, not definitive answers, can begin to emerge.

While we are all individually accountable for our actions, the effort to understand sexuality is not solely an individual task; we have a responsibility to create collectively the tools for this investigation. As Code suggests:

> Thinking individuals have a responsibility to monitor and watch over shifts in, changes in, and efforts to preserve good intellectual practice. . . . In principle, everyone is responsible, to the best of his or her ability, for the quality of cognitive practice in a community.[25]

Such a community can be difficult to form and maintain. Pressures from the dominant ideology, combined with the routine human failings, can make the task seem overwhelming. My experience is that there are different levels of community at which different levels of conversation can happen. I have done most of this work in a fairly small group that includes a core of five to ten trusted friends, colleagues, and students (fellow students when I was in graduate school, and on rare occasions now, students whom I meet as a professor). Beyond that, I sometimes meet others with similar interests and convictions with whom I have important, though perhaps not ongoing, conversations. There is no recipe for how these conversations develop and no criteria for whom I connect with. The conversations cross lines of, among other things, gender, race, age, and sexual orientation, though not without great effort and occasional stress.

But one thing that is constant for me in these conversations is an understanding—sometimes stated but often simply understood—that we won't have sex, now or in the foreseeable future. These kinds of conversations can involve strong emotions and physical responses, and it is easy to want to channel that energy into sex. Also, there are ways in which talking-about-sex can be a type of having-sex. It takes constant monitoring to reject patriarchy's rule and not engage in sex. But I believe it is essential to resist the imperative to have sex because we do not always learn more about our desire by acting on it. I believe that having sex and talking-having sex in my core epistemic community would undermine progress. It would erode trust, not just between the people involved in the sex but in the whole community, and would make it difficult, if not impossible, for the conversation to continue.[26] Such activity suggests that no matter how much one tries to redefine sexuality or talks about change, in the end we're all just interested in fucking each other.

Beyond those small communities in which we are likely to feel most safe in searching to understand sexuality, important conversations can, and must, go on in a larger context. This essay is one attempt to create an epistemic community; implicit (and now explicit) is an invitation for others to engage me in conversation. My search for community at this level happens at conferences, in the classroom, in anti-pornography and anti-rape public presentations, and in conversations with a variety of people I meet. Most often, I am sharing things I have learned in my core community with others and asking for feedback. These conversations are unpredictable but always, in some sense, productive for me.[27]

THE WORK OF WOMEN AND MEN

In her discussion of epistemic responsibility, Code asserts that "knowing well" is of considerable moral significance.[28] On matters of sexuality, knowing well requires attention not just to what our desires are but to where those desires come from. To simply *know*, "This is what arouses me," without attempting to understand *why* it does is epistemically irresponsible. Code reminds us that it can be easier "to believe that a favorite theory is true and to suppress nagging doubts than to pursue the implications of those doubts and risk having to modify the theory."[29] Being epistemically responsible requires that we investigate those nagging doubts.

In this and other work, I tend to focus on the objectification, aggression, and violence that is central to the dominant construction of male sexuality in this culture. I believe this focus is proper, especially because I am a man and I work from my experience as a man. However, these questions about the construction of our sexuality are as crucial for women as men.[30] This does not mean I claim the right to tell women what their sexuality should look like. It means that we all must acknowledge that, to varying degrees, our lives have been shaped by patriarchy and men's values, and that we must examine the effects.

An example: While having sex, a man finds it sexy to put a woman's arms behind her head and hold them down at the wrists, rendering her fairly immobile and intensifying the experience of intercourse for him. The man should consider: How did he come to develop this practice? What is it about rendering a woman immobile that feels sexy? Why does having control over a woman in such a manner intensify his orgasm? All of those questions are central to epistemic responsibility; to act morally, he needs to know. But what if the woman in that scenario also finds the practice exciting? What if the sensation of being unable to move her arms while having intercourse intensifies her sexual response? What is it about being immobile that feels sexy?

I believe women have the same epistemic responsibility as men. However, in a society where women are often blamed for being in some way responsible for the injuries that men inflict on them, such a call for epistemic responsibility can appear to be asking women to blame themselves for the ways in which they may have internalized patriarchy's values. But this is not about blame or guilt; it is about the search for understanding, for freedom. Just as pornography teaches men to rape, romance novels teach women to be rape victims. Just as fathers often instill rapist values in sons, mothers often teach daughters how to submit to the boys. I believe there are compelling moral and political arguments for men to change. It also seems clear that to survive, women must change.

HETERO AND HOMO

By the way, I am gay. I lived most of my thirty-eight years as a heterosexual. I was once married, and I have a son. I am out, although what exactly that means for me—beyond a public rejection of heterosexuality and its institutions—is unclear at the moment. But gay-or-straight doesn't much matter. The question of resistance to patriarchal sex is just as important in the gay male world as it is for straight men. As far as I can tell, the majority of gay men fuck in about the same way as straight men do. We all received pretty much the same training. In fact, the term "fucking" is thrown around in many gay male conversations with frequency and ease, in a celebratory way. Fucking is taken to be the thing that gay men do; some might even argue that if you aren't fucking, you aren't gay.

If that's the case, then I'm not gay. And I'm not straight. I'm trying to live in the cracks in the concrete.

IMAGINING NOT-SEX

In early versions of this essay, I wrote about the task of imagining what a new kind of sex, a nonpatriarchal sex, might look like. I suggested that one of the main problems in this project of resistance is that we lack a language in which to imagine what that sex might be. I felt the need to imagine things beyond our experience, in words that we have yet to find.

I still believe that we lack the vocabulary to talk about this and that creative imagination is at the center of this project. But I no longer think that imagining a new kind of sex is crucial, or even helpful, at this point. I fear that a rush to fill the void left when one starts to disengage from patriarchal sex can ultimately keep us from moving forward; we risk trying to reconstruct before we have adequately deconstructed, before we understand enough about how the norms of patriarchal sex live in our bodies. Obviously, this is not like the flushing of a system to get the toxins out, not a mechanical task that has a dear beginning and end. I expect to struggle for the rest of my life to understand how patriarchy has shaped my identity and sexuality. If I waited for the magic moment of pure clarity to begin a reconstruction project, I would be waiting forever. But I want to guard against beginning the reconstruction process prematurely.

There is an important lesson in my rush to want to fill the void with new imagined conceptions of nonpatriarchal sex. Although I claimed to have been willing to stop having sex for some period of time, my first instinct was to rush toward a reconstruction. That is, in trying to resist the imperative to have sex, I gave in to the imperative to create a new kind of sex so that I could have it. I told myself that because we are humans with bodies and needs for intimacy, that the task of imagining something new was crucial. I do have a body, and I need love and intimacy. But the question remains: Would any sex I could imagine at this moment really be nonpatriarchal? Have I disentangled myself from patriarchy enough to even begin that task?

The answer for me is clearly no, that I am not in a good position to imagine something new. That is my judgment about myself, and I don't pretend to have the answer for others. I come to this moment with a specific history that shapes what is possible for me. I do not know what is possible for others, and I expect that many men who share the values I describe decide to take other paths toward a similar goal. My point is not to persuade everyone that not-sex is their only option, but to suggest that it is a relevant question for everyone—that it is an option and that there is a compelling argument to be made for that choice. If we want to leave behind patriarchal sex, not only must we confront the likelihood that we might need to stop having sex for some period of time, but we must be willing to accept that we may not have any idea of what will take the place of patriarchal sex for quite some time. In other words, we have to be willing to live a life without sex for the sake of justice, for the sake of ourselves.

So, for the time being, I want to imagine not-sex. I reject sex in the hope that someday, maybe in my lifetime and maybe not, I can find a way to be physically intimate outside of patriarchy. Maybe we will call it sex, maybe not. At this point, it's not a terribly important question for me.

This move to embrace not-sex may seem a drastic, or even silly, rhetorical move. But I think the gravity of the situation justifies the deployment of new language. As Susan Cole puts it:

> We have a long way to go before we uncover the full extent of the damage. We may not see the full repair in our lifetimes and it may not be possible to chart the entire course for change.[31]

I no longer trust myself to chart the course for change, to refashion sex into something I can trust. So, I seek not-sex, something different than what "sex" means in the dominant culture. I want intimacy, trust, and respect from other people, and I hope that it is possible for those things to be expressed physically. But I don't want sex.[32]

To say that I don't want sex is not to deny my sexuality or cut myself off from my erotic power, as Audre Lorde uses that term.[33] Lorde talks about the way in which women's erotic power is falsely cordoned off in the bedroom, made into "plasticized sensation," and confused with the pornographic.[34] For Lorde, the erotic is a life-force, a creative energy:

> those physical, emotional, and psychic expressions of what is deepest and strongest and richest within each of us, being shared: the passions of love, in its deepest meanings.[35]

Lorde writes about expressing her erotic power in some ways that the culture does not define as sexual and others that the culture might call sexual; she writes of the erotic power flowing both in the act of writing a good poem and in "moving into sunlight against the body of a woman I love." My expression of the erotic at this point in my life need not include such movement against the body of another. What is crucial is not channeling my erotic energy into sex, but finding other ways to feel that power. Lorde writes:

> Recognizing the power of the erotic within our lives can give us the energy to pursue genuine change within our world, rather than merely settling for a shift of characters in the same weary drama.[36]

To be more specific, what does it mean to say that in my intimate (broadly defined) relationships I want to tap my erotic power while practicing not-sex? Does it mean a ban on touch that produces an erection for me? A ban on touch of another person's body in areas that are typically sexualized (genitals, breasts, buttocks)? Is there any way to achieve not-sex intimacy that involves touch?

For me, not-sex is intimacy that resists or transcends oppression. In practice, that has meant different things with different people, depending on my relationship with them and the level of trust. For example, one female friend and I hug frequently, and I feel as if that touch is not-sex and a loving intimacy. A gay male friend and I tend to hug when we greet and say goodbye, and each of us knows that if the other needed emotionally supportive not-sex physical contact we would provide it. But we are not routinely physical out of a commitment to not-sex. In both relationships, there is an erotic element; in neither case is it made sexual.

Masturbation is a more difficult issue for me in thinking through not-sex. I sometimes do it, though I am aware that the fantasies that fuel that masturbation are almost exclusively scripted by patriarchy. There is a difference between self-touch that is motivated by self-love, and self-touch that is rooted in those scripts. My struggle with this issue (not to be confused with adolescent guilt over masturbation) remains unresolved, and is one reminder that perhaps I am further from imagining a nonpatriarchal sex than I once thought.

Jim Koplin once said to me that it is at the moment when a man can no longer achieve an erection—when all the old ways of sparking sexual pleasure have failed—that something new is possible. That moment, he said, may be the most creative point in our lives. "Impotence" becomes not a failure or a problem, but the point from which something new becomes possible. In this sense, I strive for impotency; that may be the point at which I am doing something more than shuffling characters in "the same weary drama."

HEAT AND LIGHT

As I have said, I am not interested in writing a recipe book for nonpatriarchal sex. I do not want to imagine new practices or create new rules for sex at this point in my life. But is there anything one can say about a new path, about where not-sex might lead me?

There is a cliché that when an argument is of little value, it produces "more heat than light." One of the ways this culture talks about sex is in terms of heat: She's hot, he's hot, we had hot sex. Sex is bump-and-grind; the friction produces the heat, and the heat makes the sex good. Fucking produces heat. Fucking is hot.

But what if our embodied connections could be less about heat and more about light? What if instead of desperately seeking hot sex, we searched for a way to produce light when we touch? What if such touch were about finding a way to create light between people so that we could see ourselves and each other better? If the goal is knowing ourselves and others like that, then what we need is not heat but light to illuminate the path. How do we touch and talk to each other to shine that light? I'm not sure. There are lots of ways to produce light in the world, and some are better than others. Light that draws its power from rechargeable solar cells, for example, is better than light that draws on throwaway batteries. Likewise, there will be lots of ways to imagine nonpatriarchal sex. Some will be better than others, depending on the values on which they are based. The task ahead is not just imagining something new, but being alert to how things that seem new can be rooted in old ideas.

A possible response to this from other men (and women): "Not-sex. Striving for impotency. Are you crazy?"

Sometimes I wonder. But I don't think I am crazy. I feel as if I may be going sane.

NOTES

1. A copy of the message was posted on several Internet discussion lists and widely circulated—and criticized—in November 1995.

2. Raquel Kennedy Bergen, "Surviving Wife Rape: How Women Define and Cope with the Violence," *Violence against Women* 1, no. 2 (1995): 125.

3. I don't use the word "fuck" without hesitation and concern. The word carries with it incredible violence, and I realize that it can feel assaultive to some people, especially women. But in this case I believe that it is the word that most accurately represents what I am trying to describe.

4. My focus will remain on heterosexual men and their sex with women, though much of what I will say here has relevance for gay men. More on that later.

5. E.g., Lorraine Code, *What Can She Know?* (Ithaca, NY: Cornell University Press, 1991), and Camilla Stivers, "Reflections on the Role of Personal Narrative in Social Science," *Signs* 18, no. 2 (1992): 408–25.

6. See also Robert Jensen, "Men's Lives and Feminist Theory," *Race, Gender and Class* 2, no. 2 (1995): 111–25.

7. Thanks specifically to Elvia Arriola, Rebecca Bennett, Donna McNamara, Nancy Potter, and Naomi Scheman for their roles in helping me understand these issues.

8. Thanks to Jim Koplin, a friend, intellectual partner, and colleague in the antipornography movement. Much of what I write here was first spoken by Jim and by me in conversation. I can no longer trace the origin of some of the ideas; many are as much Jim's as mine. His affection, support, and wisdom inform this essay.

9. There is another kind of fear that I believe most, if not all, men live with: the fear of not meeting the imagined standard of masculinity, of never being a skilled enough sexual performer to be a "real" man—the stud, the man in total control. That fear is real, as is the alienation from self and partner that results. However, the fear I am describing here is a deeper fear, a realization of how thoroughly sexuality in this culture eroticizes domination and subordination. More on that later.

10. Robert Jensen, "Knowing Pornography," *Violence against Women* 2, no. 1 (1996): 82–102, "Pornographic Lives," *Violence against Women* 1, no. 1 (1995): 32–54, "Pornographic Novels and the Ideology of Male Supremacy," *Howard Journal of Communications* 5, nos. 1–2 (1994): 92–107, and "Pornography and the Limits of Experimental Research," in *Gender, Race and Class in Media; A Text-Reader*, ed. Gail Dines and Jean M. Humez (Thousand Oaks, CA: Sage, 1994), pp. 298–306.

11. This has proved to be the case in other parts of my life. I live without a car, a television, or meat. At earlier times in my life, I would have thought that impossible. Now I find my life immeasurably enriched by the absence of those things.

12. Catherine A. MacKinnon, *Toward a Feminist Theory of the State* (Cambridge, MA: Harvard University Press, 1989), p. 124.

13. Marilyn Frye, *Willful Virgin* (Freedom, CA: Crossing Press, 1992), p. 113.

14. Jensen, "Knowing Pornography."

15. Susan Cole, *Pornography and the Sex Crisis* (Toronto: Amanita, 1989); Andrea Dworkin, *Pornography: Men Possessing Women* (New York: Perigee, 1981), *Intercourse* (New York: Free Press, 1987), and *Letters from a War Zone* (London: Secker and Warburg, 1988); Sheila Jeffreys, *Anticlimax: A Feminist Perspective on the Sexual Revolution* (New York: New York University Press, 1990); Catherine MacKinnon, *Feminism Unmodified: Discourses on Life and Law* (Cambridge, MA: Harvard University Press, 1987), and *Toward a Feminist Theory of the State*; Diane E. H. Russell, ed., *Making Violence Sexy: Feminist Views on Pornography* (New York: Teachers College Press, 1993).

16. Dworkin, *Intercourse*, p. 63.

17. Dworkin, *Pornography: Men Possessing Women* and *Letters from a War Zone*; MacKinnon, *Feminism Unmodified*; Catharine MacKinnon, *Only Words* (Cambridge, MA: Harvard University Press, 1993).

18. Andrea Dworkin, *Our Blood* (New York: Harper & Row, 1976) p. 46.

19. John Stoltenberg, *Refusing to Be a Man: Essays on Sexual Justice* (Portland, OR: Brettenbush Books, 1989).

20. MacKinnon, *Toward a Feminist Theory of the State*.

21. Timothy Beneke, *Men on Rape* (New York: St. Martin's Press, 1982), p. 16.

22. One popular female writer argues that such "victim feminism" needs to be replaced with "power feminism" (Naomi Wolf, *Fire with Fire: The New Female Power and How It Will Change the 21st Century* [New York: Random House, 1993]). Another claims that radical feminists, or "gender feminists," have hijacked the women's movement and betrayed the real interests of women (Christina Hoff Sommers, *Who Stole Feminism? How Women Have Betrayed Women* [New York: Simon and Schuster, 1994]).

23. Andrea Dworkin, "Women-Hating Right and Left," in *The Sexual Liberals and the Attack on Feminism* (New York: Pergamon Press, 1990), pp. 38–39.

24. Lorraine Code, *Epistemic Responsibility* (Hanover, NH: University Press of New England, 1987), p. 165.

25. Ibid., p. 245.

26. This is especially true when the sex happens across differences in status that reflect potential power imbalances, such as a large age gap, significant wealth or class gaps, and gender. Most devastating, I believe, is sexual contact between people in institu-

tionalized roles of unequal power, such as student/teacher, client/therapist, parish-ioner/clergy, etc. I believe that sexual activity in such situations is always wrong.

27. I don't want to appear naive about this wider community. As troubling and divi-sive as these investigations can be in communities committed to feminism and liberatory politics, they can be dangerous in mainstream and reactionary political circles, where people may want to ignore or undermine a feminist analysis. My goal, and the goal of the feminists whose work informs my analysis, is the exploration and celebration of diversity, but the goal of those to the right is often the suppression of diversity. These political real-ities are important to consider. The kind of open discussion that is crucial to expanding our understanding may be safe in some contexts but not in others, and more safe for some than others. But it is important that the conversation continue.

28. Code, *Epistemic Responsibility*.

29. Ibid., p. 59. This is not to say that every individual in every situation need engage in discussions about these matters. People whose sexuality is under attack by the estab-lished social structure—lesbians, gay men, and, in some sense, many heterosexual women—might feel that social conditions make it unsafe to engage in such open discus-sion. For example, a lesbian high school teacher in a small town may not be able to be part of a discussion about sexual practices in that community. Still, the idea of epistemic responsibility does suggest we should make whatever efforts are possible to pursue knowledge about sexuality and its social construction.

30. Thanks to Rebecca Bennett for reminding me of the importance of discussing this.

31. Cole, *Pornography and the Sex Crisis*, p. 132.

32. In response to a draft of this essay, Jim Koplin suggested that labeling this "not-sex" is reactive rather than inventive and offered alternative terms such as "body-play," "body-connection," or "creative touch." I understand his point, but I think that at this stage in my project I want to hold onto a clear break from sex. At some point in the future, I may shift to such language, but my gut tells me it is too early for me to do that.

33. See also Carter Heyward, *Touching Our Strength: The Erotic as Power and the Love of God* (San Francisco: Harper & Row, 1989).

34. Audre Lorde, "Uses of the Erotic: The Erotic as Power," in *Sister Outsider* (Freedom, CA: Crossing Press, 1984), p. 54.

35. Ibid., p. 56.

36. Ibid., p. 59.

33.

QUEERNESS, DISABILITY, AND
THE VAGINA MONOLOGUES

Kim Q. Hall

In 1998 Eve Ensler published *The Vagina Monologues*, a collection of various vaginal facts and stories told from the perspective of women from diverse racial, regional, sexual, and age backgrounds. Before publishing the book, Ensler staged one-woman performances of the monologues. These events led to the development of V-Day, an organization that seeks to raise money for the prevention and consciousness of violence against women (Ensler 2000, 130). In addition to other programs, the organization launched the V-Day College Initiative, a program in which colleges and universities are invited to stage performances of *The Vagina Monologues* and to contribute the proceeds to local organizations opposing violence against women. The event has become hugely popular and has even attracted the interest of celebrities such as Glenn Close and Oprah Winfrey, who have joined the ranks of countless women across the nation in performing Ensler's work. While some campus administrators continue to balk at the thought of sponsoring and advertising a program with 'vagina' in the title, it sometimes seems as if many women and men just can't get enough of *The Vagina Monologues*. In fact, Ensler's text has become so popular that it seems safe to say that it is teetering on the edges of (if it has not already entered) the mainstream of popular culture in the United States.

Reprinted by permission from *Hypatia* 20, no. 1 (Winter 2005) © by Kim Q. Hall.

Eve Ensler decided to write *The Vagina Monologues* because she was worried about vaginas; I am also worried about vaginas. However, while Ensler is primarily concerned "about what we think about vaginas, and even more worried that we don't think about them" (Ensler 1998, 3), I am also concerned about how the vagina enters the realm of intelligibility in both patriarchal and feminist discourses. In particular, I am concerned about how *The Vagina Monologues* establishes the vagina as a sign of feminist embodiment, subjectivity, and ultimately empowerment for women. I share Ensler's desire for a feminist vaginal politics that will move women beyond shame, contempt, embarrassment, and unfamiliarity with what's "down there" in order to make the vagina a part of the body again on women's own terms. However, I also want to question the connection between vaginas and feminist embodiment in Ensler's text and to consider the ways in which the text both challenges and reinscribes (albeit unintentionally) systems of patriarchy, compulsory heterosexuality, and ableism. Rather than dismiss *The Vagina Monologues* as hopelessly flawed, I hope to show how the text offers theorists and activists in feminist, queer, and disability communities an invaluable opportunity to understand how power operates in both dominant discourses that degrade vaginas and strategies of feminist resistance that seek to reclaim and celebrate them.

Judith Butler's discussion of abject bodies as the constitutive outside for that which is intelligible as a sexed (or raced or classed or enabled) body offers an interesting and constructive perspective from which to consider *The Vagina Monologues.* This is especially so in light of the recent criticism of Ensler's text and performance by the Intersex Society of North America (ISNA),[1] a criticism that became known as V-Day Challenge 2002. ISNA's Web site offers the following explanation for the mobilization of their V-Day Challenge: "While we find most of *The Vagina Monologues* funny, insightful, and empowering, we were disturbed by the wide *disparity* between how the play depicts the cutting of young women's genitals in Africa ('female genital mutilation,' or FGM) versus the cutting of young intersex people's genitals in the United States ('intersex genital mutilation,' or IGM)" (ISNA 2002, www.isna.org/events/vday). ISNA's critique informs my consideration of how the vagina is materialized in Ensler's text. Elizabeth Grosz notes that the bodies of both conjoined twins and intersexed people have been considered "monstrous" and "freakish," outside the realm of the human in dominant ideas about the "natural," "normal" body (1996, 55–56). To the extent that Ensler's reclamation and celebration of the vagina marginalizes intersexed bodies, it reinforces heteropatriarchal regulatory norms that have historically infused the vagina with the very meanings Ensler wishes to critique.

In what follows, I will seek to answer the following questions: In what sense, if any, do some human beings have female bodies? If the meaning of sex, like gender, is an effect of discourse, what are feminists to make of attempts to reclaim and celebrate the female body? Is it possible to celebrate the female body without reinforcing the terms of sexual difference at the core of heteropatriarchal structures of oppression? And, to quote a well-known feminist health book, in what sense, if any, are our bodies our selves (Boston Women's Health Collective 1984)? I will compare *The Vagina Monologues* with some examples from feminist body art and the feminist health movement and argue that in order to avoid reproducing structures of oppression, feminist attempts to reclaim the female body will have to adopt a strategy of disidentification.[2]

TOWARD A QUEER FEMINIST STRATEGY OF DISIDENTIFICATION

My approach to the theoretical conundrum posed by Enlser's text, ISNA's critique, and the mainstream appeal of V-Day performances takes seriously Michel Foucault's insight that power is constitutive, and thus informs the claiming of resistant identities as well as the oppressive forces that contain, immobilize, and defuse the resistant identities and practices that threaten existing hierarchies (Foucault 1978, 101–102). While some feminist theorists have questioned the political usefulness of Foucault's concept of power, others have critically appropriated Foucault to construct a nonfoundational feminist and antiracist identity politics.[3] In commenting on the implications that a Foucauldian strategy of disidentification has for queer activism, David Halperin stresses the fact that Foucault's understanding of sexuality as a strategic position rather than a foundational nature has made room for "the possibility of a *queer politics* defined not by the struggle to liberate a common, repressed, preexisting nature but by an ongoing process of self-constitution and self-transformation—a queer politics anchored in the perilous and shifting sands of non-identity, positionality, discursive reversibility, and collective invention" (Halperin 1995, 122). Thus, identity matters politically, but not because it is a foundational ground that unites members of an oppressed group across their differences. Rather identity is politically useful to the extent that it is a continually negotiated site for the disarticulation of historical and cultural forces that have shaped its meaning, as well as a consciously forged site of shared struggle against oppression.

For Judith Butler it is just as important to "mobilize identity categories . . . in the service of a political goal" as it is to persistently disidentify "with those regulatory norms by which sexual difference is materialized" (1993, 4). Disidentification as a queer feminist political strategy enables a reconceptualization of bodies and a space for the emergence of bodies that have not yet been considered (such as intersexed bodies) (1993, 4). Some might object that Butler's claims are too abstract, too removed from women's lived experience to be politically bene-ficial for feminists. These critics might assert that most women in the world think of themselves as women and do not spend their time wondering whether women have vaginas. Following this critique, Ensler's text is politically useful for feminists because it utilizes women's experiences of their bodies to provide an avenue for many women to reclaim and learn to love and celebrate their female bodies. However, when one considers ISNA's critique of *The Vagina Monologues*, one can begin to understand the political significance of queer feminist critiques of the body's materiality.

ISNA's Critique

ISNA's critique of Ensler's text focuses specifically on three passages. Given the centrality of these passages for their critique and for my own analysis, I will quote them at length. In the first passage, Ensler offers the following "Vaginal Fact" about female genital mutilation: "In the eighteenth century, girls who learned to develop orgasmic capacity by masturbation were regarded as medical problems. Often they were 'treated' or 'corrected' by amputation or cautery of the clitoris or 'miniature chastity belts,' sewing the vaginal lips together to put the cli-toris out of reach, and even castration by surgical removal of the ovaries" (Ensler 1998, 61). In the second passage, Ensler notes, "Genital mutilation has been inflicted on 80 [million] to 100 million girls and young women. In countries where it is practiced, mostly African, about 2 million youngsters a year can expect the knife—or the razor or a glass shard—to cut their clitoris or remove it altogether, [and] to have part or all of the labia . . . sewn together with catgut or thorns" (63).

In her presentation of these vaginal facts, Ensler can be read as building on the insights of feminists of color such as Audre Lorde (1984), Chandra Mohanty (1991), Trinh T. Minh-Ha (1989), and others, who have criticized Western femi-nism's characterization of "Third World women" as victims of worse forms of patriarchal harms than "Western women" and who are thus unable to be the sub-jects of feminist discourse. Rather than contribute to colonialist notions of "Third World women" as more oppressed or the "Third World" as the land fem-inism forgot, Ensler locates female genital mutilation in both the Western and non-Western world.

Nonetheless, when Ensler comments on genital mutilation in the West, she locates this form of violence against women in the past, as if genital mutilation in the West ended after the nineteenth century. Thus, because Enlser's discussion of genital mutilation presents a West that has moved beyond this practice while the non-Western world is construed as remaining trapped in a more patriarchal past, her account contributes to colonialist conceptions of non-Western women.[4] As a result, *The Vagina Monologues* mobilizes a colonialist discourse, a discourse in which the experience of "Third World women" and the category 'Third World women' are deployed in a way that, as Chandra Mohanty notes, "enables and sustains the Western woman" as the norm and center of reference (1991, 73–74).

Ensler's discussion of genital mutilation is not confined to the two pages discussed above, and perhaps the full meaning and impact of these vaginal facts about female genital mutilation can be understood only by considering them in relation to Ensler's discussion of the woman in Oklahoma who was born without a vagina and who didn't realize it until she was fourteen.

> She was playing with her girlfriend. They compared their genitals and she realized hers were different, something was wrong. She went to the gynecologist with her father, the parent she was close to, and the doctor discovered that in fact she did not have a vagina or a uterus. Her father was heartbroken, trying to repress his tears and sadness so his daughter would not feel bad. On the way home from the doctor, in a noble attempt to comfort her, he said, "Don't worry, darlin'. This is all gonna be just fine. As a matter of fact, it's gonna be great. We're gonna get you the best homemade pussy in America. And when you meet your husband, he's gonna know we had it made specially for him." (1998, 83–84)

At the end of recounting this story, the only comment Ensler makes is, "And they did get her a new pussy, and she was relaxed and happy and when she brought her father back two nights later, the love between them melted me" (84).

Although Ensler's comment is brief, much can be said about this passage. First, the fact that the "discovery" of the missing vagina was made during play with a girlfriend is never discussed in the text. Instead, Ensler, the doctor, and the father all assume (and ultimately enforce) the fourteen-year-old girl's heterosexuality. After all, the girl's future husband's happiness is the justification for vaginal construction and the sign of its success. Perhaps Ensler is simply representing the story as it was conveyed to her; however, Ensler could have made more observations than she did at the end of the story. To merely say, "the love between them melted me" does not, to put it mildly, say enough. In the context of a book and performance that attempt to make visible the oppressive forces that have estranged women from their bodies, the omission of any further comment on the woman's story is glaring.

Ensler's discussion of female genital mutilation also disregards a form of ongoing genital mutilation in the West, particularly the genital mutilation of intersexed children. In *The Vagina Monologues* intersexed bodies are situated at the periphery of the "normal" female body, a body that is defined by a vagina. In the story of the woman born without a vagina, the genital mutilation of inter-sexed young people is portrayed as a loving gesture of a father who wants his daughter to be happy and who understands her future happiness to necessitate both surgical construction of an aesthetically and functionally 'normal' vagina and heterosexuality. As told by Ensler, the only real harm and tragedy in the woman's story seems to be the fact that she was born without a vagina. Indeed, throughout Ensler's description, the father is described as "noble" and caring. He wants the best for his "little girl," and the best in this case is a vagina that will make her future husband happy.

Throughout *The Vagina Monologues*, Ensler stresses the fact that patriarchal violence has established distance between women and their vaginas, and thus has fragmented and alienated women. One of the hallmarks of oppression is the way it often makes those who are oppressed perceive their bodies as separate from, and alien to, their selves (Young 1990; Bartky 1990, 1998; Fanon 1967; DuBois 1989). As the euphemism "down there" makes clear, women and girls have felt detached from, ambivalent about, fearful of, and even disgusted by their genitals, feelings that have been conditioned by a long history of misogynistic messages about female bodies (Bartky 1990, 23).

According to *The Vagina Monologues*, the measure of patriarchal violence is the extent to which women are unable to think of their vaginas *as* themselves. In many respects, Ensler's point is very well taken. Patriarchal violence harms many women and girls around the world every day, and as a result of "the bad things that happen to women's vaginas" (Ensler 1998, xxii) many women and girls experience shame, disgust, terror, and a decreased ability or an inability to enjoy sexual intimacy. In this context of patriarchal violence, *The Vagina Monologues* contributes to healing, survival, and resistance. Ensler reports that after an initial reluctance to talk about their vaginas, many of the women she interviewed reported feeling better after telling their story (1998, 5 and 30).

Ensler and others who have seen performances of *The Vagina Monologues* often stress the empowerment *and* sisterhood they felt in a room packed with women and men. These accounts portray the vagina as a common bond between women, that which unites women across our many differences. Stories of menstruation become a "wild, collective song"(Ensler 1998, 33). And in the more recent V-Day edition of the text she writes, "women and men faint during the shows. It happens a lot. Always at the exact same place in the script" (2001, xxix). Even Katha Pollitt commented on the sense of vaginal unity generated by *The Vagina Monologues* when she wrote, "Besides being a wonderful night at the theater, it reminded me that after all the feminist debates (and splits) and all the books and the Theory and the theories, in the real world there are still such people as women, who share a common biology and much else besides. . . . Sisterhood-is-powerful feminism may feel out of date to the professoriat, but there's a lot of new music still to be played on those old bones. Besides, if feminists don't talk about sex in a fun, accessible, inspiring, nonpuritanical way, who will?" (Pollitt 2001, 10). While I share Pollitt's desire for fun, accessible, inspiring, nonpuritanical feminist conversations about sex, those conversations must be informed by an awareness of intersexed people and their embodied experiences. Feminist conversations about sex must also be informed by the critiques that feminists of color have directed at premature white feminist assumptions and celebrations of a global "sisterhood." As Chandra Mohanty exclaims, "Beyond sisterhood there are still racism, colonialism, and imperialism" (1991, 68). To this list, I would add heterosexism and ableism.

Feminist appeals to the vagina's power to unite women across our differences, while compelling, nonetheless ignore the responses of many intersexed people to performances of *The Vagina Monologues*. Comparing the struggles of intersexed people with the struggles of incest survivors, Emi Koyama, a member of ISNA, reports in her "Open Letter to V-Day Participants," "Many of us intersex people and our friends, family members, and allies went to see the play in the past, and came out upset, hurt, angry, and/or in tears, walking through a crowd of women talking to each other about how empowered they felt. We felt invisible, it presented horror stories about genital mutilation occurring in other continents, as if we do not experience them here" (http://isna.org/events/vday-email.html). For many intersexed people the genital surgeries and hormone treatments that are routinely used to "correct" intersexed bodies are experienced as acts of institutional violence used to maintain the interrelated patriarchal myths of genital dimorphism and a two-gendered society. In their V-Day challenge ISNA points out that both IGM and FGM are routinely performed in an effort to "correct" or "normalize" unruly bodies (that is, bodies that do not conform to cultural norms of gendered bodies); both are routinely performed without the consent of young people; and both are performed in order to make bodies conform to dominant ideals of bodily appearance and function without consideration of the effects the procedures can have on future experiences of sexual pleasure, health, or for the sexual self-confidence of those who undergo the surgeries and treatments (Dreger 1998; Walker and Parmar 1993). Thus, according to ISNA, both IGM and FGM are acts of gender violence that need to be criticized by feminists.

It is crucial to increase awareness of violence against intersexed people. Nonetheless, ISNA, like Ensler, seems to universalize patriarchy in their comparison between IGM and FGM.[5] In other words, both ISNA and Ensler fail to develop a critique of female genital mutilation that is informed by the historical and cultural specificity of its occurrence; for both, female genital mutilation remains a form of patriarchal violence that happens in a monolithic Africa. Chandra Mohanty argues that these universalizing notions of violence against women are characteristic of a colonialist feminism that assumes the coherency of the group "women" in advance and ignores the specific contexts in which patriarchal violence, for example, has meaning (1991, 58).

ISNA's Additive Solution

Because ISNA casts the problem as the invisibility of violence against intersexed people in *The Vagina Monologues*, the solution to this problem is understood to be additive. In other words, if Ensler's text has contributed to the erasure of intersexed people's experiences, the text can be improved by the addition of intersex monologues. Anticipating criticism of her exclusion of some women's experiences, Ensler offers the following explanation in the V-Day edition of *The Vagina Monologues*: "Whenever I have tried to write a monologue to serve a politically correct agenda, for example, it always fails. Note the lack of monologues about menopause or transgendered women. I tried. *The Vagina Monologues* is about attraction, not promotion" (2001, xxvi–xxvii). From this perspective, the only flaw in the text is the fact that it does not contain monologues that represent women from all social, cultural, and economic groups, but this is forgivable since it would be unreasonable to expect Ensler to represent all experiences in her text. After all, does one have to do everything in order to do one thing well (in this case, reclaim vaginas and raise awareness of and money to combat violence against women)? Does drawing attention to the invisibility of violence against intersexed people diminish the obviously profound way in which many women have identified with Ensler's text?

In response to ISNA's criticism, V-Day endorsed the V-Day Challenge by encouraging people who stage performances of *The Vagina Monologues* to distribute information about intersexuality and violence against intersexed people and to consider making donations to the Intersex Society of North America. While I agree that there needs to be more awareness of intersex genital mutilation and while I am heartened by V-Day's endorsement of ISNA's V-Day Challenge, I don't think the problem targeted by the V-Day Challenge is only a problem of the invisibility of intersex experience, which can be adequately addressed by the addition of intersex monologues or by the distribution of information about intersex genital mutilation at performances. Rather, the absence of any intersex experiences is an effect of the gendered bodily norms operating in Ensler's text. In fact, it is precisely its celebration of the normative vagina that has contributed to the mainstream appeal and success of *The Vagina Monologues*.

The idea that women are ultimately beings with vaginas despite other differences among women appeases a mainstream society and a feminist movement that have been challenged by transgender and intersex theory and activism.

In response to my concerns, some might argue that the play's fluidity and multiplicity destabilize the meaning of the vagina with each unique perform-ance. In other words, because *The Vagina Monologues* can be performed by many different women all over the world, the meanings of the vagina are transformed in every performance of Ensler's text, and thus, there is no single story of the "normal" vagina. The meaning of the vagina remains open to endless possibility because *The Vagina Monologues* is a point of departure, an invitation to women and girls to create their own stories and find their own voices.

V-Day has done very important work and their V-Day campaigns have raised a lot of money for antiviolence organizations all over the world. In 2001, performances of *The Vagina Monologues* raised an estimated seven million dol-lars. Both ISNA and V-Day have done a great deal to end gender violence, and I don't mean to suggest that their work has been useless. Still, the fact that many women all over the world are able to perform *The Vagina Monologues* when Ensler releases the copyright does not automatically mean that dominant mean-ings of the vagina are subverted.[6]

Consider the hybridity of cultural meanings of sperm. In her article on how cultural notions of masculinity shape scientific narratives of sperm, Lisa Jean Moore critiques the notion that the malleability of masculinity opens the possi-bility for a counterhegemonic masculinity. On the contrary, she claims that the very hegemony of dominant masculinity is based on its ability to appropriate nondominant masculinities, an ability that makes it possible for dominant mas-culinity to adapt to changing historical circumstances and continue to legitimate male privilege in a patriarchal society. In fact, Moore asserts,

> As patriarchy faces crises in legitimation, HM [hegemonic masculinity] must be able to respond by being malleable enough to incorporate new aspects of newly redefined maleness. Most significantly, HM can adapt styles of subordinated men and emotionality and neutralize any counterhegemonic potential. Within the scientific community, empowerment of men through the creation of previ-ously unopened avenues of reproductive agency is the primary means of per-petuating the gendered order and hegemonic masculine practices. (Moore 2002, 95–96)

Moore's point about hegemonic masculinity is similar to what critical race theo-rists have noted about whiteness. The dominant force of whiteness is buttressed both by its status as an unmarked racial category and by its ability to appropriate aspects of nonwhite cultures. As such, whiteness (like white, class-privileged citizens of the United States) is able to freely cross cultural and national borders and bring back souvenirs of cultural and racial difference, while "nonwhiteness" is forced to remain fixed in its authenticity (Frankenberg 1993; Minh-Ha 1989). Thus, Madonna and Eminem are rewarded for appropriating cultures of color, but Chris Ofili, an Afro-British artist, is chastised for daring to depict a black Virgin Mary (Roediger 2002, 27–43).[7] The "fluidity" of that which is "American" means that McDonald's can offer a new "McArabia" sandwich in Baghdad,[8] while Arabs and Arab-Americans in the United States are harassed, arrested, and deported. The normativity of "Western," "American," and "white" is secured, not disrupted, by their ability to appropriate nondominant difference. Similarly, the narrative force of *The Vagina Monologues* is the ability of the normative vagina to appropriate different women's experiences and yet still produce the same story of the "normal" female body as a body with a vagina.

It is not accidental that Ensler ends the text with an account of witnessing the birth of her granddaughter. In this story the process of reproduction is naturalized as Ensler looks into her daughter-in-law's vagina and marvels at the birthing process. There is only a room in which the birth takes place; the social, political, and economic conditions that determine the limits of women's reproductive freedom are erased in this story. Readers are asked to marvel at the power of women to reproduce without asking the difficult questions that beg to be answered, such as whether this can be considered a power at all in a society that denies many women access to affordable abortion and other forms of choice regarding reproduction. Moore asks, "What type of social order is being invented or resurrected in this rendering of human sexual reproduction? How is it that when real men are attacked, sperm are enabled to be triumphant?" (2002, 109). I wonder how it is that when the notion of "real" women is attacked by transgender, transsexual, and intersex existence and activism, the vagina is celebrated as an avenue of feminist empowerment?

Ultimately, the visibility of the vagina as the center and ground of female identity is made possible by the *visibility* (not the invisibility) of the intersexed woman's story. In *The Vagina Monologues* the woman from Oklahoma who was born without a vagina is visible as an exception, an alternative to the general rule that women have vaginas. Robert McRuer uses Adrienne Rich's concept of compulsory heterosexuality to argue that both compulsory heterosexuality and compulsory able-bodiedness are sustained and unsettled by the invisibility *and* the visibility of the "alternative identities" they produce (2002, 88–89, 97). Intersexed bodies certainly unsettle dominant systems, systems that rely on the notion that a seamless connection between genitals, gender identity, and heterosexual desire and practice are fixed in nature, and thus normal.

In writing about the feminine body, Rosemarie Garland-Thomson suggests that while patriarchal narratives have marked the female body as abnormal in relation to the universal, normal, male body, the very normality of the feminine body is made possible by the abnormality of the unfeminine body (1997, 287). Similarly, the normality of female bodies with vaginas is made possible by the abnormality of female bodies without vaginas. In fact, "abnormal" bodies reveal what "normal" bodies are and how they should function (Dreger 1998, 6). As Anne Fausto-Sterling and many others have noted, the biological foundation of sex is also a medical construction influenced by male dominance, heteronormativity, and able-bodied norms (Fausto-Sterling 1993; Hubbard 1990; Kessler 1998; Dreger 1998). The assumption of the normalcy of "feminine," heterosexual female bodies and masculine, heterosexual male bodies is evident in the reasons surgeons offer for "correcting" the genitals of intersexed young people. For example, the success of vaginal reconstruction is frequently measured by the ability of the reconstructed vagina to accommodate a "normal size" penis during heterosexual intercourse (Kessler 1998, 107). In the words of one surgeon, "Without a vagina, a woman is not normal. It's like having a nose. You can breathe fine without a nose, but you look funny without a nose" (quoted in Kessler 1998, 107).

As Esther Morris, author of "The Missing Vagina Monologue," notes, "Being born without a vagina was not my problem. Having to get one was the real problem. . . . The standard normal we aim for is imaginary. We alter women's bodies when our attitudes need adjusting. . . . Women shouldn't have to endure emotional and physical pain to perform one sexual act when so many options are available. . . . Identity shouldn't be centered around body parts—missing, constructed, or removed" (http://isna.org/library/missingvagina/html). As "The Missing Vagina Monologue" makes clear, the relation between having a vagina and being a woman is not fixed in nature, and women who are born without vaginas are not fragmented women. Vaginas establish women as the counterpart of men, enabling both differentiation between male and female bodies and participation in heterosexual, reproductive activity.

FEMINIST BODY ART

Given this critique of Ensler's text, is it possible to reclaim the female body without reinforcing patriarchal conceptions of sexual difference that make sexed bodies meaningful? What would a feminist anatomy look like? As Merleau-Ponty points out, consciousness is inseparable from our embodied experiences within particular social, cultural, and historical situations (1962). Iris Young extends Merleau-Ponty's analysis to consider what female embodiment reveals about patriarchal oppression. In her discussion of breasted experience Young observes, "However alienated male-dominated culture makes us from our bodies, however much it gives us instruments of self-hatred and oppression, still our bodies are ourselves. . . . If we love ourselves at all, we love our bodies" (1990, 192).

The Vagina Monologues is perhaps the most recent incarnation of feminist art that seeks to represent women's bodies on women's own terms in an attempt to critique misogynistic portrayals of female bodies and women in patriarchal culture. In the 1970s this art attempted to redefine the female body from the ground of women's experiences, to transform the female body from being a passive object of male consumption to being a speaking, empowered agent (Broude and Garrard 1994, 22). Judy Chicago's *The Dinner Party* (1979), Carolee Schneemann's *Interior Scroll* performance (1975), the goddess movement in feminist art, and Tee Corinne's *Cunt Coloring Book* (1974) are some examples of feminist attempts to reconceptualize the female body.

Of course, these innovations challenged and continue to challenge Western patriarchal sensibility, according to which women ought to be silent and discreet regarding their sexual anatomies. Indeed, women's epistemic authority regarding the female body has been denied. The threatening difference of feminist representations of female bodies is that feminists are defining the form and function of female bodies from the ground of women's experiences.

Each of the thirty-nine place settings in Judy Chicago's *The Dinner Party* included a hand-painted plate. Chicago explained that the brightly colored images on the plates were butterflies, symbols of transition and change (Aptheker 1989, 148). However, as Bettina Aptheker observes, "Most viewers . . . looked at the butterflies and saw vaginas" (148). Nor were all of the plates emblazoned with brightly colored butterfly-vulvas; the place setting for Sojourner Truth consisted of a plate with three faces. In her review of *The Dinner Party*, Alice Walker wondered why a white feminist artist found it difficult to imagine that black women have vaginas:

> I was gratified . . . to learn that in the "Dinner Party" there was a place "set," as it were, for black women. The illumination came when I stood in front of it. All the other plates are creatively imagined vaginas. . . . The Sojourner Truth plate is the only one in the collection that shows—instead of a vagina—a face. In fact, *three* faces. . . . It occurred to me that perhaps white women feminists, no less than white women generally, cannot imagine that black women have vaginas. However, to think of black women as women is impossible if you cannot imagine them with vaginas. (quoted in Aptheker 1989, 152)

As Walker's criticism indicates, despite her intention of honoring women who have been erased in patriarchal accounts of Western history, Chicago nonetheless contributes to the erasure of black women *as* women. Still, Walker's response contributes to the naturalization of women as beings/bodies with vaginas. Readers of Walker's review are asked to remember that Sojourner Truth was a woman because she had a vagina through which children emerged into the world. It certainly is problematic that Chicago could not imagine the genital anatomy of a black woman, and I share Walker's criticism of *The Dinner Party*. However, the problem of naturalizing the relationship between having a vagina and being female is not addressed by either Judy Chicago or Alice Walker.

In her *Interior Scroll* performance, Carolee Schneemann stood on a table, painted her naked body with mud, and read from a scroll while removing it from her vagina. Schneemann explains, "I thought of the vagina in many ways—physically, conceptually: as a sculptural form, an architectural referent, the sources of sacred knowledge, ecstasy, birth passage, transformation. I saw the vagina as a translucent chamber of which the serpent was the outward model: enlivened by its passage from the visible to the invisible, a spiraled coil ringed with the shape of desire and generative mysteries, attributes of both female and male sexual power" (http://www.caroleeschneemann.com/interiorscroll.html). While Schneemann sought to celebrate the "interior knowledge" of the vagina as part of "Goddess worship," she draws on conventional narratives of genital anatomies and sexual difference in her description. For example, in Leonardo da Vinci's drawings of heterosexual intercourse created between 1493 and 1500, the vagina was represented as having the shape of an interior, invisible penis, thus contributing to the view that heterosexual intercourse was natural because the penis was the key that fit into the lock of the vagina (Gilman 1989, 91–94). Da Vinci's drawings present the "natural" design of male and female bodies as a sign of "natural" heterosexuality. By imagining the scroll as the visible, male model of that which is invisible and female, Schneemann ultimately reinforces the assumption of naturalized sexual difference and its corresponding heterosexuality that are the ideological foundations of patriarchal structures.

Some feminist goddess art has also appropriated the image of the Sheela Na Gig. Sheela Na Gigs are stone carvings of bald, old women who are squatting, often grinning, and displaying their vaginas. These figures are found on many very old churches throughout Ireland and are considered to be images of female power and evidence of original pagan sites on which churches were later constructed.[9] Sheela Na Gigs are very interesting figures, and their appearance on patriarchal churches is certainly a mystery; however, feminist appropriation of these figures is problematic to the extent that it reinforces the idea of the vagina as central to female embodiment.

Tee Corinne's *Cunt Coloring Book* is another example of feminist attempts to reclaim and reimagine female genitalia. As Tee Corinne explains her decision to begin drawing women's genitals in 1974, "I know that whatever we don't have names for and images of, we are likely to label crazy and bad. Images of women's genitals, although available to men in porn magazines, had been denied to women. Part of the early seventies Women's Movement was a reclamation of our bodies which included using speculums to looks at our cervixes and mirrors to look at our labia" (Corinne 1992, 4). The *Cunt Coloring Book* was never as popular as *The Vagina Monologues*. Tee Corrine's project presents a range of female genitalia and invites the reader to color (and thus reinvent) them as she wishes. Implicit in the *Cunt Coloring Book* is the understanding that genitalia are infinitely various. By contrast, *The Vagina Monologues* presents stories that cannot be altered in performance and within which all women are expected to be able to find themselves.

The feminist health movement strives to empower women by providing information about their bodies. What is interesting about the feminist health movement for the purposes of this paper is not only its efforts to provide information that empowers those who have been disempowered and pathologized by medical authority, but also its efforts to redefine the female body by creating feminist anatomies. In their study of clitoral anatomy, Lisa Jean Moore and Adele E. Clarke consider "how anatomists have represented, labeled, and narrated various 'female parts,' focusing especially on what (if anything) counts as 'the clitoris'" (1995, 256). Their research led them to consider feminist reconceptualizations of the clitoris (262).

For example, in their 1981 book, *New View of a Woman's Body*, the Federation of Feminist Women's Health Centers discussed and represented many different kinds of clitorises, thus challenging the patriarchal narrative of the clitoris as an unchanging and ultimately insignificant part of female genital anatomy (280, 290). The Federation of Feminist Women's Health Centers renarrated female genital anatomy in ways that completely decentered, if not entirely eliminated, the vagina. As Moore and Clarke observe, the clitoris is the main character of female genital anatomy in *New View of a Woman's Body* (1995, 279). In fact, the federation's representations of female genital anatomy include references such as the "clitoral opening of the vagina" and "the inner lips of the clitoris." Indeed, there the vagina is represented as one, noncentral part of female genital anatomy—the vaginal canal (1981, 34). While some might object that their decision to subordinate the vagina to the clitoris is a mere reversal of dominant discourse, I share Moore's and Clarke's suspicion that something much more politically interesting and transgressive is occurring. The federation's view of female genitalia does not challenge patriarchal representations of women's bodies because it highlights the clitoris as opposed to the vagina, a move that would simply make the clitoris rather than the vagina central to having a female body. "Rather, the Federation challenges patriarchal representations of women's bodies because the drawings of female genitalia in *New View of a Woman's Body* reimagine the clitoris and thereby expose the arbitrary, political nature of 'truths' about anatomy and sexual difference" (Moore and Clarke 1995, 283–84). Perhaps the best way to understand the significance of the federation's re-vision of female sexual anatomy is to consider it in the context of Monique Wittig's claim that she does not have a vagina.

Wittig is famous among feminist and queer theorists for her claim that "lesbians are not women" (Wittig 1992, 32), thereby emphasizing that *woman* has meaning only within a heterosexual economy. For Wittig, *woman* is not a natural category; *woman* is a political class because "what makes a woman is a specific social relation to a man, a relation that we have previously called 'servitude,' a relation which implies personal and physical obligation as well as economic obligation . . . a relation which lesbians escape by refusing to become or to stay heterosexual" (20). Given her observations about the meaning of the category *woman*, it makes sense that Wittig claimed not to have a vagina. To say that the category of sex is socially, historically, and economically determined is to say that both the category of woman and what is considered to be the biology or materiality of sex is also socially produced. To naturalize either is to naturalize and legitimate relations of oppression when it is those relations of oppression that mark otherwise neutral physical features as determinants of sex (11). Such naturalizations of inequality are reinforced by sexist pronouncements of the inevitability of patriarchy and by feminist celebrations of women's "natural" bodies.

The vagina, like the category 'woman', is a political category. That is, the vagina is made intelligible to the extent that it perpetuates the notion that the (biological) capacity to give birth is what makes one a woman (Wittig 1992, 10). Thus, within a heteropatriarchal society, having a vagina is what makes one a biological woman. So, to engage in the project of reclaiming the vagina without simultaneously adopting a strategy of disidentification regarding the reality of the vagina does not challenge the social, political, historical, and economic context that imbues the vagina with meaning. Wittig says that she does not have a vagina because

> what we believe to be a physical and direct perception is only a sophisticated and mythic construction, an "imaginary formation," which reinterprets physical features (in themselves as neutral as any others but marked by the social system) through the network of relationships in which they are perceived. (They are seen *as black*, therefore they *are* black; they are seen *as women*, therefore, they *are* women. But before being *seen* that way, they first had to be *made* that way.) (1992, 11–12)

One does not have to adopt a nominalism regarding race and gender to accept Wittig's claim. Because, as so many feminist theorists have convincingly argued, feminists need the category of woman in order to make visible women's oppression, there is a sense in which women exist just as there is a sense in which vaginas exist. The categories *woman* and *vagina* enable feminists to name the bad things that happen to those who are perceived as women and to that which is perceived as a vagina. Female body parts and women are real in the sense that they are lived effects of power in a sexist, racist, classist, ableist, heterosexist society. The answer, then, is not for feminists to abandon all reference to vaginas or women or race. Rather, feminists must adopt strategies of resistance that have the potential to change our relationship to the female body and the category woman. Linda Martín Alcoff argues that understanding gender as positionality is a political strategy that both recognizes the constructed nature of gender and the reality of lived experiences of sexism (1995). Similarly, an effective feminist body politics would adopt a strategy of disidentification regarding the relation between being a woman and having a female body, a strategy that reveals both the constructed nature of the female body and the reality of embodied experiences of sexism. Such a strategy would be informed by Alcoff's understanding of identity as positionality and would emphasize the extent to which an effective feminist politics of disidentification would have to recognize how women are positioned as women in a patriarchal society while simultaneously striving to reveal the fiction of the identity "woman."

Two Core Beliefs

So what does this mean for *The Vagina Monologues*? Should feminists be in the business of promoting or opposing these performances? Rather than answer this question, I have attempted to articulate a problem that I hope will inspire further dialogue. Identities and bodies are sites of perpetual struggle for meaning. Because we are compelled to be our bodies and our bodies are compelled to reveal our selves, our bodies are, in a sense, battlegrounds (Kruger 1989). Any queer feminist politics that emerge from these struggles will be forged, by necessity, in the context of communities that are in constant states of transformation. Following the example of the Federation of Feminist Women's Health Centers, performances of *The Vagina Monologues* could (though I doubt Ensler would change the performance restrictions) make apparent the ultimately arbitrary and self-defeating nature of grounding identity in anatomy and raise questions about strategies of identification in general. In other words, performances could make explicit the problem while understanding a need to name and organize against violence against women. A guerrilla grrrls intervention would be very interesting![10]

If the visibility of intersexed bodies both sustains and unsettles systems of oppression, *The Vagina Monologues,* V-Day, and the V-Day Challenge will need to do more than simply add new monologues and distribute educational materials at performances. They will also have to constantly critique rather than assume the connection between vaginas and female embodiment. We do not challenge dominant systems by emphasizing the normality or naturalism of bodies and body parts and their relation to identity. As disability studies demonstrate, such pretensions of the normal are always based on exclusion, marginalization, and pathologization of those bodies defined as abnormal. In order to effectively resist patriarchal devaluations of vaginas and women, *The Vagina Monologues* will also have to challenge two core beliefs that sustain the institutions of patriarchy, compulsory heterosexuality, and compulsory ablebodiedness: (1) the belief that genitals are prediscursive and thus natural (Butler 1990, 7) and (2) the belief that the vagina is an essential part of normal female embodiment. Without these challenges, the narrative reconstruction of the vagina offered in *The Vagina Monologues* is yet another narrative rehabilitation of the norms of heteropatriarchal female embodiment.

Kim Q. Hall is Associate Professor of Philosophy and member of the Women's Studies Program at Appalachian State University. She is the editor of the *NWSA Journal* special issue on Feminist Disability Studies (2002), and she coedited, with Chris Cuomo, *Whiteness: Feminist Philosophical Reflections* (Rowman & Littlefield, 1999), hallki@appstate.edu.

NOTES

I am grateful to many friends and colleagues for their helpful comments and suggestions on various drafts of this paper, especially Rosemarie Garland-Thomson, Robert McRuer, Bente Meyer, Jill Ehnenn, Kathryn Kirkpatrick, Rosemary Horowitz, Martha McCaughey, Sue Schweik, Sheila Lintott, and Beth Carroll.

1. The Intersex Society of North America (ISNA) is an activist and educational organization that provides information about intersex issues and opposes violence and other forms of discrimination against intersexed people. ISNA has been very vocal in its opposition to surgeries and hormonal treatments designed to "normalize" and "correct" the bodies of intersexed young people.

2. My use of disidentification to describe a queer feminist political strategy is influ-

enced by José Muñoz and Judith Butler. Butler uses the term in *Gender Trouble* to describe the contestation that enables a democratization of queer and feminist politics (4:227). Muñoz uses the term to describe a strategy utilized in the performance politics of queers of color to generate "new social relations" (1999, 5). For Muñoz, disidentification is part of intersectional politics (8). A strategy of disidentification is Foucauldian in its recognition that both oppression and resistance are conditioned by processes of subjection, processes that produce subjects.

3. For example, Nancy Hartsock questions whether Foucault's notion of power actually disempowers feminist strategies of resistance to the extent that it fails to provide feminists a politically useful theory of power (Hartsock 1990). And, while she is critical of Foucault's failure to consider the harms of patriarchal oppression of women (1996), Linda Martín Alcoff also uses Foucault (and Merleau-Ponty) as a point of departure for her development of a nuanced and politically useful concept of racial identity and embodiment (1999). Ladelle McWhorter also provides an insightful, moving account of how reading Foucault helped her to claim a lesbian identity while maintaining a critical sense of the complexities of identification (1999).

4. Another example of colonialist discourse in *The Vagina Monologues* is a more recent monologue titled "Under the Burqua." This monologue purports to address the violence experienced by Afghan women under Taliban rule. When I first saw this monologue performed, I was struck by the references to the "darkness" of Afghan women's lives. As opposed to other monologues that claim to present the experiences of different women, "Under the Burqua" presents an Afghan woman who is at the same time *all* Afghan women. Ultimately, the monologue fixes Afghan women in despair, "darkness," and violence. This monologue is especially problematic at a time when the Bush administration has disregarded the United Nations, world, and national opposition and declared war against Iraq and all other countries it considers to be harboring potential terrorist threats. Bush attempted to justify war in Afghanistan by expressing outrage at the Taliban's treatment of Afghan women; however, the US war in Afghanistan was certainly never about liberating Afghan women, and the lives of Afghan women have not been improved by the US presence in Afghanistan. There is another paper to be written about vaginas and the nation.

5. In raising this critique of ISNA I do not wish to diminish the importance of their efforts to raise awareness of violence against intersexed people. Their work has been and continues to be crucial, and I share their desire to eliminate this violence. My critique of both *The Vagina Monologues* and ISNA's V-Day Challenge is offered in the spirit of furthering queer feminist efforts to eliminate all forms of violence against oppressed people.

6. In fact, those who perform *The Vagina Monologues* are permitted to change neither the words nor the order of the text, thus underscoring the notion that these stories really are stories by, for, and about "all of us."

7. New York City Mayor Rudolph Giuliani famously accused Ofili of "smearing" elephant dung on the image of the Virgin Mary and thus "desecrating somebody else's religion" (Roediger 2002, 29). As David Roediger points out, however, Ofili, who is also a Catholic, represented a black Virgin Mary. Far from attacking "somebody else's religion," Ofili drew from traditions of Catholicism nonwhite cultures and representations of black

women in popular culture in order to critically comment on the position of black women in white supremacy and in rap music (29). Contrary to Giuliani's claim, no elephant dung was "smeared" on the face of the Virgin Mary; one of her breasts was constructed of elephant dung, and the painting was placed on two balls of elephant dung rather than hung on the wall.

8. Reported on National Public Radio on Monday, March 10, 2003.

9. I am grateful to Georgia Rhoades, Kathryn Kirkpatrick, and Jill Ehnenn for providing helpful information about Sheela Na Gigs.

10. Thanks to Martha McCaughey for this suggestion.

References

Alcoff, Linda Martín. 1988/1995. "Cultural feminism versus post-structuralism: The identity crisis in feminist theory." In *Feminism and philosophy: Essential readings in theory, reinterpretation and application*, ed. Nancy Tuana and Rosemarie Tong. Boulder, CO: Westview Press.

———. 1996. "Dangerous pleasures: Foucault and the politics of pedophilia." In *Feminist interpretations of Michel Foucault*, ed. Susan J. Hekman. University Park: Pennsylvania State University Press.

———. 1999. "Towards a phenomenology of racial embodiment." *Radical Philosophy* 95 (May/June): 15–26.

Aptheker, Bettina. 1989. *Tapestries of life: Women's work, women's consciousness, and the meaning of daily experience*. Amherst: University of Massachusetts Press.

Bartky, Sandra. 1990. *Femininity and domination: Studies in the phenomenology of oppression*. New York: Routledge.

———. 1998. "Skin deep: Femininity as disciplinary regime." In *Daring to be good: Essays in feminist ethico-politics*, ed. Bat-Ami Bar On and Ann Ferguson. New York: Routledge.

Boston Women's Health Collective. 1984. *The new our bodies, ourselves*. New York: Simon and Schuster.

Broude, Norma, and Mary D. Garrard. 1994. "Introduction: Feminism and art in the twentieth century." In *The power of feminist art*, ed. Norma Broude and Mary D. Garrard. New York: Harry N. Abrams.

Butler, Judith. 1990. *Gender trouble: Feminism and the subversion of identity*. New York: Routledge.

———. 1993. *Bodies that matter: On the discursive limits of "sex."* New York: Routledge.

Chicago, Judy. 1979. *The dinner party* (installation).

Corinne, Tee. 1974/1988. *The cunt coloring book*. San Francisco: Last Gasp.

———. 1992. *Tee Corinne twenty-two years: 1970–1992*. Self-published.

Dreger, Alice. 1998. *Hermaphrodites and the medical invention of sex*. Cambridge, MA: Harvard University Press.

Du Bois, W. E. B. 1903/1989. *The souls of black folk*. New York: Penguin.

Ensler, Eve. 2001. 1998. *The vagina monologues.* New York: Villard.

———. *The vagina monologues, The v-day edition.* New York: Villard.

Fanon, Frantz. 1967. *Black skin, white masks,* trans. Charles Lam Markmann. New York: Grove.

Fausto-Sterling, Anne. 1993. The five sexes. *Sciences* (March/April): 20–24.

Federation of Feminist Women's Health Centers. 1981. *A new view of a woman's body: A fully illustrated guide.* New York: Touchstone.

Foucault, Michel. 1978/1990. *The history of sexuality: An introduction,* vol. 1, trans. Robert Hurley. New York: Vintage.

Frankenberg, Ruth. 1993. *White women, race matters: The social construction of whiteness.* Minneapolis: University of Minnesota Press.

Garland-Thomson, Rosemarie. 1997. "Feminist theory, the body and the disabled figure." In *The disability studies reader,* ed. Lennard J. Davis. New York: Routledge.

Gilman, Sander L. 1989. *Sexuality: An illustrated history.* New York: John Wiley and Sons.

Grosz, Elizabeth. 1996. "Intolerable ambiguity: Freaks as/at the limit." In *Freakery: Cultural spectacles of the extraordinary body,* ed. Rosemarie Garland-Thomson. New York: New York University Press.

Halperin, David. 1995. *Saint Foucault: Towards a gay hagiography.* New York: Oxford University Press.

Hartsock, Nancy. 1990. "Foucault on power: A theory for women?" In *Feminism/Postmodernism,* ed. Linda Nicholson. New York: Routledge.

Hubbard, Ruth. 1990. *The politics of women's biology.* New Brunswick, NJ: Rutgers University Press.

The Interior Scroll. http://www.caroleeschneemann.com/interiorscroll.html.

Intersex Society of North America. 2002. V-Day challenge. http://www.isna.org/events/vday (accessed February 2002).

Kessler, Suzanne J. 1998. *Lessons from the intersexed.* New Brunswick, NJ: Rutgers University Press.

Koyama, Emi. 2002. "Open letter to v-day organizers." http://www.isna.org/events/vday/vday-email.html.

Kruger, Barbara. 1989. Untitled (your body is a battleground).

Lorde, Audre. 1984. *Sister outsider.* Freedom, CA: Crossing Press.

McRuer, Robert. 2002. "Compulsory ablebodiedness and queer/disabled existence." In *Disability studies: Enabling the humanities,* ed. Sharon L. Snyder, Brenda Jo Brueggemann, and Rosemarie Garland-Thomson. New York: Modern Language Association of America.

McWhorter, Ladelle. 1999. *Bodies and pleasures: Foucault and the politics of sexual normalization.* Bloomington: Indiana University Press.

Merleau-Ponty, Maurice. 1962. *Phenomenology of perception,* trans. Colin Smith. Atlantic Heights, NJ: Humanities Press.

Minh-Ha, Trinh T. 1989. *Woman, native, other: Writing postcoloniality and feminism.* Bloomington: Indiana University Press.

Mohanty, Chandra Talpade. 1991. "Under Western eyes: Feminist scholarship and colonial discourse." In *Third world women and the politics of feminism,* ed. Chandra Talpade Mohanty, Ann Russo, and Lourdes Torres. Bloomington: Indiana University Press.

Moore, Lisa Jean. 2002. "Extracting men from semen: Masculinity in scientific representations of sperm." *Social Text* 20 (4): 91–119.

Moore, Lisa Jean, and Adele E. Clarke. 1995. "Clitoral conventions and transgressions: Graphic representations in anatomy texts, c. 1900–1991." *Feminist Studies* 21 (2): 255–301.

Morris, Esther. 2002. "The missing vagina monologue." http://www.isna.org/library/missingvagina/html.

Muñoz, José Esteban. 1999. *Disidentifications: Queers of color and the performance of politics.* Minneapolis: University of Minnesota Press.

Pollitt, Katha. 2001. "Vaginal politics." *Nation,* February 15.

Roediger, David R. 2002. *Colored white: Transcending the racial past.* Berkeley and Los Angeles: University of California Press.

Schneemann, Carolee. 1975. *Interior scroll* (performance).

Walker, Alice, and Pratibha Parmar. 1993. *Warrior marks: Female genital mutilation and the sexual blinding of women.* New York: Harcourt Brace.

Wittig, Monique. 1992. *The straight mind and other essays.* Boston: Beacon.

Young, Iris Marion. 1990. *Throwing like a girl and other essays in feminist philosophy and social theory.* Bloomington: Indiana University Press.

34.

ABUSIVE IMAGES BELITTLE WOMEN, MEN, AND SEX

Robert Jensen

Pornography is an industrial media product primarily sold to men in a male-dominant culture for use as a masturbation facilitator.

With that simple sentence, we can dispatch with a lot of the knee-jerk defenses of pornography.

First, today's producers of sexually explicit material aren't interested in creating a space for artists exploring the mysteries of sexuality. Pornographers make good money by churning out a rigidly formatted product that minimizes creativity and maximizes profit.

Second, despite all the talk about "couples-friendly" pornography and the rise in women's porn consumption, the overwhelming majority of consumers of heterosexual pornography are men. Not surprisingly in a male-dominant society, the material reflects a hyper-masculine sexual imagination rooted in a conventional conception of masculinity: sex as conquest and the acquisition of pleasure through the taking of women.

Third, men don't encounter this toxic definition of sex as a rational argument to be evaluated critically but through masturbation leading to orgasm—a

Taken from *Irish Examiner* (Dublin), June 7, 2007, p. 10. Reprinted by permission. Robert Jensen's articles can be found online at http://uts.cc.utexas.edu/~rjensen/index.html.

powerful method for delivering the woman-hating message of the genre, reinforced in virtually every other institution of the society.

Evidence from laboratory studies and in-depth interviews indicates that men's habitual use of media material that sexually degrades women (1) heightens the risk of sexual violence for women and (2) leads to women's dissatisfaction with male partners in many relationships.

The evidence makes it even clearer that this pornographic culture is also destructive for men.

This doesn't mean the harms of pornography are borne equally by all; in male-dominant societies, women bear the brunt of the damage from the sexualizing of a domination/subordination dynamic, which is so central to pornography. Nor does it mean that all people experience pornography the same way.

But while human behavior is variable, there are patterns we can observe. From nearly 20 years of research on the issue, I have concluded that one of the most damaging aspects of pornography (along with much of pop culture) is not only that it objectifies women but that it also encourages men to objectify ourselves, to cut ourselves off from the rich, complex experience of sexuality and intimacy. Pornography provides men a quick and easy orgasm, producing physical pleasure with little or no emotional engagement. But to do that, what are we doing to ourselves?

In hundreds of formal interviews and informal discussions with men, I repeatedly hear them describe going emotionally numb when viewing pornography and masturbating, a state of being "checked out." In my own use of pornography as a child and young man, I remember how completely I would shut down during the experience.

So, to enter into the pornographic world and experience that intense sexual rush, many men have to turn off some of the emotional reactions typically connected to a sexual experience with a real person—a sense of the other's humanity, an awareness of being present with another person, the recognition of something outside our own bodies, as well as a deeper connection to oneself. Many of those same men report that in intimate relationships with another person, this same emotionally shut-down response to sexual stimulation kicks in.

In short: Pornography helps train men not to feel during an experience that is most about feeling.

Compounding the problem is the way in which pornography intensifies men's sense of control, over self and others. In pornography, men—the actors on the screen and the viewers at home—control everything. For viewers, technology has allowed more control of the sexual experience, first with the fast-forward button on a VCR to speed past a particular scene that may be less exciting. DVDs offer the same feature, enhanced further by the segmenting of movies by performer or type of sex acts; on many DVDs, one can click to be taken directly to anal penetration, for example.

So, men turn women into objects in order to turn ourselves into objects, splitting off loving emotion from body, in search of a sexual experience in which we don't have to feel and can stay in complete control. Coming full circle, this is not only destructive for men but dangerous for women. Because sex is always more than a physical act, men seeking this split-off state often find themselves having uncontrollable emotional reactions that can get channeled easily into violence and cruelty, increasing the risk to women.

Despite this, the pornography industry continues to tell us that their products represent the ultimate in sexual liberation. But the only thing being liberated is our cash, into their pockets.

In the end, I believe men should reject pornography and resist the pornifying of the culture for two reasons. First is an argument from justice, a principled concern for the welfare of women. Second is an argument from self-interest.

Do we want to be shut down and cut off from one of the great mysteries of life? Do we want to trade our humanity for a quick, cheap thrill that ends up costing us all more than we may realize?

35.

SURVIVING SEXUAL VIOLENCE

A Philosophical Perspective

Susan J. Brison

This is an unorthodox philosophy article, in both style and subject matter. Its primary aim is not to defend a thesis by means of argumentation, but rather to give the reader imaginative access to what is, for some, an unimaginable experience, that of a survivor of rape. The fact that there is so little philosophical writing about violence against women results not only from a lack of understanding of its prevalence and of the severity of its effects, but also from the mistaken view that it is not a properly philosophical subject. I hope in this essay to illuminate the nature and extent of the harm done by sexual violence and to show why philosophers should start taking this problem more seriously.[1]

On July 4, 1990, at 10:30 in the morning, I went for a walk along a peaceful-looking country road in a village outside Grenoble, France. It was a gorgeous day, and I didn't envy my husband, Tom, who had to stay inside and work on a manuscript with a French colleague of his. I sang to myself as I set out, stopping to pet a goat and pick a few wild strawberries along the way. About an hour and a half later, I was lying face down in a muddy creek bed at the bottom of a dark ravine, struggling to stay alive. I had been grabbed from behind,

First published in the *Journal of Social Philosophy* 24, no. 1 (Spring 1993). Reprinted by permission of the *Journal of Social Philosophy*.

pulled into the bushes, beaten, and sexually assaulted. Feeling absolutely helpless and entirely at my assailant's mercy, I talked to him, calling him "sir." I tried to appeal to his humanity, and, when that failed, I addressed myself to his self-interest. He called me a whore and told me to shut up. Although I had said I'd do whatever he wanted, as the sexual assault began I instinctively fought back, which so enraged my attacker that he strangled me until I lost consciousness. When I awoke, I was being dragged by my feet down into the ravine. I had often, while dreaming, thought I was awake, but now I was awake and convinced I was having a nightmare. But it was no dream. After ordering me, in a gruff, Gestapo-like voice, to get on my hands and knees, my assailant strangled me again. I wish I could convey the horror of losing consciousness while my animal instincts desperately fought the effects of strangulation. This time, I was sure I was dying. But I revived, just in time to see him lunging toward me with a rock. He smashed it into my forehead, knocking me out, and eventually, after another strangulation attempt, he left me for dead.

After my assailant left, I managed to climb out of the ravine, and was rescued by a farmer who called the police, a doctor, and an ambulance. I was taken to emergency at the Grenoble hospital, where I underwent neurological tests, x-rays, blood tests, and a gynecological exam. Leaves and twigs were taken from my hair for evidence, my fingernails were scraped, and my mouth was swabbed for samples. I had multiple head injuries, my eyes were swollen shut, and I had a fractured trachea, which made breathing difficult. I was not permitted to drink or eat anything for the first thirty hours, though Tom, who never left my side, was allowed to dab my blood-encrusted lips with a wet towel. The next day, I was transferred out of emergency and into my own room. But I could not be left alone even for a few minutes. I was terrified my assailant would find me and finish the job. When someone later brought in the local paper with a story about my attack, I was greatly relieved that it referred to me as *Mlle. M. R.* and didn't mention that I was an American. Even when I left the hospital, eleven days later, I was so concerned about my assailant tracking me down that I put only my lawyer's address on the hospital records.

Although fears for my safety may have initially explained why I wanted to remain anonymous, by that time my assailant had been apprehended, indicted for rape and attempted murder, and incarcerated without possibility of bail. Still, I didn't want people to know that I had been sexually assaulted. I don't know whether this was because I could still hardly believe it myself, because keeping this information confidential was one of the few ways I could feel in control of my life, or because, in spite of my conviction that I had done nothing wrong, I felt ashamed.

When I started telling people about the attack, I said, simply, that I was the victim of an attempted murder. People typically asked, in horror, "What was the motivation? Were you mugged?" and when I replied "No, it started as a sexual assault," most inquirers were satisfied with that as an explanation of why some man wanted to murder me. I would have thought that a murder attempt *plus a* sexual assault would require more, not less, of an explanation than a murder attempt by itself. (After all, there are *two* criminal acts to explain here.)

One reason sexual violence is taken for granted by many is because it is so very prevalent. The FBI, notorious for underestimating the frequency of sex crimes, notes that, in the United States, a rape occurs on an average of every six minutes.[2] But this figure covers only the reported cases of rape, and some researchers claim that only about 10 percent of all rapes get reported.[3] Every fifteen seconds, a woman is beaten.[4] The everydayness of sexual violence, as evidenced by these mind-numbing statistics, leads many to think that male violence against women is natural, a given, something not in need of explanation, and not amenable to change. And yet, through some extraordinary mental gymnastics, while most people take sexual violence for granted, they simultaneously manage to deny that it really exists—or, rather, that it could happen to them. We continue to think that we—and the women we love—are immune to it, provided, that is, that we don't do anything "foolish." How many of us have swallowed the potentially lethal lie that "If you don't do anything wrong, if you're just careful enough, you'll be safe?" How many of us have believed its damaging, victim-blaming corollary: "If you are attacked, it's because *you* did something wrong?" These are lies, and in telling my story I hope to expose them, as well as to help bridge the gap between those of us who have been victimized and those who have not.

But what, you may be thinking, does this have to do with philosophy? Why tell my story in this academic forum? Judging from the virtual lack of philosophical writing on sexual violence, one might well conclude there is nothing here of interest to philosophers. Certainly, I came across nothing in my search for philosophical help with explaining what had happened to me and putting my shattered world back together.[5] Yet sexual violence and its aftermath raise numerous philosophical issues in a variety of areas in our discipline. The disintegration of the self experienced by victims of violence challenges our notions of personal identity over time, a major preoccupation of metaphysics. A victim's seemingly justified skepticism about everyone and everything is pertinent to epistemology, especially if the goal of epistemology is, as Wilfrid Sellars put it, that of feeling at home in the world. In aesthetics—as well as in philosophy of law—the discussion of sexual violence in—or as—art could use the illumination provided by a victim's perspective. Perhaps the most important issues posed by sexual violence are in the areas of social, political, and legal philosophy, and insight into these, as well, requires an understanding of what it's like to be a victim of such violence.

One of the very few articles written by philosophers on violence against women is Ross Harrison's "Rape: A Case Study in Political Philosophy."[6] In this article Harrison argues that not only do utilitarians need to assess the harmfulness of rape in order to decide whether the harm to the victim outweighs the benefit to the rapist, but even on a rights-based approach to criminal justice we need to be able to assess the benefits and harms involved in criminalizing and punishing violent acts such as rape. On his view, it is not always the case, contra Ronald Dworkin, that rights trump considerations of utility, so, even on a rights-based account of justice, we need to give an account of why, in the case of rape, the pleasure gained by the perpetrator (or by multiple perpetrators, in the case of gang-rape) is always outweighed by the harm done to the victim. He points out the peculiar difficulty most of us have in imagining the pleasure a rapist gets out of an assault, but, he asserts confidently, "There is no problem imagining what it is like to be a victim. . . ."[7] To his credit, he acknowledges the importance, to political philosophy, of trying to imagine others' experience, for otherwise we could not compare harms and benefits, which he argues must be done even in cases of conflicts of rights in order to decide which of competing rights should take priority. But imagining what it is like to be a rape victim is no simple matter, since much of what a victim goes through is unimaginable. Still, it's essential to try to convey it.

In my efforts to tell the victim's story—my story, our story—I've been inspired and instructed not only by feminist philosophers who have refused to accept the dichotomy between the personal and the political, but also by critical race theorists such as Patricia Williams, Mari Matsuda, and Charles Lawrence who have incorporated first-person narrative accounts into their discussions of the law. In writing about hate speech, they have argued persuasively that one cannot do justice to the issues involved in debates about restrictions on speech without listening to the victims' stories.[8] In describing the effects of racial harassment on victims, they have departed from the academic convention of speaking in the impersonal, "universal," voice and related incidents they themselves experienced. In her ground-breaking book, *The Alchemy of Race and Rights*, Williams describes how it felt to learn about her great-great-grandmother who was purchased at age eleven by a slave owner who raped and impregnated her the following year. And in describing instances of everyday racism she herself has lived through, she gives us imaginative access to what it's like to be the victim of racial discrimination. Some may consider such first-person accounts in academic writing to be self-indulgent, but I consider them a welcome antidote to the arrogance of those who write in a magisterial voice that in the guise of "universality" silences those who most need to be heard.

Philosophers are far behind legal theorists in acknowledging the need for a diversity of voices. We are trained to write in an abstract, universal voice and to shun first-person narratives as biased and inappropriate for academic discourse. Some topics, however, such as the impact of racial and sexual violence on victims, cannot even be broached unless those affected by such crimes can tell of their experiences in their own words. Unwittingly further illustrating the need for the victim's perspective, Harrison writes, elsewhere in his article on rape, "What principally distinguishes rape from normal sexual activity is the consent of the raped woman."[9] There is no parallel to this in the case of other crimes, such as theft or murder. Try "What principally distinguishes theft from normal gift-giving is the consent of the person stolen from." We don't think of theft as "gift-giving minus consent." We don't think of murder as "assisted suicide minus consent." Why not? In the latter case, it could be because assisted suicide is relatively rare (even compared with murder) and so it's odd to use it as the more familiar thing to which we are analogizing. But in the former case, gift-giving is presumably more prevalent than theft (at least in academic circles) and yet it still sounds odd to explicate theft in terms of gift-giving minus consent. In the cases of both theft and murder, the notion of violation seems built into our conceptions of the physical acts constituting the crimes, so it is inconceivable that one could consent to the act in question. Why is it so easy for a philosopher such as Harrison to think of rape, however, as "normal sexual activity minus consent"? This may be because the nature of the violation in the case of rape hasn't been all that obvious. Witness the phenomenon of rape jokes, the prevalence of pornography glorifying rape, the common attitude that, in the case of women, "no" means "yes," that women really want it.[10]

Since I was assaulted by a stranger, in a "safe" place, and was so visibly injured when I encountered the police and medical personnel, I was, throughout my hospitalization and my dealings with the police, spared the insult, suffered by so many rape victims, of not being believed or of being said to have asked for the attack. However, it became clear to me as I gave my deposition from my hospital bed that this would still be an issue in my assailant's trial. During my deposition, I recalled being on the verge of giving up my struggle to live when I was galvanized by a sudden, piercing image of Tom's future pain on finding my corpse in that ravine. At this point in my deposition, I paused, glanced over at the police officer who was typing the transcript, and asked whether it was appropriate to include this image of my husband in my recounting of the facts. The *gendarme* replied that it definitely was and that it was a very good thing I mentioned my husband, since my assailant, who had confessed to the sexual assault, was claiming I had provoked it. As serious as the occasion was, and as much as it hurt to laugh, I couldn't help it—the suggestion was so ludicrous. Could it have been those baggy Gap jeans I was wearing that morning? Or was it the heavy sweat-shirt? My maddeningly seductive jogging shoes? Or was it simply my walking along minding my own business that had provoked his murderous rage?

After I completed my deposition, which lasted eight hours, the police officer asked me to read and sign the transcript he'd typed to certify that it was accurate. I was surprised to see that it began with the words, "*Comme je suis sportive . . .*"—Since I am athletic . . .—added by the police to explain to the court just what possessed me to go for a walk by myself that fine morning. I was too exhausted by this point to protest "no, I'm not an athlete, I'm a philosophy professor," and I figured the officer knew what he was doing, so I let it stand. That evening, my assailant confessed to the assault. I retained a lawyer, and met him along with the investigating magistrate, when I gave my second deposition toward the end of my hospitalization. Although what occurred was officially a crime against the state, not against me, I was advised to pursue a civil suit in order to recover unreimbursed medical expenses, and, in any case, I needed an advocate to explain the French legal system to me. I was told that since this was an "easy" case, the trial would occur within a year. In fact, the trial took place two-and-a-half years after the assault, due to the delaying tactics of my assailant's lawyer, who was trying to get him off on an insanity defense. According to Article 64 of the French criminal code, if the defendant is determined to have been insane at the time, then, legally, there was "*ni crime, ni délit*"—neither crime nor offense. The jury, however, did not accept the insanity plea and found my assailant guilty of rape and attempted murder, sentencing him to ten years in prison.

As things turned out, my experience with the criminal justice system was better than that of most sexual assault victims. I did, however, occasionally get glimpses of the humiliating insensitivity victims routinely endure. Before I could be released from the hospital, for example, I had to undergo a second forensic examination at a different hospital. I was taken in a wheelchair out to a hospital van, driven to another hospital, taken to an office where there were no receptionists and where I was greeted by two male doctors I had never seen before. When they told me to take off my clothes and stand in the middle of the room, I refused. I had to ask for a hospital gown to put on. For about an hour the two of them went over me like a piece of meat, calling out measurements of bruises and other assessments of damage, as if they were performing an autopsy. This was just the first of many incidents in which I felt as if I was experiencing things posthumously. When the inconceivable happens, one starts to doubt even the most mundane, realistic perceptions. Perhaps I'm not really here, I thought, perhaps I did die in that ravine. The line between life and death, once so clear and sustaining, now seemed carelessly drawn and easily erased.

For the first several months after my attack, I led a spectral existence, not quite sure whether I had died and the world went on without me, or whether I was alive but in a totally alien world. Tom and I returned to the States, and I continued to convalesce, but I felt as though I'd somehow outlived myself. I sat in our apartment and stared outside for hours, through the blur of a detached vitreous, feeling like Robert Lowell's newly widowed mother, described in one of his poems as mooning in a window "as if she had stayed on a train / one stop past her destination."[11]

My sense of unreality was fed by the massive denial of those around me—a reaction I learned is an almost universal response to rape. Where the facts would appear to be incontrovertible, denial takes the shape of attempts to explain the assault in ways that leave the observers' worldview unscathed. Even those who are able to acknowledge the existence of violence try to protect themselves from the realization that the world in which it occurs is their world and so they find it hard to identify with the victim. They cannot allow themselves to imagine the victim's shattered life, or else their illusions about their own safety and control over their lives might begin to crumble. The most well-meaning individuals, caught up in the myth of their own immunity, can inadvertently add to the victim's suffering by suggesting that the attack was avoidable or somehow her fault. One victims' assistance coordinator, whom I had phoned for legal advice, stressed that she herself had never been a victim and said that I would benefit from the experience by learning not to be so trusting of people and to take basic safety precautions like not going out alone late at night. She didn't pause long enough during her lecture for me to point out that I was attacked suddenly, from behind, in broad daylight.

We are not taught to empathize with victims. In crime novels and detective films, it is the villain, or the one who solves the murder mystery, who attracts our attention; the victim, a merely passive pretext for our entertainment, is conveniently disposed of—and forgotten—early on. We identify with the agents' strength and skill, for good or evil, and join the victim, if at all, only in our nightmares. Though one might say, as did Clarence Thomas, looking at convicted criminals on their way to jail, "but for the grace of God, there go I,"[12] a victim's fate prompts an almost instinctive "it could never happen to me." This may explain why there is, in our criminal justice system, so little concern for justice for victims—especially rape victims. They have no constitutionally protected rights qua victims. They have no right to a speedy trial or to compensation for damages (though states have been changing this in recent years), or to privacy vis-à-vis the press. As a result of their victimization, they often lose their jobs, their homes, their spouses—in addition to losing a great deal of money, time, sleep, self-esteem, and peace of mind. The rights to "life, liberty, and the pursuit of happiness," possessed, in the abstract, by all of us, are of little use to victims who can lose years of their lives, the freedom to move about in the world without debilitating fear, and any hope of returning to the pleasures of life as they once knew them.

People also fail to recognize that if a victim could not have anticipated an attack, she can have no assurance that she will be able to avoid one in the future. More to reassure themselves than to comfort the victim, some deny that such a thing could happen again. One friend, succumbing to the gambler's fallacy, pointed out that my having had such extraordinary bad luck meant that the odds of my being attacked again were now quite slim (as if fate, though not completely benign, would surely give me a break now, perhaps in the interest of fairness). Others thought it would be most comforting to pretend nothing had happened. The first card I received from my mother, while I was still in the hospital, made no mention of the attack or of my pain and featured the "bluebird of happiness," sent to keep me ever cheerful. The second had an illustration of a bright, summery scene with the greeting: "Isn't the sun nice? Isn't the wind nice? Isn't everything nice?" Weeks passed before I learned, what I should have been able to guess, that after she and my father received Tom's first call from the hospital they held each other and sobbed. They didn't want to burden me with their pain—a pain which I now realize must have been greater than my own.

Some devout relatives were quick to give God all the credit for my survival but none of the blame for what I had to endure. Others acknowledged the suffering that had been inflicted on me, but as no more than a blip on the graph of God's benevolence—a necessary, fleeting evil, there to make possible an even greater show of good. An aunt, with whom I have been close since childhood, did not write or call at all until three months after the attack, and then sent a belated birthday card with a note saying that she was sorry to hear about my "horrible experience" but pleased to think that as a result I "will become stronger and will be able to help so many people. A real blessing from above for sure." Such attempts at a theodicy discounted the horror I had to endure. But I learned that everyone needs to try and make sense, in however inadequate a way, of such senseless violence. I watched my own seesawing attempts to find something for which to be grateful, something to redeem the unmitigated awfulness: I was glad I didn't have to reproach myself (or endure others' reproaches) for having done something careless, but I wished I had done something I could consider reckless so that I could simply refrain from doing it in the future. I was glad I did not yet have a child, who would have to grow up with the knowledge that even the protector could not be protected, but I felt an inexpressible loss when I recalled how much Tom and I had wanted a baby and how joyful were our attempts to conceive. It is difficult, even now, to imagine getting pregnant, because it is so hard to let even my husband near me, and because it would be harder still to let a child leave my side.

It might be gathered, from this litany of complaints, that I was the recipient of constant, if misguided, attempts at consolation during the first few months of my recovery. This was not the case. It seemed to me that the half-life of most people's concern was less than that of the sleeping pills I took to ward off flashbacks and nightmares—just long enough to allow the construction of a comforting illusion that lulls the shock to sleep. During the first few months after my assault, most of the aunts, uncles, cousins, and friends of the family notified by my parents almost immediately after the attack didn't phone, write, or even send a get well card, in spite of my extended hospital stay. These are all caring, decent people who would have sent wishes for a speedy recovery if I'd had, say, an appendectomy. Their early lack of response was so striking that I wondered whether it was the result of self-protective denial, a reluctance to mention something so unspeakable, or a symptom of our society's widespread emotional illiteracy that prevents most people from conveying any feeling that can't be expressed in a Hallmark card.

In the case of rape, the intersection of multiple taboos—against talking openly about trauma, about violence, about sex—causes conversational gridlock, paralyzing the would-be supporter. We lack the vocabulary for expressing appropriate concern, and we have no social conventions to ease the awkwardness. Ronald de Sousa has written persuasively about the importance of grasping paradigm scenarios in early childhood in order to learn appropriate emotional responses to situations.[13] We do not learn—early or later in life—how to react to a rape. What typically results from this ignorance is bewilderment on the part of victims and silence on the part of others, often the result of misguided caution. When, on entering the angry phase of my recovery period, I railed at my parents: "Why haven't my relatives called or written? Why hasn't my own brother phoned?" They replied, "They all expressed their concern to us, but they didn't want to remind you of what happened." Didn't they realize I thought about the attack every minute of every day and that their inability to respond made me feel as though I had, in fact, died and no one had bothered to come to the funeral?

For the next several months, I felt angry, scared, and helpless, and I wished I could blame myself for what had happened so that I would feel less vulnerable, more in control of my life. Those who haven't been sexually violated may have difficulty understanding why women who survive assault often blame themselves, and may wrongly attribute it to a sex-linked trait of masochism or lack of self-esteem. They don't know that it can be less painful to believe that you did something blameworthy than it is to think that you live in a world where you can be attacked at any time, in any place, simply because you are a woman. It is hard to go on after an attack that is both random—and thus completely unpredictable—and not random, that is, a crime of hatred towards the group to which you happen to belong. If I hadn't been the one who was attacked on that road in France, it would have been the next woman to come along. But had my husband walked down that road instead, he would have been safe.

Although I didn't blame myself for the attack, neither could I blame my attacker. Tom wanted to kill him, but I, like other rape victims I came to know, found it almost impossible to get angry with my assailant. I think the terror I still felt precluded the appropriate angry response. It may be that experiencing anger toward an attacker requires imagining oneself in proximity to him, a prospect too frightening for a victim in the early stages of recovery to conjure up. As Aristotle observed in the *Rhetoric*, Book I, "no one grows angry with a person on whom there is no prospect of taking vengeance, and we feel comparatively little anger, or none at all, with those who are much our superiors in power."[14] The anger was still there, however, but it got directed toward safer targets: my family and closest friends. My anger spread, giving me painful shooting signs that I was coming back to life. I could not accept what had happened to me. What was I supposed to do now? How could everyone else carry on with their lives when women were dying? How could Tom go on teaching his classes, seeing students, chatting with colleagues . . . and why should he be able to walk down the street when I couldn't?

The incompatibility of fear of my assailant and appropriate anger toward him became most apparent after I began taking a women's self-defense class. It became clear that the way to break out of the double bind of self-blame versus powerlessness was through empowerment—physical as well as political. Learning to fight back is a crucial part of this process, not only because it enables us to experience justified, healing rage, but also because, as Iris Young has observed in her essay "Throwing Like a Girl," "women in sexist society are physically handicapped," moving about hesitantly, fearfully, in a constricted lived space, routinely underestimating what strength we actually have.[15] We have to learn to feel entitled to occupy space, to defend ourselves. The hardest thing for most of the women in my self-defense class to do was simply to yell 'No!' Women have been taught not to fight back when being attacked, to rely instead on placating or pleading with one's assailant—strategies that researchers have found to be least effective in resisting rape."[16]

The instructor of the class, a survivor herself; helped me through the difficult first sessions, through the flashbacks and the fear, and showed me I could be tougher than ever. As I was leaving after one session, I saw a student arrive for the next class—with a guide dog. I was furious that, in addition to everything else this woman had to struggle with, she had to worry about being raped. I thought I understood something of her fear since I felt, for the first time in my life, like I had a perceptual deficit—not the blurred vision from the detached vitreous, but, rather, the more hazardous lack of eyes in the back of my head. I tried to compensate for this on my walks by looking over my shoulder a lot and punctuating my purposeful, straight-ahead stride with an occasional pirouette, which must have made me look more whimsical than terrified.

The confidence I gained from learning how to fight back effectively not only enabled me to walk down the street again, it gave me back my life. But it was a changed life. A paradoxical life. I began to feel stronger than ever before, and more vulnerable, more determined to fight to change the world, but in need of several naps a day. News that friends found distressing in a less visceral way—the trials of the defendants in the Central Park jogger case, the controversy over *American Psycho*, the Gulf war, the Kennedy rape case, the Tyson trial, the fatal stabbing of law professor Mary Jo Frug near Harvard Square, the ax murders of two women graduate students at Dartmouth College—triggered debilitating flashbacks in me. Unlike survivors of wars or earthquakes, who inhabit a common shattered world, rape victims face the cataclysmic destruction of their world alone, surrounded by people who find it hard to understand what's so distressing. I realized that I exhibited every symptom of post-traumatic stress disorder—dissociation, flashbacks, hypervigilance, exaggerated startle response, sleep disorders, inability to concentrate, diminished interest in significant activities, and a sense of a foreshortened future.[17] I could understand why children exposed to urban violence have such trouble envisioning their futures. Although I had always been career-oriented, always planning for my future, I could no longer imagine how I would get through each day, let alone what I might be doing in a year's time. I didn't think I would ever write or teach philosophy again.

The American Psychiatric Association's *Diagnostic and Statistical Manual* defines post-traumatic stress disorder, in part, as the result of "an event that is outside the range of usual human experience."[18] Because the trauma is, to most people, inconceivable, it's also unspeakable. Even when I managed to find the words—and the strength—to describe my ordeal, it was hard for others to hear about it. They would have preferred me to just "buck up," as one friend urged me to do. But it's essential to talk about it, again and again. It's a way of remastering the trauma, although it can be retraumatizing when people refuse to listen. In my case, each time someone failed to respond it felt as though I were alone again in the ravine, dying, screaming. And still no one could hear me. Or, worse, they heard me, but refused to help.

I now know they were trying to help, but that recovering from trauma takes time, patience, and, most of all, determination on the part of the survivor. After about six months, I began to be able to take more responsibility for my own recovery, and stopped expecting others to pull me through. I entered the final stage of my recovery, a period of gradual acceptance and integration of what had happened. I joined a rape survivors' support group, I got a great deal of therapy, and I became involved in political activities, such as promoting S.15: the Violence against Women Act of 1991. . . .[19] Gradually, I was able to get back to work.

When I resumed teaching at Dartmouth in the fall of 1991, the first student who came to see me in my office during freshman orientation week told me that she had been raped. Last spring four Dartmouth students reported sexual assaults to the local police. In the aftermath of these recent reports, the women students on my campus have been told to use their heads, lock their doors, not go out after dark without a male escort. They have been advised: just don't do anything stupid.

Although colleges are eager to "protect" women by limiting their freedom of movement or providing them with male escorts, they continue to be reluctant to teach women to protect themselves. After months of lobbying the administration at my college, we were able to convince them to offer a women's self-defense and rape prevention course. It was offered last winter as a physical education course, and nearly one hundred students and employees signed up for it. Shortly after the course began, I was informed that the women students were not going to be allowed to get P.E. credit for it, since the administration had determined that it discriminated against men. I was told that granting credit for the course was in violation of Title IX, which prohibits sex-discrimination in education programs receiving federal funding—even though granting credit to men for being on the football team was not, even though Title IX law makes an explicit exception for P.E. classes involving substantial bodily contact, and even though every term the college offers several martial arts courses, for credit, that are open to men, geared to men's physiques and needs, and taken predominantly by men. I was told by an administrator that, even if Title IX permitted it, offering a women's self-defense course for credit violated "the College's nondiscrimination clause—a clause which, I hope, all reasonable men and women support as good policy." The implication that I was not a "reasonable woman" didn't sit well with me as a philosopher, so I wrote a letter to the appropriate administrative committee criticizing my college's position that single-sex sports, male-only fraternities, female-only sororities, and pregnancy leave policies are not discriminatory, in any invidious sense, while a women's self-defense class is. The administration has finally agreed to grant P.E. credit for the course, but shortly after that battle was over, I read in the *New York Times* that "a rape prevention ride service offered to women in the city of Madison and on the University of Wisconsin campus may lose its university financing because it discriminates against men."[20] The dean of students at Wisconsin said that this group—the Women's Transit Authority—which has been providing free nighttime rides to women students for nineteen years—must change its policy to allow male drivers and passengers. These are, in my view, examples of the application of what Catharine MacKinnon refers to as "the stupid theory of equality."[21] To argue that rape prevention policies for women discriminate against men is like arguing that money spent making university buildings more accessible to disabled persons discriminates against those able-bodied persons who do not benefit from these improvements.[22]

Sexual violence victimizes not only those women who are directly attacked, but *all* women. The fear of rape has long functioned to keep women in their place. Whether or not one agrees with the claims of those, such as Susan Brownmiller, who argue that rape is a means by which *all* men keep *all* women subordinate,[23] the fact that all women's lives are restricted by sexual violence is indisputable. The authors of *The Female Fear*, Margaret Gordon and Stephanie Riger, cite studies substantiating what every woman already knows—that the fear of rape prevents women from enjoying what men consider to be their birthright. Fifty percent of women never use public transportation after dark because of fear of rape. Women are eight times more likely than men to avoid walking in their own neighborhoods after dark, for the same reason.[24] In the seminar I taught last spring on Violence against Women, the men in the class were stunned by the extent to which the women in the class took precautions against assault every day—locking doors and windows, checking the back seat of the car, not walking alone at night, looking in closets on returning home. And this is at a 'safe' rural New England campus.

Although women still have their work and leisure opportunities unfairly restricted by their relative lack of safety, paternalistic legislation excluding women from some of the 'riskier' forms of employment (e.g., bartending[25]) has, thankfully, disappeared, except, that is, in the military. We are still debating whether women should be permitted to engage in combat, and the latest rationale for keeping women out of battle is that they are more vulnerable than men to sexual violence. Those wanting to limit women's role in the military are now using the reported indecent assaults on the two female American prisoners of war in Iraq as evidence for women's unsuitability for combat.[26] One might as well argue that the fact that women are much more likely than men to be sexually assaulted on college campuses is evidence that women are not suited to post-secondary education. No one, to my knowledge, has proposed returning Ivy League colleges to their former all-male status as a solution to the problem of campus rape. Some have, however, seriously proposed enacting after-dark curfews for women, in spite of the fact that men are the perpetrators of the assaults. This is yet another indication of how natural it still seems to many people to address the problem of sexual violence by curtailing women's lives. The absurdity of this approach becomes apparent once one realizes that a woman can be sexually assaulted anywhere, at any time—in 'safe' places, in broad daylight, even in her own home.

For months after my assault, I was afraid of people finding out about it—afraid of their reactions and of their inability to respond. I was afraid that my professional work would be discredited, that I would be viewed as 'biased,' or, even worse, not properly 'philosophical.' Now I am no longer afraid of what might happen if I speak out about sexual violence. I'm much more afraid of what *will* continue to happen if I don't. Sexual violence is a problem of catastrophic proportions—a fact obscured by its mundanity, by its relentless occurrence, by the fact that so many of us have been victims of it. Imagine the moral outrage, the emergency response we would surely mobilize, if all of these everyday assaults occurred at the same time or were restricted to one geographical region? But why should the spatiotemporal coordinates of the vast numbers of sexual assaults be considered to be morally relevant? From the victim's point of view, the fact that she is isolated in her rape and her recovery, combined with the ordinariness of the crime that leads to its trivialization, makes the assault and its aftermath even more traumatic.

As devastating as sexual violence is, however, I want to stress that it is possible to survive it, and even to flourish after it, although it doesn't seem that way at the time. Whenever I see a survivor struggling with the overwhelming anger and sadness, I'm reminded of a sweet, motherly woman in my survivors' support group who sat silently throughout the group's first meeting. At the end of the hour she finally asked, softly, through tears: "Can anyone tell me if it ever stops hurting?" At the time I had the same question, and wasn't satisfied with any answer. Now I can say, yes, it does stop hurting, at least for longer periods of time. A year ago, I was pleased to discover that I could go for fifteen minutes without thinking about my attack. Now I can go for hours at a stretch without a flashback. That's on a good day. On a bad day, I may still take to my bed with lead in my veins, unable to find one good reason to go on.

Our group facilitator told us that first meeting: "You will never be the same. But you can be better." I protested that I had lost so much: my security, my self-esteem, my love, and my work. I had been happy with the way things were. How could they ever be better now? As a survivor, she knew how I felt, but she also knew that, as she put it, "When your life is shattered, you're forced to pick up the pieces, and you have a chance to stop and examine them. You can say 'I don't want this one anymore' or 'I think I'll work on that one.' I have had to give up more than I would ever have chosen to. But I have gained important skills and insights, and I no longer feel tainted by my victimization. Granted, those of us who live through sexual assault aren't given ticker tape parades or the keys to our cities, but it's an honor to be a survivor. Although it's not exactly the sort of thing I can put on my résumé, it's the accomplishment of which I'm most proud.

Now, more than two years after the assault, I can acknowledge the good things that have come from the recovery process—the clarity, the confidence, the determination, the many supporters and survivors who have brought meaning back into my world. This is not to say that the attack and its aftermath were, on balance, a good thing or, as one aunt put it, "a real blessing from above." I would rather not have gone down that road. It's been hard for me, as a philosopher, to learn the lesson that knowledge isn't always desirable, that the truth doesn't always set you free. Sometimes, it fills you with incapacitating terror and, then, uncontrollable rage. But I suppose you should embrace it anyway, for the reason Nietzsche exhorts you to love your enemies: if it doesn't kill you, it makes you stronger.

People ask me if I'm recovered now, and I reply that it depends on what that means. If they mean "am I back to where I was before the attack"? I have to say, no, and I never will be. I am not the same person who set off, singing, on that sunny Fourth of July in the French countryside. I left her—and her trust, her innocence, her *joie de vivre*—in a rocky creek bed at the bottom of a ravine. I had to in order to survive. I now understand what a friend described to me as a Jewish custom of giving those who have outlived a brush with death new names. The trauma has changed me forever, and if I insist too often that my friends and family acknowledge it, that's because I'm afraid they don't know who I am.

But if recovery means being able to incorporate this awful knowledge into my life and carry on, then, yes, I'm recovered. I don't wake each day with a start, thinking: "this can't have happened to me!" It happened. I have no guarantee that it won't happen again, although my self-defense classes have given me the confidence to move about in the world and to go for longer and longer walks—with my two dogs. Sometimes I even manage to enjoy myself. And I no longer cringe when I see a woman jogging alone on the country road where I live, though I may still have a slight urge to rush out and protect her, to tell her to come inside where she'll be safe. But I catch myself, like a mother learning to let go, and cheer her on, thinking, may she always be so carefree, so at home in her world. She has every right to be.

NOTES

1. I would like to thank the North American Society for Social Philosophy for inviting me to give this paper as a plenary address at the Eighth International Social Philosophy Conference, Davidson College, August 1, 1992. I am also grateful to the Franklin J. Matchette Foundation for sponsoring this talk.

2. Federal Bureau of Investigation, *Uniform Crime Reports for the United States* (1989), p. 6.

3. Robin Warshaw notes that "[g]overnment estimates find that anywhere from three to ten rapes are committed for every one rape reported. And while rapes by strangers are still underreported, rapes by acquaintances are virtually nonreported. Yet, based on intake observations made by staff at various rape counseling centers (where victims come for treatment, but do not have to file police reports), 70–80 percent of all rape crimes are acquaintance rapes." See Robin Warshaw, *I Never Called It Rape* (New York: Harper & Row, 1988), p. 12.

4. National Coalition against Domestic Violence, fact sheet, in "Report on Proposed Legislation S.15: The Violence against Women Act," p. 9. On file with the Senate Judiciary Committee.

5. After I presented this paper at Davidson College, Iris Young drew my attention to Jeffner Allen's discussion of her rape in Jeffner Allen, *Lesbian Philosophy: Explorations* (Palo Alto, CA: Institute of Lesbian Studies, 1986).

6. Another, much more perceptive, article is Lois Pineau's "Date Rape: A Feminist Analysis," *Law and Philosophy* 8 (1989): 217–43. In addition, an excellent book on the causes of male violence was written by a scholar trained as a philosopher, Myriam Miedzian. See Myriam Miedzian, *Boys Will Be Boys: Breaking the Link between Masculinity and Violence* (New York: Doubleday, 1991). Philosophical discussions of the problem of evil, even recent ones such as that in Robert Nozick, *The Examined Life: Philosophical Meditations* (New York: Touchstone Books, 1989), don't mention the massive problem of sexual violence. Even Nell Noddings's book, *Women and Evil* (Berkeley and Los Angeles: University of California Press, 1989), which is an "attempt to describe evil from the per-spective of women's experience," mentions rape only twice, briefly, and in neither instance from the victim's point of view.

7. Ross Harrison, "Rape—A Study in Political Philosophy," in *Rape: An Historical and Cultural Inquiry*, ed. Sylvana Tomaselli and Roy Porter (New York: Basil Blackwell, 1986), p. 51.

8. See especially Patricia Williams's discussion of the Ujaama House incident in *The Alchemy of Race and Rights* (Cambridge, MA: Harvard University Press, 1991), pp. 110–16; Mari Matsuda, "Public Response to Racist Speech: Considering the Victim's Story," *Michigan Law Review* 87, no. 8 (1989): 2320–81; and Charles Lawrence, "If He Hollers, Let Him Go: Regulating Racist Speech on Campus," *Duke Law Journal* (1990): 481–83.

9. Harrison, "Rape," p. 52.

10. As the authors of *The Female Fear* note: "The requirement of proof of the victim's nonconsent is unique to the crime of forcible rape. A robbery victim, for example, is usu-ally not considered as having 'consented' to the crime if he or she hands money over to an assailant [especially if there was use of force or threat of force]." See Margaret T. Gordon and Stephanie Riger, *The Female Fear: The Social Cost of Rape* (Chicago: Univer-sity of Illinois Press, 1991), p. 59.

11. Robert Lowell, *Selected Poems* (New York: Farrar, Straus and Giroux, 1977), p. 82.

12. Quoted in the *New York Times*, September 13, 1991, p. A-18. Although Judge Thomas made this statement during his confirmation hearings, Justice Thomas's actions while on the Supreme Court have belied his professed empathy with criminal defendants.

13. Ronald de Souza, *The Rationality of Emotion* (Cambridge, MA: MIT Press, 1987).

14. In Jonathan Barnes, ed., *The Complete Works of Aristotle* (Princeton: Princeton University Press, 1984), 2: 2181–82. I thank John Cooper for drawing my attention to this aspect of Aristotle's theory of the emotions.

15. Iris Marion Young, *Throwing Like a Girl and Other Essays in Feminist Philosophy and Social Theory* (Indianapolis: Indiana University Press, 1990), p. 153.

16. See Pauline B. Bart and Patricia H. O'Brien, "Stopping Rape: Effective Avoidance Strategies," *Signs* 10, no. 1 (1984): 83–101.

17. For a clinical description of Post-Traumatic Stress Disorder (or PTSD), see the *Diagnostic and Statistical Manual*, 3rd ed., rev. (American Psychiatric Association, 1987). Excellent discussions of the recovery process undergone by rape survivors can be found in Morton Bard and Dawn Sangrey, *The Crime Victim's Book* (New York: Brunner/Mazel, 1986); Helen Benedict, *Recovery: How to Survive Sexual Assault—for Women, Men, Teenagers, Their Friends and Families* (Garden City, NY: Doubleday, 1985); Judith Lewis Herman, *Trauma and Recovery* (New York: Basic Books, 1992); and Ronnie Janoff-Bulman, *Shattered Assumptions: Towards a New Psychology of Trauma* (New York: Free Press, 1992). I have also found it very therapeutic to read first-person accounts by rape survivors such as Susan Estrich, *Real Rape* (Cambridge, MA: Harvard University Press, 1987), and Nancy Ziegenmeyer, *Taking Back My Life* (New York: Summit Books, 1992).

18. *Diagnostic and Statistical Manual*, 3rd ed., rev. (Washington, DC: American Psychiatric Association, 1987), p. 247.

19. S.15, sponsored by Sen. Joseph Biden (D-Del.), was drafted largely by Victoria Nourse, Special Counsel for Criminal Law, Office of the Senate Judiciary Committee. I am particularly interested in Title III, which would reclassify gender-motivated assaults as bias crimes. From the victim's perspective this reconceptualization is important. What was most difficult for me to recover from was the knowledge that some man wanted to kill me simply because I am a woman. This aspect of the harm inflicted in hate crimes (or bias crimes) is similar to the harm caused by hate speech. One cannot make a sharp distinction between physical and psychological harm in the case of PTSD sufferers. Most of the symptoms are physiological. I find it odd that in philosophy of law, so many theorists are devoted to a kind of Cartesian dualism that most philosophers of mind rejected long ago.

20. *New York Times*, April 19, 1992, p. 36.

21. She characterized a certain theory of equality in this way during the discussion after a Gauss seminar she gave at Princeton University, April 9, 1992.

22. For an illuminating discussion of the ways in which we need to treat people differently in order to achieve genuine equality, see Martha Minnow, *Making All the Difference: Inclusion, Exclusion, and American Law* (Ithaca, NY: Cornell University Press, 1990).

23. See Susan Brownmiller, *Against Our Will: Men, Women, and Rape* (New York: Bantam Books, 1975).

24. Gordon and Riger, *The Female Fear*.

25. As recently as 1948, the United States Supreme Court upheld a state law prohibiting the licensing of any woman as a bartender (unless she was the wife or daughter of the bar owner where she was applying to work). *Goesaert v. Cleary*, 335 U.S. 464 (1948).

26. *New York Times*, June 19, 1992, pp. 1, A-13.

36.

MEN IN GROUPS
Collective Responsibility for Rape
Larry May and Robert Strikwerda

As teenagers, we ran in a crowd that incessantly talked about sex. Since most of us were quite afraid of discovering our own sexual inadequacies, we were quite afraid of women's sexuality. To mask our fear, of which we were quite ashamed, we maintained a posture of bravado, which we were able to sustain through mutual reinforcement when in small groups or packs. Riding from shopping mall to fast food establishment, we would tell each other stories about our sexual exploits, stories we all secretly believed to be pure fictions. We drew strength from the camaraderie we felt during these experiences. Some members of our group would yell obscenities at women on the street as we drove by. Over time, conversation turned more and more to group sex, especially forced sex with women we passed on the road. To give it its proper name, our conversation turned increasingly to rape. At a certain stage, we tired of it all and stopped associating with this group of men, or perhaps they were in most ways still boys. The reason we left was not that we disagreed with what was going on, but, if this decision to leave was reasoned at all, it was that the posturing (the endless attempts to impress one another by our daring ways) simply became very tiresome. Only much later in life did we think that there was anything wrong, morally, socially,

Originally published in *Hypatia* 9, no. 2 (Spring 1994). © by Larry May and Robert Strikwerda. Reprinted with permission of the authors.

or politically, with what went on in that group of adolescents who seemed so
ready to engage in rape. Only later still did we wonder whether we shared in
responsibility for the rapes that are perpetrated by those men who had similar
experiences to ours.[1]

Catharine MacKinnon has recently documented the link between violence
and rape in the war in Bosnia. Young Serbian soldiers, some with no previous
sexual experience, seemed quite willing to rape Muslim and Croatian women as
their reward for "winning" the war. These young men were often encouraged in
these acts by groups of fellow soldiers, and even sometimes by their commanding
officers. Indeed, gang rape in concentration camps, at least at the beginning of
the war, seems to have been common.[2] The situation in Bosnia is by no means
unique in the history of war.[3] But rape historically has never been considered a
war crime. MacKinnon suggests that this is because "Rape in war has so often
been treated as extracurricular, as just something men do, as a product rather
than a policy of war."[4]

War crimes are collective acts taken against humanity; whereas rape has
almost always been viewed as a despicable "private" act. In this essay we wish to
challenge the view that rape is the responsibility only of the rapists by challenging the notion that rape is best understood as an individual, private act. This
is an essay about the relationship between the shared experiences of men in
groups, especially experiences that make rape more likely in Western culture, and
the shared responsibility of men for the prevalence of rape in that culture. The
claim of the essay is that in some societies men are collectively responsible for
rape in that most (if not all) men contribute in various ways to the prevalence of
rape, and as a result these men should share in responsibility for rape.

Most men do very little at all to oppose rape in their societies; does this make
them something like co-conspirators with the men who rape? In Canada, a
number of men have founded the "White Ribbon Campaign." This is a program
of fund-raising, consciousness-raising, and symbolic wearing of white ribbons
during the week ending on December 6, the anniversary of the murder of fourteen women at a Montreal engineering school by a man shouting "I hate feminists." Should men in US society start a similar campaign? If they do not, do they
deserve the "co-conspirator" label? If they do, is this symbolic act enough to
diminish their responsibility? Should men be speaking out against the program
of rape in the war in Bosnia? What should they tell their sons about such rapes,
and about rapes that occur in their home towns? If men remain silent, are they
not complicitous with the rapists?

We will argue that insofar as male bonding and socialization in groups contributes to the prevalence of rape in Western societies, men in those societies
should feel responsible for the prevalence of rape and should feel motivated to

counteract such violence and rape. In addition, we will argue that rape should be seen as something that men, as a group, are collectively responsible for, in a way, which parallels the collective responsibility of a society for crimes against humanity perpetrated by some members of their society. Rape is indeed a crime against humanity, not merely a crime against a particular woman. And rape is a crime perpetrated by men as a group, not merely by the individual rapist.

To support our claims we will criticize four other ways to understand responsibility for rape. First, it is sometimes said that only the rapist is responsible since he alone intentionally committed the act of rape. Second, it is sometimes said that no one is responsible since rape is merely a biologically oriented response to stimuli that men have little or no control over. Third, it is sometimes said that everyone, women and men alike, contribute to the violent environment which produces rape, so both women and men are equally responsible for rape, and hence it is a mistake to single men out. Fourth, it is sometimes said that it is "patriarchy," rather than individual men or men as a group, which is responsible for rape.[5] After examining each of these views we will conclude by briefly offering our own positive reasons for thinking that men are collectively responsible for the prevalence of rape in Western society.

1. The Rapist as Loner or Demon

Joyce Carol Oates has recently described the sport of boxing, where men are encouraged to violate the social rule against harming one another, as "a highly organized ritual that violates taboo."

> The paradox of the boxer is that, in the ring, he experiences himself as a living conduit for the inchoate, demonic will of the crowd: the expression of their collective desire, which is to pound another human being into absolute submission.[6]

Oates makes the connection here between boxing and rape. The former boxing heavyweight champion of the world, Mike Tyson, epitomizes this connection both because he is a convicted rapist, and also because, according to Oates, in his fights he regularly used the pre-fight taunt "I'll make you into my girlfriend," clearly the "boast of a rapist."[7]

Just after being convicted of rape, Mike Tyson gave a twisted declaration of his innocence:

> I didn't rape anyone. I didn't hurt anyone—no black eyes, no broken ribs. When I'm in the ring, I break their ribs, I break their jaws. To me, that's hurting someone.[8]

In the ring, Tyson had a license to break ribs and jaws; and interestingly he understood that this was a case of hurting another person. It was just that in the ring it was acceptable. He knew that he was not supposed to hurt people outside the ring. But since he didn't break any ribs or jaws, how could anyone say that he hurt his accuser, Desiree Washington? Having sex with a woman could not be construed as having hurt her, for Tyson apparently, unless ribs or jaws were broken.

Tyson's lawyer, attempting to excuse Tyson's behavior, said that the boxer grew up in a "male-dominated world." And this is surely true. He was plucked from a home for juvenile delinquents and raised by boxing promoters. Few American males had been so richly imbued with male tradition, or more richly rewarded for living up to the male stereotype of the aggressive, indomitable fighter. Whether or not he recognized it as a genuine insight, Tyson's lawyer points us toward the heart of the matter in American culture: misbehavior, especially sexual misbehavior of males toward females is, however mixed the messages, something that many men condone. This has given rise to the use of the term "the rape culture" to describe the climate of attitudes that exists in the contemporary American male-dominated world.[9]

While noting all of this, Joyce Carol Oates ends her *Newsweek* essay on Tyson's rape trial by concluding that "no one is to blame except the perpetrator himself." She absolves the "culture" at large of any blame for Tyson's behavior. Oates regards Tyson as a sadist who took pleasure in inflicting pain both in and out of the boxing ring. She comes very close to demonizing him when, at the end of her essay, she suggests that Tyson is an outlaw or even a sociopath. And while she is surely right to paint Tyson's deed in the most horrific colors, she is less convincing when she suggests that Tyson is very different from other males in our society. In one telling statement in her essay, however, Oates opens the door for a less individualistic view of rape by acknowledging that the boxing community had built up in Tyson a "grandiose sense of entitlement, fueled by the insecurities and emotions of adolescence."[10]

Rape is normally committed by individual men; but, in our view, rape is not best understood in individualistic terms. The chief reasons for this are that individual men are more likely to engage in rape when they are in groups, and men receive strong encouragement to rape from the way they are socialized as men, that is, in the way they come to see themselves as instantiations of what it means to be a man. Both the "climate" that encourages rape and the "socialization" patterns which instill negative attitudes about women are difficult to understand or assess when one focuses on the isolated individual perpetrator of a rape. There are significant social dimensions to rape that are best understood as group-oriented.

As parents, we have observed that male schoolchildren are much more likely to misbehave (and subsequently to be punished by being sent to "time out") than are female schoolchildren. This fact is not particularly remarkable, for boys are widely believed to be more active than girls. What is remarkable is that school-teachers, in our experience, are much more likely to condone the misbehavior of boys than the misbehavior of girls. "Boys will be boys" is heard as often today as it was in previous times.[11] (See Robert Lipsyte's essay about the Glen Ridge, New Jersey, rape trial where the defense attorney used just these words to defend the star high school football players who raped a retarded girl.) From their earliest experience with authority figures, little boys are given mixed signals about mis-behavior. Yes, they are punished, but they are also treated as if their misbehavior is expected, even welcome. It is for some boys, as it was for us, a "badge of honor" to be sent to detention or "time out." From older boys and from their peers, boys learn that they often will be ostracized for being "too goody-goody." It is as if part of the mixed message is that boys are given a license to misbehave.

And which of these boys will turn out to be rapists is often as much a matter of luck as it is a matter of choice. Recent estimates have it that in the first few months of the war "30,000 to 50,000 women, most of them Muslim" were raped by Serbian soldiers.[12] The data on date rape suggest that young men in our society engage in much more rape than anyone previously anticipated. It is a serious mistake in psychological categorization to think that all of these rapes are committed by sadists. (Studies by Amir show that the average rapist is not psy-chologically "abnormal."[13]) Given our own experiences and similar reports from others, it is also a serious mistake to think that those who rape are significantly different from the rest of the male population. (Studies by Smithyman indicate that rapists "seemed not to differ markedly from the majority of males in our culture."[14]) Our conclusion is that the typical rapist is not a demon or sadist, but, in some sense, could have been many men.

Most of those who engage in rape are at least partially responsible for these rapes, but the question we have posed is this: are those who perpetrate rape the *only* ones who are responsible for rape? Contrary to what Joyce Carol Oates con-tends, we believe that it is a serious mistake to think that only the perpetrators are responsible. The interactions of men, especially in all-male groups, con-tribute to a pattern of socialization that also plays a major role in the incidence of rape. In urging that more than the individual perpetrators be seen as respon-sible for rape, we do not mean to suggest that the responsibility of the perpe-trator be diminished. When responsibility for harm is shared, it need not be true that the perpetrators of harm find their responsibility relieved or even dimin-ished. Rather, shared responsibility for harms merely means that the range of people who are implicated in these harms is extended. (More will be said on this point in the final section.)

II. The Rapist As Victim of Biology

The most recent psychological study of rape is that done by Randy Thornhill and Nancy Wilmsen Thornhill, "The Evolutionary Psychology of Men's Coercive Sexuality."[15] In this work, any contention that coercion or rape may be socially or culturally learned is derisively dismissed, as is any feminist argument for changing men's attitudes through changing especially group-based socialization. The general hypothesis they support is that

> sexual coercion by men reflects a sex-specific, species-typical psychological adaptation to rape: Men have certain psychological traits that evolved by natural selection specifically in the context of coercive sex and made rape adaptive during human evolution.[16]

They claim that rape is an adaptive response to biological differences between men and women.

Thornhill and Thornhill contend that the costs to women to engage in sex ("nine months of pregnancy") greatly exceed the costs to men ("a few minutes of time and an energetically cheap ejaculate"). As a result women and men come very early in evolutionary time to adapt quite differently sexually.

> Because women are more selective about mates and more interested in evaluating them and delaying copulation, men, to get sexual access, must often break through feminine barriers of hesitation, equivocation, and resistance.[17]

Males who adapted by developing a proclivity to rape and thus who "solved the problem" by forcing sex on a partner, were able to "out-reproduce" other, more passive males and gain an evolutionary advantage.

In one paragraph, Thornhill and Thornhill dismiss feminists who support a "social learning theory of rape" by pointing out that males of several "species with an evolutionary history of polygyny" are also "more aggressive, sexually assertive and eager to copulate." Yet, in "the vast majority of these species there is no sexual training of juveniles by other members of the group." This evidence, they conclude, thoroughly discredits the social learning theory and means that such theories "are never alternatives to evolutionary hypotheses about psychological adaptation."[18] In response to their critics, Thornhill and Thornhill go so far as to say that the feminist project of changing socialization patterns is pernicious.

> The sociocultural view does seem to offer hope and a simple remedy in that it implies that we need only fix the way that boys are socialized and rape will disappear. This naive solution is widespread. . . . As Hartung points out, those who

feel that the social problem of rape can be solved by changing the nature of men through naive and arbitrary social adjustments should "get real about rape" because their perspective is a danger to us all.[19]

According to the Thornhills, feminists and other social theorists need to focus instead on what are called the "cues that affect the use of rape by adult males."[20] The evolutionary biological account of rape we have rehearsed above would seemingly suggest that no one is responsible for rape. After all, if rape is an adaptive response to different sexual development in males and females, particular individuals who engage in rape are merely doing what they are naturally adapted to do. Rape is something to be controlled by those who control the "cues" that stimulate the natural rapist instincts in all men. It is for this reason that the Thornhills urge that more attention be given to male arousal and female stimulation patterns in laboratory settings.[21] Notice that even on the Thornhills' own terms, those who provide the cues may be responsible for the prevalence of rape, even if the perpetrators are not. But Thornhill and Thornhill deny that there are any normative conclusions that follow from their research and criticize those who wish to draw out such implications as committing the "naturalistic fallacy."[22]

In contrast to the Thornhills, a more plausible sociobiological account is given by Lionel Tiger. Tiger is often cited as someone who attempted to excuse male aggression. In his important study he defines aggression as distinct from violence, but nonetheless sees violence as one possible outcome of the natural aggressive tendencies, especially in men.

> Aggression occurs when an individual or group see their interest, their honor, or their job bound up with coercing the animal, human, or physical environment to achieve their own ends rather than (or in spite of) the goals of the object of their action. Violence may occur in the process of interaction.[23]

For Tiger, aggression is intentional behavior which is goal-directed and based on procuring something which is necessary for survival. Aggression is a "'normal' feature of the human biologically based repertoire."[24] Violence, "coercion involving physical force to resolve conflict,"[25] on the other hand, is not necessarily a normal response to one's environment, although in some circumstances it may be. Thus, while human males are evolutionarily adapted to be aggressive, they are not necessarily adapted to be violent.

Tiger provided an account that linked aggression in males with their biological evolution.

> Human aggression is in part a function of the fact that hunting was vitally important to human evolution and that aggression is typically undertaken by

> males in the framework of a unisexual social bond of which participants are aware and with which they are concerned. It is implied, therefore, that aggression is 'instinctive' but also must occur within an explicit social context varying from culture to culture and to be learned by members of any community. . . . Men in continuous association aggress against the environment in much the same way as men and women in continuous association have sexual relations.[26]

And while men are thus predisposed to engage in aggression, in ways that women are not, it is not true in Tiger's view that a predisposition to engage in violent acts is a normal part of this difference.

Thornhill and Thornhill fail to consider Tiger's contention that men are evolutionarily adapted to be aggressive, but not necessarily to be violent. With Tiger's distinction in mind it may be said that human males, especially in association with other males, are adapted to aggress against women in certain social environments. But this aggressive response need not lead to violence, or the threat of violence, of the sort epitomized by rape; rather it may merely affect noncoercive mating rituals. On a related point, Tiger argues that the fact that war has historically been "virtually a male monopoly" is due to both male bonding patterns and evolutionary adaptation.[27] Evolutionary biology provides only part of the story since male aggressiveness need not result in such violent encounters as occur in war or rape. After all, many men do not rape or go to war; the cultural cues provided by socialization must be considered at least as important as evolutionary adaptation.

We side with Tiger against the Thornhills in focusing on the way that all-male groups socialize their members and provide "cues" for violence. Tiger has recently allied himself with feminists such as Catharine MacKinnon and others who have suggested that male attitudes need to be radically altered in order to have a major impact on the incidence of rape (see the preface to the second edition of *Men in Groups*). One of the implications of Tiger's research is that rape and other forms of male aggressive behavior are not best understood as isolated acts of individuals. Rather than simply seeing violent aggression as merely a biologically predetermined response, Tiger places violent aggressiveness squarely into the group dynamics of men's interactions—a result of his research not well appreciated.

In a preface to the second edition of his book, Tiger corrects an unfortunate misinterpretation of his work.

> One of the stigmas which burdened this book was an interpretation of it as an apology for male aggression and even a potential stimulus of it—after all, boys will be boys. However I clearly said the opposite: "This is not to say that . . . hurtful and destructive relations between groups of men are inevitable. . . . It may be possible, as many writers have suggested, to alter social conceptions of

maleness so that gentility and equivocation rather than toughness and more or less arbitrary decisiveness are highly valued."[28]

If Tiger is right, and the most important "cues" are those which young boys and men get while in the company of other boys and men, then the feminist project of changing male socialization patterns may be seen as consistent with, rather than opposed to, the sociobiological hypotheses. Indeed, other evidence may be cited to buttress the feminist social learning perspective against the Thornhills. Different human societies have quite different rates of rape. In her anthropological research among the Minangkabau of West Sumatra, Peggy Reeves Sanday has found that this society is relatively rape-free. Rape does occur, but at such a low rate—28 per 3 million in 1981–82, for example—as to be virtually nonexistent.[29] In light of such research, men, rather than women, are the ones who would need to change their behavior. This is because it is the socialization of men by men in their bonding-groups, and the view of women that is engendered, that provides the strongest cues toward rape. Since there may indeed be something that males could and should be doing differently that would affect the prevalence of rape, it does not seem unreasonable to continue to investigate the claim that men are collectively responsible for the prevalence of rape.

III. THE RAPIST AS VICTIM OF SOCIETY

It is also possible to acknowledge that men are responsible for the prevalence of rape in our society but nonetheless to argue that women are equally responsible. Rape is often portrayed as a sex crime perpetrated largely by men against women. But importantly, rape is also a crime of violence, and many factors in our society have increased the prevalence of violence. This prevalence of violence is the cause of both rape and war in Western societies. Our view, that violence of both sorts is increased in likelihood by patterns of male socialization which then creates collective male responsibility, may be countered by pointing out that socialization patterns are created by both men and women, thereby seemingly implicating both men and women in collective responsibility for rape and war.

Sam Keen has contended that it is violence that we should be focusing on rather than sex or gender, in order to understand the causes and remedies for the prevalence of rape. According to Keen,

> Men are violent because of the systematic violence done to their bodies and spirits. Being hurt they become hurters. In the overall picture, male violence toward women is far less than male violence toward other males . . . these outrages are a structural part of a warfare system that victimizes both men and women.[30]

Keen sees both men and women conspiring together to perpetuate this system of violence, especially in the way they impart to their male children an acceptance of violence.

Women are singled out by Keen as those who have not come to terms with their share of responsibility for our violent culture. And men have been so guilt-tripped on the issue of rape that they have become desensitized to it. Keen thinks that it is a mistake to single out men, and not women also, as responsible for rape.

> Until women are willing to weep for and accept equal responsibility for the systematic violence done to the male body and spirit by the war system, it is not likely that men will lose enough of their guilt and regain enough of their sensitivity to accept responsibility for women who are raped.[31]

Even though women are equally responsible for the rape culture, in Keen's view, women should be singled out because they have not previously accepted their share of responsibility for the creation of a violent society.

Keen is at least partially right insofar as he insists that issues of rape and war be understood as arising from the same source, namely the socialization of men to be violent in Western cultures. We agree with Keen that rape is part of a larger set of violent practices that injure both men and women. He is right to point out that men are murdering other men in our society in increasing numbers, and that this incidence of violence probably has something to do with the society's general condoning, even celebrating, of violence, especially in war.

Keen fails to note though that it is men, not women, who are the vast majority of both rapists and murderers in our society. And even if some women do act in ways which trigger violent reactions in men, nevertheless, in our opinion this pales in comparison with the way that men socialize each other to be open to violence. As Tiger and others have suggested, aggressive violence results primarily from male-bonding experiences. In any event, both fathers and mothers engage in early childhood socialization. Men influence the rape culture both through early childhood socialization and through male-bonding socialization of older male children. But women only contribute to this culture, when they do, through individual acts of early childhood socialization. For this reason Keen is surely wrong to think that women share responsibility *equally* with men for our rape culture.

In our view, some women could prevent some rapes; and some women do contribute to the patterns of socialization of both men and women that increase the incidence of rape. For these reasons, it would not be inappropriate to say that women share responsibility for rape as well as men. But we believe that it is a mistake to think that women share equally in this responsibility with men. For one thing, women are different from men in that they are, in general, made worse off by the prevalence of rape in our society. As we will next see, there is a sense in which men, but not women, benefit from the prevalence of rape, and this fact means that men have more of a stake in the rape culture, and hence have more to gain by its continued existence.

In general, our conclusion is that women share responsibility, but to a far lesser extent than men, for the prevalence of rape. We do not support those who try to "blame the victim" by holding women responsible for rape because of not taking adequate precautions, or dressing seductively, etc. Instead, the key for us is the role that women, as mothers, friends, and lovers, play in the overall process of male socialization that creates the rape culture. It should come as no surprise that few members of Western society can be relieved of responsibility for this rape culture given the overwhelming pervasiveness of that culture. But such considerations should not deter us from looking to men, first and foremost, as being collectively responsible for the prevalence of rape. The women who do contribute to aggressive male socialization do so as individuals; women have no involvement parallel to the male-bonding group.

IV. THE RAPIST AS GROUP MEMBER

Popular literature tends to portray the rapist as a demonic character, as the "Other." What we find interesting about the research of Thornhill and Thornhill is that it operates unwittingly to support the feminist slogan that "all men are rapists," that the rapist is not male "Other" but male "Self." What is so unsettling about the tens of thousands of rapes in Bosnia is the suggestion that what ordinary men have been doing is not significantly different from what the "sex-fiends" did. The thesis that men are adapted to be predisposed to be rapists, regardless of what else we think of the thesis, should give us pause and make us less rather than more likely to reject the feminist slogan. From this vantage point, the work of Tiger as well as Thornhill and Thornhill sets the stage for a serious reconsideration of the view that men are collectively responsible for rape.

There are two things that might be meant by saying that men are collectively responsible for the prevalence of rape in Western culture. First, seeing men as collectively responsible may mean that men as a group are responsible in that they form some sort of super-entity that causes, or at least supports, the prevalence of rape. When some feminists talk of "patriarchy," what they seem to mean is a kind of institution that operates through, but also behind, the backs of individual men to oppress women. Here it may be that men are collectively responsible for the prevalence of rape and yet no men are individually responsible. We call this *nondistributive collective responsibility* [italics added]. Second, seeing men as collectively responsible may mean that men form a group in which there are so many features that the members share in common, such as attitudes or dispositions to engage in harm, that what holds true for one man also holds true for all other men. Because of the common features of the members of the group of men, when one man is responsible for a particular harm, other men are implicated. Each member of the group has a share in the responsibility for a harm such as rape. We call this *distributive collective responsibility* [italics added].[32] In what follows we will criticize the first way of understanding men's collective responsibility, and offer reasons to support the second.

When collective responsibility is understood in the first (nondistributive) sense, this form of responsibility is assigned to those groups that have the capacity to act. Here there are two paradigmatic examples: the corporation and the mob.[33] The corporation has the kind of organizational structure that allows for the group to form intentions and carry out those intentions, almost as if the corporation were itself a person. Since men, qua men, are too amorphous a group to be able to act in an organized fashion, we will not be interested in whether they are collectively responsible in this way. But it may be that men can act in the way that mobs act, that is, not through a highly organized structure but through something such as like-mindedness. If there is enough commonality of belief, disposition, and interest of all men, or at least all men within a particular culture, then the group may be able to act just as a mob is able to respond to a commonly perceived enemy.

It is possible to think of patriarchy as the oppressive practices of men coordinated by the common interests of men, but not organized intentionally. It is also productive to think of rape as resulting from patriarchy. For if there is a "collective" that is supporting or creating the prevalence of rape it is not a highly organized one, since there is nothing like a corporation that intentionally plans the rape of women in Western culture. If the current Serbian army has engaged in the systematic and organized rape of Muslim women as a strategy of war, then this would be an example of nondistributive responsibility for rape. But the kind of oppression characterized by the prevalence of rape in most cultures appears to be systematic but not organized. How does this affect our understanding of whether men are collectively responsible for rape?

If patriarchy is understood merely as a system of coordination that operates behind the backs of individual men, then it may be that no single man is responsible for any harms that are caused by patriarchy. But if patriarchy is understood as something which is based on common interests, as well as common benefits, extended to all or most men in a particular culture, then it may be that men are collectively responsible for the harms of patriarchy in a way which distributes out to all men, making each man in a particular culture at least partially responsible for the harms attributable to patriarchy. This latter strategy is consistent with our own view of men's responsibility for rape. In the remainder of this essay we will offer support for this conceptualization of the collective responsibility of men for the prevalence of rape.

Our positive assessment, going beyond our criticism of the faulty responses in earlier sections of our paper, is that men in Western culture are collectively responsible in the distributive sense, that is, they each share responsibility, for the prevalence of rape in that culture. This claim rests on five points: (1) Insofar as most perpetrators of rape are men, then these men are responsible, in most cases, for the rapes they committed. (2) Insofar as some men, by the way they interact with other (especially younger) men, contribute to a climate in our society where rape is made more prevalent, then they are collaborators in the rape culture and for this reason share in responsibility for rapes committed in that culture. (3) Also, insofar as some men are not unlike the rapist, since they would be rapists if they had the opportunity to be placed into a situation where their inhibitions against rape were removed, then these men share responsibility with actual rapists for the harms of rape. (4) In addition, insofar as many other men could have prevented fellow men from raping, but did not act to prevent these actual rapes, then these men also share responsibility along with the rapists. (5) Finally, insofar as some men benefit from the existence of rape in our society, these men also share responsibility along with the rapists.

It seems to us unlikely that many, if any, men in our society fail to fit into one or another of these categories. Hence, we think that it is not unreasonable to say that men in our society are collectively responsible (in the distributive sense) for rape. We expect some male readers to respond as follows:

> I am adamantly opposed to rape, and though when I was younger I might have tolerated rape-conductive comments from friends of mine, I don't now, so I'm not a collaborator in the rape culture. And I would never be a rapist whatever the situation, and I would certainly act to prevent any rape that I could. I'm pretty sure I don't benefit from rape. So how can I be responsible for the prevalence of rape?

In reply we would point out that nearly all men in a given Western society meet the third and fifth conditions above (concerning similarity and benefit). But women generally fail to meet either of these conditions, or the first. So, the involvement of women in the rape culture is much less than is true for men. In what follows we will concentrate on these similarity and benefit issues.

In our discussion above, we questioned the view that rapists are "other." Diane Scully, in her study of convicted rapists, turns the view around, suggesting that it is women who are "other." She argues that rapists in America are not pathological; but instead that men who rape have something to tell us about the cultural roots of sexual violence. . . . They tell us that some men use rape as a means of revenge and punishment. Implicit in revenge rape is the collective liability of women. In some cases, victims are substitutes for significant women on whom men desire to take revenge. In other cases, victims represent all women. . . . In either case, women are seen as objects, a category, but not as individuals with rights. For some men, rape is an afterthought or bonus they add to burglary or robbery. In other words, rape is "no-big deal." . . . Some men rape in groups as a male bonding activity—for them it's just something to do. . . . Convicted rapists tell us that in this culture, sexual violence is rewarding . . . these men perceived rape as a rewarding, low-risk act.[34]

It is the prevalent perception of women as "other" by men in our culture that fuels the prevalence of rape in American society.

Turning to the issue of benefit, we believe that Lionel Tiger's work illustrates the important source of strength that men derive from the all-male groups they form. There is a strong sense in which men benefit from the all-male groups that they form in our culture. What is distinctly lacking is any sense that men have responsibility for the social conditions, especially the socialization of younger men, which diminishes inhibitions toward rape that are created in those groups. Male bonding is made easier because there is an "Other" that males can bond "against." And this other is the highly sexualized stereotype of the "female." Here is a benefit for men in these groups—but there is a social cost: from the evidence we have examined there is an increased' prevalence of rape. Men need to consider this in reviewing their own role in a culture that supports so much rape.

There is another sense in which benefit is related to the issue of responsibility for rape. There is a sense in which many men in our society benefit from the prevalence of rape in ways many of us are quite unaware. Consider this example:

> Several years ago, at a social occasion in which male and female professors were present, I asked off-handedly whether people agreed with me that the campus was looking especially pretty at night these days. Many of the men responded positively. But all of the women responded that this was not something that they had even thought about, since they were normally too anxious about being on campus at night, especially given the increase in reported rapes recently.[35]

We men benefited in that, relative to our female colleagues, we were in an advantageous position vis-à-vis travel around campus. And there were surely other comparative benefits that befell us as a result of this advantage concerning travel, such as our ability to gain academically by being able to use the library at any hour we chose.

In a larger sense, men benefit from the prevalence of rape in that many women are made to feel dependent on men for protection against potential rapists. It is hard to overestimate the benefit here for it potentially affects all aspects of one's life. One study found that 87 percent of women in a borough of London felt that they had to take precautions against potential rapists, with a large number reporting that they never went out at night alone.[36] Whenever one group is made to feel dependent on another group, and this dependency is not reciprocal, then there is a strong comparative benefit to the group that is not in the dependent position. Such a benefit, along with the specific benefits mentioned above, supports the view that men as a group have a stake in perpetuating the rape culture in ways that women do not. And just as the benefit to men distributes throughout the male population in a given society, so the responsibility should distribute as well.

V. CONCLUSIONS

When people respond to conflict with violence, they coerce one another and thereby fail to treat one another with respect as fellow autonomous beings. Rape and murder, especially in war, victimize members of various groups simply because they are group members. These two factors combine to create a form of dehumanization that can warrant the charge of being a crime against humanity. What makes an act of violence more than just a private individual act in wartime is that killing and rape are perpetrated not against the individual for his or her unique characteristics, but solely because the individual instantiates a group characteristic, for example, being Jewish, or Muslim, or being a woman. Such identification fails to respect what is unique about each of us.

Our point is not that all men everywhere are responsible for the prevalence of rape. Rather, we have been arguing that in Western societies, rape is deeply embedded in a wider culture of male socialization. Those who have the most to do with sustaining that culture must also recognize that they are responsible for the harmful aspects of that culture.[37] And when rape is conjoined with war, especially as an organized strategy, then there is a sense that men are collectively responsible for the rapes that occur in that war,[38] just as groups of people are held responsible for the crimes of genocide, where the victims are persecuted simply because they fall into a certain category of low-risk people who are ripe for assault.

Rape, especially in times of war, is an act of violence perpetrated against a person merely for being an instantiation of a type. Insofar as rape in times of war is a systematically organized form of terror, it is not inappropriate to call rape a war crime, a crime against humanity. Insofar as rape in times of peace is also part of a pattern of terror against women to the collective benefit of men, then rape in times of peace is also a crime against humanity.[39] Rape, in war or in peace, is rarely a personal act of aggression by one person toward another person. It is an act of hostility and a complete failure to show basic human respect.[40] And more than this, rape is made more likely by the collective actions, or inactions, of men in a particular society. Insofar as men in a particular society contribute to the prevalence of rape, they participate in a crime against humanity for which they are collectively responsible.

The feminist slogan "all men are rapists" seems much stronger than the claim "all men contribute to the prevalence of rape." Is the feminist slogan merely hyperbole? It is if what is meant is that each time a rape occurs, every man did it, or that only men are ever responsible for rape. But, as we have seen, each time a rape occurs, there is a sense in which many men could have done it, or made it less likely to have occurred, or benefited from it. By direct contribution, or by negligence or by similarity of disposition, or by benefiting, most (if not all) men do share in each rape in a particular society. This is the link between being responsible for the prevalence of rape and being responsible, at least to some extent, for the harms of each rape.

The purpose of these arguments has been to make men aware of the various ways that they are implicated in the rape culture in general as well as in particular rapes. And while we believe that men should feel some shame for their group's complicity in the prevalence of rape, our aim is not to shame men but rather to stimulate men to take responsibility for resocializing themselves and their fellow men. How much should any particular man do? Answering this question would require another paper, although participating in the Canadian White Ribbon Campaign, or in anti-sexism education programs, would be a good first step.[41] Suffice it to say that the status quo, namely doing nothing, individually or as a group, is not satisfactory, and will merely further compound our collective and shared responsibility for the harms caused by our fellow male members who engage in rape.[42]

NOTES

1. This paragraph is based on Larry May's experiences growing up in an upper-middle-class suburban US society. While our experiences differ somewhat in this respect, these experiences are so common that we have referred to them in the first person plural.

2. Tony Post et al., "A Pattern of Rape," *Newsweek*, January 4, 1993, pp. 32–36.

3. Susan Brownmiller, "Making Female Bodies the Battlefield," *Newsweek*, January 4, 1993, p. 37.

4. Catherine A. MacKinnon, "Turning Rape into Pornography: Postmodern Genocide," *Ms.*, July/August 1993, p. 30.

5. There is a fifth response, namely, that women alone are somehow responsible for being raped. This response will be largely ignored in our essay since we regard it as merely another case of "blaming the victim." See Diana Scully, *Understanding Sexual Violence* (Boston: Unwin Hyman, 1990) for a critical discussion of this response. Undoubtedly there are yet other responses. We have tried to focus our attention on the most common responses we have seen in the literature on rape.

6. Joyce Carol Oates, "Rape and the Boxing Ring," *Newsweek*, February 24, 1992, p. 60.

7. Ibid., p. 61.

8. *St. Louis Post-Dispatch*, March 27, 1992, p. 20A.

9. See Susan Griffin, "Rape: The All-American Crime," *Ramparts*, September 1971, pp. 26–35; reprinted in *Women and Values: Readings in Feminist Philosophy*, ed. Marilyn Pearsall (Belmont, CA: Wadsworth, 1986).

10. Oates, "Rape and the Boxing Ring," p. 61.

11. Robert Lipsyte, "An Ethics Trial: Must Boys Always Be Boys?" *New York Times*, March 12, 1993, p. B-11.

12. Post et al., "A Pattern of Rape," p. 32.

13. Cited in Griffin, "Rape: The All-American Crime," p. 178.

14. Cited in Scully, *Understanding Sexual Violence*, p. 75.

15. *Behavioral and Brain Sciences* 15 (1992): 36–75.

16. Ibid., p. 363.

17. Ibid., p. 366.

18. Ibid., p. 364.

19. Ibid., p. 416.

20. Ibid.

21. Ibid., p. 375.

22. Ibid., p. 407.

23. Lionel Tiger, *Men in Groups*, 2nd ed. (New York: Marion Boyars Publishers, 1984), pp. 158–59. (The first edition appeared in 1969.)

24. Ibid., p. 159.

25. Ibid.

26. Ibid., pp. 159–60.

27. Ibid., p. 81.

28. Ibid., p. 191.

29. Peggy Reeves Sanday, "Rape and the Silencing of the Feminine," in *Rape: An Historical and Social Enquiry*, ed. Sylvana Tomaselli and Roy Porter (Oxford: Basil Blackwell, 1986), p. 85; and Sanday, "Androcentric and Matrifocal Gender Representation in Minangkabau Ideology," in *Beyond the Second Sex*, ed. Peggy Reeves Sanday and Ruth Gallagher Goodenough (Philadelphia: University of Pennsylvania Press, 1990). See also Maria Lepowsky, "Gender in an Egalitarian Society," in *Beyond the Second Sex*.

30. Sam Keen, *Fire in the Belly* (New York: Bantam Books, 1991), p. 47.

31. Ibid.

32. Larry May, *The Morality of Groups*, chap. 2 (Notre Dame, IN: University of Notre Dame Press, 1987).

33. Ibid., chapters 2 and 4.

34. Scully, *Understanding Sexual Violence*, pp. 162–63.

35. In his fascinating study of the climate of rape in American culture, Timothy Beneke also reports as one of his conclusions that the fear of rape at night "inhibits the freedom of the eye, hurts women economically, undercuts women's independence, destroys solitude, and restricts expressiveness." Such curtailments of freedom, he argues, "must be acknowledged as part of the crime." Timothy Beneke, *Men on Rape* (New York: St. Martin's Press, 1982), p. 170.

36. See Jill Radford, "Policing Male Violence, Policing Women," in *Women, Violence, and Social Control*, ed. Valna Hammer and Mary Maynard (Atlantic Highlands, NJ: Humanities Press, 1987), p. 33.

37. Roy Porter, "Does Rape Have a Historical Meaning?" in *Rape: An Historical and Social Enquiry*, pp. 222–23.

38. The European Community's preliminary investigation into the reports of wide-spread Bosnian rapes of Muslim women by Serbian soldiers concluded that "Rape is part of a pattern of abuse, usually perpetrated with the conscious intention of demoralizing and terrorizing communities, driving them from their homes and demonstrating the power of the invading forces. Viewed in this way, rape cannot be seen as incidental to the main purpose of the aggression but as serving a strategic purpose in itself." *St. Louis Post-Dispatch*, January 9, 1993, p. 8A.

39. See Claudia Card, "Rape as a Terrorist Institution," in *Violence, Terrorism, and Justice*, ed. R. G. Frey and Christopher Morris (New York: Cambridge University Press, 1991).

40. See Carolyn M. Shafer and Marilyn Frye, "Rape and Respect, " in *Feminism and Philosophy*, ed. Mary Vetterling-Braggin, Frederick Elliston, and Jane English (Totowa, NJ: Littlefield Adams, 1977).

41. We would also recommend recent essays by philosophers who are trying to come to terms with their masculinity. See our essay on friendship as well as the essay by Hugh LaFollette in our anthology *Rethinking Masculinity*, ed. Larry May and Robert Strikwerda (Lanham, MD: Rowen & Littlefield, 1992).

42. We would like to thank Virginia Ingram, Jason Clevenger, Victoria Davion, Karen Warren, Duane Cady, and Marilyn Friedman for providing us with critical comments on earlier drafts of this essay.

37.

IS THERE A HISTORY OF SEXUALITY?

David M. Halperin

Sex has no history.[1] It is a natural fact, grounded in the functioning of the body, and, as such, it lies outside of history and culture. Sexuality, by contrast, does not properly refer to some aspect or attribute of bodies. Unlike sex, sexuality is a cultural production: it represents the *appropriation* of the human body and of its physiological capacities by an ideological discourse.[2] Sexuality is not a somatic fact; it is a cultural effect. Sexuality, then, does have a history—though (as I shall argue) not a very long one.

To say that, of course, is not to state the obvious—despite the tone of assurance with which I just said it—but to advance a controversial, suspiciously fashionable, and, perhaps, a strongly counterintuitive claim. The plausibility of such a claim might seem to rest on nothing more substantial than the prestige of the brilliant, pioneering, but largely theoretical work of the late French philosopher Michel Foucault.[3] According to Foucault, sexuality is not a thing, a natural fact, a fixed and immovable element in the eternal grammar of human subjectivity, but is instead a "set of effects produced in bodies, behaviors, and social relations by a certain deployment" of "a complex political technology."[4] "Sexuality," Foucault insists in another passage,

First published in *History and Theory* 28, no. 3 (1989). Reprinted by permission of the author.

must not be thought of as a kind of natural given which power tries to hold in check, or as an obscure domain which knowledge tries gradually to uncover. It is the name that can be given to a historical construct [*dispositif*]: not a furtive reality that is difficult to grasp, but a great surface network in which the stimulation of bodies, the intensification of pleasures, the incitement to discourse, the formation of special knowledges, the strengthening of controls and resistances, are linked to one another, in accordance with a few major strategies of knowledge and power.[5]

Is Foucault right? I believe he is, but I also believe that more is required to establish the historicity of sexuality than the mere weight of Foucault's authority. To be sure, a great deal of work, both conceptual and empirical, has already been done to sustain Foucault's central insights and to carry forward the historicist project that he did so much to advance.[6] But much more needs to be accomplished if we are to fill in the outlines of the picture that Foucault had time only to sketch—hastily and inadequately, as he was the first to admit[7]—and if we are to demonstrate that sexuality is indeed, as he claimed, a uniquely modern production.

The study of classical antiquity has a special role to play in this historical enterprise. The sheer interval of time separating the ancient from the modern world spans cultural changes of such magnitude that the contrasts to which they give rise cannot fail to strike anyone who is on the lookout for them. The student of classical antiquity is inevitably confronted in the ancient record by a radically unfamiliar set of values, behaviors, and social practices, by ways of organizing and articulating experience that challenge modern notions about what life is like, and that call into question the supposed universality of "human nature" as we currently understand it. Not only does this historical distance permit us to view ancient social and sexual conventions with particular sharpness; it also enables us to bring more clearly into focus the ideological dimension—the purely conventional and arbitrary character—of our own social and sexual experiences.[8] One of the currently unquestioned assumptions about sexual experience which the study of antiquity calls into question is the assumption that sexual behavior reflects or expresses an individual's "sexuality."

Now that would seem to be a relatively harmless and unproblematic assumption to make, empty of all ideological content, but what exactly do we have in mind when we make it? What, in particular, do we understand by our concept of "sexuality"? I think we understand "sexuality" to refer to a positive, distinct, and constitutive feature of the human personality, to the characterological seat within the individual of sexual acts, desires, and pleasures—the determinate source from which all sexual expression proceeds. "Sexuality" in this sense is not a purely descriptive term, a neutral representation of some objective state of affairs or a simple recognition of some familiar facts about us; rather, it is a distinctive way of constructing, organizing, and interpreting those "facts," and it performs quite a lot of conceptual work.

First of all, sexuality defines itself as a separate, sexual domain within the larger field of human psychophysical nature. Second, sexuality effects the conceptual demarcation and isolation of that domain from other areas of personal and social life that have traditionally cut across it, such as carnality, venery, libertinism, virility, passion, amorousness, eroticism, intimacy, love, affection, appetite, and desire—to name but a few of the older claimants to territories more recently staked out by sexuality. Finally, sexuality generates sexual identity: it endows each of us with an individual sexual nature, with a personal essence defined (at least in part) in specifically sexual terms; it implies that human beings are individuated at the level of their sexuality, that they differ from one another in their sexuality and, indeed, belong to different types or kinds of being by virtue of their sexuality.

These, at least, appear to me to be some of the significant ramifications of "sexuality," as it is currently conceptualized. I shall argue that the outlook it represents is alien to the recorded experience of the ancients. Two themes, in particular, that seem intrinsic to the modern conceptualization of sexuality but that hardly find an echo in ancient sources will provide the focus of my investigation: the autonomy of sexuality as a separate sphere of existence (deeply implicated in other areas of life, to be sure, but distinct from them and capable of acting on them at least as much as it is acted on by them), and the function of sexuality as a principle of individuation in human natures. In what follows, I shall take up each theme in turn, attempting to document in this fashion the extent of the divergence between ancient and modern varieties of sexual experience.

First, the autonomy of sexuality as a separate sphere of existence. The basic point I should like to make has already been made for me by Robert Padgug in a now-classic essay on conceptualizing sexuality in history. Padgug argues that

> what we consider "sexuality" was, in the pre-bourgeois world, a group of acts and institutions not necessarily linked to one another, or, if they were linked, combined in ways very different from our own. Intercourse, kinship, and the family, and gender, did not form anything like a "field" of sexuality. Rather, each group of sexual acts was connected directly or indirectly—that is, formed part of—institutions and thought patterns which we tend to view as political, economic, or social in nature, and the connections cut across our idea of sexuality as a thing, detachable from other things, and as a separate sphere of private existence.[9]

The ancient evidence amply supports Padgug's claim. In classical Athens, for example, sex did not express inward dispositions or inclinations so much as it served to position social actors in the places assigned to them, by virtue of their political standing, in the hierarchical structure of the Athenian polity. Let me expand this formulation.

In classical Athens a relatively small group made up of the adult male citizens held a virtual monopoly of social power and constituted a clearly defined elite within the political and social life of the city-state. The predominant feature of the social landscape of classical Athens was the great divide in status between this superordinate group, composed of citizens, and a subordinate group, composed of women, children, foreigners, and slaves—all of whom lacked full civil rights (though they were not all equally subordinate). Sexual relations not only respected that divide but were strictly polarized in conformity with it.

Sex is portrayed in Athenian documents not as a mutual enterprise in which two or more persons jointly engage but as an action performed by a social superior upon a social inferior. Consisting, as it was held to do, of an asymmetrical gesture—the penetration of the body of one person by the body (and, specifically, by the phallus)[10] of another—sex effectively divided and distributed its participants into radically distinct and incommensurable categories ("penetrator" versus "penetrated"), categories which in turn were wholly congruent with superordinate and subordinate social categories. For sexual penetration was thematized as domination: the relation between the insertive and the receptive sexual partner was taken to be the same kind of relation as that obtaining between social superior and social inferior.[11] Insertive and receptive sexual roles were therefore necessarily isomorphic with superordinate and subordinate social status; an adult male citizen of Athens could have legitimate sexual relations *only* with statutory minors (his inferiors not in age but in social and political status): the proper targets of his sexual desire included, specifically, women of any age, free males past the age of puberty who were not yet old enough to be citizens (I'll call them "boys," for short), as well as foreigners and slaves of either sex.[12]

Moreover, the physical act of sex between a citizen and a statutory minor was stylized in such a way as to mirror in the minute details of its hierarchical arrangement the relation of structured inequality that governed the wider social interaction of the two lovers. What an Athenian did in bed was determined by the differential in status that distinguished him or her from his or her sexual partner; the (male) citizen's superior prestige and authority expressed themselves in his sexual precedence—in his power to initiate a sexual act, his right to obtain pleasure from it, and his assumption of an insertive rather than a receptive sexual role. Different social actors had different sexual roles: to assimilate both the superordinate and the subordinate member of a sexual relationship to the same "sexuality" would have been as bizarre, in Athenian eyes, as classifying burglar as an "active criminal," his victim as a "passive criminal," and the two of them alike as partners in crime—it would have been to confuse what, in reality, were supposedly separate and distinct identities.[13] Each act of sex was no doubt an expression of real, personal desire on the part of the sexual actors involved, but their very desires had already been shaped by the shared cultural definition of sex as an activity that generally occurred only between a citizen and a noncitizen, between a person invested with full civil status and a statutory minor.

The "sexuality" of the classical Athenians, then, far from being independent of "politics" (each construed as an autonomous sphere) *was constituted by the very principles* on which Athenian public life was organized. In fact, the correspondences in classical Athens between sexual norms and social practices were so strict that an inquiry into Athenian "sexuality" *per se* would be nonsensical: such an inquiry could only obscure the phenomenon it was intended to elucidate, for it would conceal the sole context in which the sexual protocols of the classical Athenians make any sense—namely, the structure of the Athenian polity. The social articulation of sexual desire in classical Athens thus furnishes a telling illustration of the interdependence in culture of social practices and subjective experiences. Indeed, the classical Greek record strongly supports the conclusion drawn (from a quite different body, of evidence) by the French anthropologist Maurice Godelier: "it is not sexuality which haunts society, but society which haunts the body's sexuality."[14]

For those inhabitants of the ancient world about whom it is possible to generalize, sexuality did not hold the key to the secrets of the human personality. (In fact, the very concept of and set of practices centering on "the human personality"—the physical and social sciences of the blank individual—belong to a much later era and bespeak the modern social and economic conditions that accompanied their rise.) In the Hellenic world, by contrast, the measure of a free male was most often taken by observing how he fared when tested in public competition against other free males, not by scrutinizing his sexual constitution. War (and other agonistic contests), not love, served to reveal the inner man, the stuff a free Greek male was made of.[15] A striking instance of this emphasis on public life as the primary locus of signification can be found in the work of Artemidorus, a master dream-interpreter who lived and wrote in the second century of our era and whose testimony, there is good reason to believe, accurately represents the sexual norms of ancient Mediterranean culture.[16] Artemidorus saw public life, not erotic life, as the principal tenor of dreams. Even sexual dreams, in Artemidorus's system, are seldom *really* about sex: rather, they are about the rise and fall of the dreamer's public fortunes, the vicissitudes of his domestic economy.[17] If a man dreams of having sex with his mother, for example, his dream signifies to Artemidorus nothing in particular about the dreamer's own sexual psychology, his fantasy life, or the history of his relations with his parents;

it's a very common dream, and so it's a bit tricky to interpret precisely, but basically it's a lucky dream: it may signify—depending on the family's circumstances at the time, the postures of the partners in the dream, and the mode of penetration—that the dreamer will be successful in politics ("success" meaning, evidently, the power to screw one's country), that he will go into exile or return from exile, that he will win his lawsuit, obtain a rich harvest from his lands, or change professions, among many other things (1.79). Artemidorus's system of dream interpretation resembles the indigenous dream-lore of certain Amazonian tribes who, despite their quite different sociosexual systems, share with the ancient Greeks a belief in the predictive value of dreams. Like Artemidorus, these Amazonian peoples reverse what modern bourgeois Westerners take to be the natural flow of signification in dreams (from images of public and social events to private and sexual meanings): in both Kagwahiv and Mehinaku culture, for example, dreaming about the female genitalia portends a wound (and so a man who has such a dream is especially careful when he handles axes or other sharp instruments the next day); dreamt wounds do not symbolize the female genitalia.[18] Both these ancient and modern dream-interpreters, then, are innocent of "sexuality": what is fundamental to their experience of sex is not anything we would regard as essentially sexual;[19] it is instead something essentially outward, public, and social. "Sexuality," for cultures not shaped by some very recent European and American bourgeois developments, is not a cause but an effect. The social body precedes the sexual body.

* * *

I now come to the second of my two themes—namely, the individuating function of sexuality, its role in generating individual sexual identities. The connection between the modern interpretation of sexuality as an autonomous domain and the modern construction of individual sexual identities has been well analyzed, once again, by Robert Padgug:

> the most commonly held twentieth-century assumptions about sexuality imply that it is a separate category of existence (like "the economy," or "the state," other supposedly independent spheres of reality), almost identical with the sphere of private life. Such a view necessitates the location of sexuality within the individual as a fixed essence, leading to a classic division of individual and society and to a variety of psychological determinisms, and, often enough, to a full-blown biological determinism as well. These in turn involve the enshrinement of contemporary sexual categories as universal, static, and permanent, suitable for the analysis of all human beings and all societies.[20]

The study of ancient Mediterranean societies clearly exposes the defects in any such essentialist conceptualization of sexuality. Because, as we have seen in the case of classical Athens, erotic desires and sexual object-choices in antiquity were generally not determined by a typology of anatomical sexes (male versus female), but rather by the social articulation of power (superordinate versus subordinate), the currently fashionable distinction between homosexuality and heterosexuality (and, similarly, between "homosexuals" and "heterosexuals" as individual types) had no meaning for the classical Athenians: there were not, so far as they knew, two different kinds of "sexuality," two differently structured psychosexual states or modes of affective orientation, but a single form of sexual experience which all free adult males shared—making due allowance for variations in individual tastes, as one might make for individual palates.[21]

Thus, in the Third Dithyramb by the classical poet Bacchylides, the Athenian hero Theseus, voyaging to Crete among the seven youths and seven maidens destined for the Minotaur and defending one of the maidens from the advances of the libidinous Cretan commander, warns him vehemently against molesting *any one* of the Athenian youths (*tin' ëitheon*: 43)—that is, any girl *or boy*. Conversely, the antiquarian *littérateur* Athenaeus, writing six or seven hundred years later, is amazed that Polycrates, the tyrant of Samos in the sixth century BCE, did not send for any boys *or women* along with the other luxury articles he imported to Samos for his personal use during his reign, "despite his passion for relations with males" (12.540c–e).[22] Now *both* the notion that an act of heterosexual aggression in itself makes the aggressor suspect of homosexual tendencies *and* the mirror-opposite notion that a person with marked homosexual tendencies is bound to hanker after heterosexual contacts are nonsensical to us, associating as we do sexual object-choice with a determinate kind of "sexuality," a fixed sexual nature, but it would be a monumental task indeed to enumerate all the ancient documents in which the alternative "boy or woman" occurs with perfect nonchalance in an erotic context, as if the two were functionally interchangeable.[23]

A particularly striking testimony to the imaginable extent of male indifference to the sex of sexual objects can be found in a marriage-contract from Hellenistic Egypt dating to 92 BCE .[24] This not-untypical document stipulates that "it shall not be lawful for Philiscus [the prospective husband] to bring home another wife in addition to Apollonia or to have a concubine *or boy-lover. . . .*"[25] The possibility that one's husband might take it into his head at some point during one's marriage to set up another household with his boyfriend evidently figured among the various potential domestic disasters that a prudent fiancée would be sure to anticipate and to indemnify herself against. A somewhat similar expectation is articulated in an entirely different context by Dio Chrysostom, a moralizing Greek orator from the late first century CE. In a speech denouncing the corrupt morals of city life, Dio asserts that even respectable women are so easy to seduce nowadays that men will soon tire of them and will turn their attention to boys instead, just as addicts progress inexorably from wine to hard drugs (7.150–152). According to Dio, then, pederasty is not simply a second best; it is not "caused," as many modern historians of the ancient Mediterranean appear to believe, by the supposed seclusion of women, by the practice (it was more likely an ideal) of locking them away in the inner rooms of their fathers' or husbands' houses and thereby preventing them from serving as sexual targets for adult men. In Dio's fantasy, at least, pederasty springs not from the insufficient but from the superabundant supply of sexually available women; the easier it is to have sex with women, on his view, the less desirable sex with women becomes, and the more likely men are to seek sexual pleasure with boys. Scholars sometimes describe the cultural formation underlying this apparent refusal by Greek males to discriminate categorically among sexual objects on the basis of anatomical sex as a bisexuality of penetration[26] or—even more intriguingly—as a heterosexuality indifferent to its object,[27] but I think it would be advisable not to speak of it as a sexuality at all but to describe it, rather, as a more generalized ethos of penetration and domination,[28] a socio-sexual discourse structured by the presence or absence of its central term: the phallus.[29] It may be worth pausing now to examine one text in particular which clearly indicates how thoroughly ancient cultures were able to dispense with the notion of sexual identity.

The document in question is the ninth chapter in the Fourth Book of the *De morbis chronicis*, a mid-fifth-century CE. Latin translation and adaptation by the African writer Caelius Aurelianus of a now largely lost work on chronic diseases by the Greek physician Soranus, who practiced and taught in Rome during the early part of the second century CE. Caelius's work is not much read nowadays, and it is almost entirely neglected by modern historians of "sexuality";[30] its date is late, its text is corrupt, and, far from being a self-conscious literary artifact, it belongs to the despised genre of Roman technical writing. But, despite all these drawbacks, it repays close attention, and I have chosen to discuss it here partly in order to show what can be learned about the ancient world from works that lie outside the received canon of classical authors.

The topic of this passage is *molles* (*malthakoi* in Greek)—that is, "soft" or unmasculine men, men who depart from the cultural norm of manliness insofar as they actively desire to be subjected by other men to a "feminine" (that is, receptive) role in sexual intercourse.[31] Caelius begins with an implicit defense of his own unimpeachable masculinity by noting how difficult it is to believe that such people actually exist;[32] he then goes on to observe that the cause of their affliction is not natural (that is, organic) but is rather their own excessive desire, which—in a desperate and foredoomed attempt to satisfy itself—drives out their sense of shame and forcibly converts parts of their bodies to sexual uses not intended by nature. These men willingly adopt the dress, gait, and other characteristics of women, thereby confirming that they suffer not from a bodily disease but from a mental (or moral) defect. After some further arguments in support of that point, Caelius draws an interesting comparison: "For just as the women called *tribades* [in Greek], because they practice both kinds of sex, are more eager to have sexual intercourse with women than with men and pursue women with an almost masculine jealousy . . . so they too [i.e., the *molles*] are afflicted by a mental disease" (132–33). The mental disease in question, which strikes both men and women alike and seems to be defined as a perversion of sexual desire, would certainly appear to be nothing other than homosexuality as it is often understood today.

Several considerations combine to prohibit that interpretation, however. First of all, what Caelius treats as a pathological phenomenon is not the desire on the part of either men or women for sexual contact with a person of the same sex; quite the contrary: elsewhere, in discussing the treatment of satyriasis (a state of abnormally elevated sexual desire accompanied by itching or tension in the genitals), he issues the following advice to those who suffer from it (*De morbis acutis*, 3.18.180–81).[33]

> Do not admit visitors and particularly young women and boys. For the attractiveness of such visitors would again kindle the feeling of desire in the patient. Indeed, *even healthy persons*, seeing them, would in many cases seek sexual gratification, stimulated by the tension produced in the parts [i.e., in their own genitals].[34]

There is nothing medically problematical, then, about a desire on the part of males to obtain sexual pleasure from contact with males—so long as the proper phallocentric protocols are observed; what is of concern to Caelius,[35] as well as to other ancient moralists,[36] is the male desire to be sexually penetrated by males, for such a desire represents a voluntary abandonment of the culturally constructed masculine identity in favor of the culturally constructed feminine one. It is sex-role reversal, or gender-deviance, that is problematized here and that also furnishes part of the basis for Caelius's comparison of unmasculine men to masculine women, who assume a supposedly masculine role in their relations with other women and actively "pursue women with an almost *masculine* jealousy."

Moreover, the ground of the similitude between these male and female gender-deviants is not that they are both homosexual but rather that they are both bisexual (in our terms), although in that respect at least they do not depart from the ancient sexual norm. The tribads "are [*relatively*] more eager to have sexual intercourse with women *than with men*" and "practice both kind of sex"—that is, they have sex with both men and women.[37] As for the *molles*, Caelius's earlier remarks about their extraordinarily intense sexual desire implies that they turn to receptive sex because, although they try, they are not able to satisfy themselves by means of more conventionally masculine sorts of sexual activity, including insertive sex with women.[38] Far from having desires that are structured differently from those of normal folk, these gender-deviants desire sexual pleasure just as most people do, but they have such strong and intense desires that they are driven to devise some unusual and disreputable (though ultimately futile) ways of gratifying them. This diagnosis becomes explicit at the conclusion of the chapter when Caelius explains why the disease responsible for turning men into *molles* is the only chronic disease that becomes stronger as the body grows older.

> For in other years when the body is still strong and can perform the normal functions of love, the sexual desire [of these persons] assumes a dual aspect, in which the soul is excited sometimes while playing a passive and sometimes while playing an active role. But in the case of old men who have lost their virile powers, all their sexual desire is turned in the opposite direction and consequently exerts a stronger demand for the feminine role in love. In fact, many infer that this is the reason why boys too are victims of this affliction. For, like old men, they do not possess virile powers; that is, they have not yet attained those powers which have already deserted the aged. [137][39]

"Soft" or unmasculine men, far from being a fixed and determinate sexual species with a specifically sexual identity, are evidently either men who once experienced an orthodoxly masculine sexual desire in the past or who will eventually experience such a desire in the future. They may well be men with a constitutional tendency to gender-deviance, according to Caelius, but they are not homosexuals: being a womanish man, or a mannish woman, after all, is not the same thing as being a homosexual. Furthermore, all the other ancient texts known to me, which assimilate both males who enjoy sexual contact with males and females who enjoy sexual contact with females to the same category, do so—in conformity with the two taxonomic strategies employed by Caelius Aurelianus—either because such males and females both *reverse* their proper sex-roles and adopt the sexual styles, postures, and modes of copulation conventionally associated with the opposite gender, or because they both *alternate* between the personal characteristics and sexual practices proper, respectively, to men and to women.[40]

Caelius's testimony makes an important historical point. Before the scientific construction of "sexuality" as a positive, distinct, and constitutive feature of individual human beings—an autonomous system within the physiological and psychological economy of the human organism—certain kinds of sexual *acts* could be individually evaluated and categorized, and so could certain sexual tastes or inclinations, but there was no conceptual apparatus available for identifying a person's fixed and determinate sexual *orientation*, much less for assessing and classifying it.[41] That human beings differ, often markedly, from one another in their sexual tastes in a great variety of ways (including sexual object-choice), is an unexceptionable and, indeed, an ancient observation[42]: Plato's Aristophanes invents a myth to explain why some men like women, why some men like boys, why some women like men, and why some women like women (*Symposium* 189c–193d). But it is not immediately evident that patterns of sexual object-choice are by their very nature more revealing about the temperament of individual human beings, more significant determinants of personal *identity*, than, for example, patterns of dietary object-choice.[43] And yet, it would never occur to us to refer a person's dietary preference to some innate, characterological disposition,[44] to see in his or her strongly expressed and even unvarying preference for the white meat of chicken the symptom of a profound psychophysical orientation, leading us to identify him or her in contexts quite removed from that of the eating of food as, say, a "pectoriphage" or a "stethovore"; nor would we be likely to inquire further, making nicer discriminations according to whether an individual's predilection for chicken breasts expressed itself in a tendency to eat them quickly, or slowly, seldom or often, alone or in company, under normal circumstances or only in periods of great stress, with a clear or a guilty conscience ("ego-dystonic pectoriphagia"), beginning in earliest childhood or originating with a gastronomic trauma suffered in adolescence. If such questions did occur to us, moreover, I very much doubt whether we would turn to the academic disciplines of anatomy, neurology, clinical psychology, genetics, or sociobiology in the hope of obtaining a clear causal solution to them. That is because (1) we regard the liking for certain foods as a matter of taste; (2) we currently lack a theory of taste; and (3) in the absence of a theory we do not normally subject our behavior to intense, scientific or aetiological, scrutiny.

In the same way, it never occurred to the ancients to ascribe a person's sexual tastes to some positive, structural, or constitutive sexual feature of his or her personality. Just as we tend to assume that human beings are not individuated at the level of dietary preference and that we all, despite many pronounced and frankly acknowledged differences from one another in dietary habits, share the same fundamental set of alimentary appetites, and hence the same "dieticity" or "edility," so most premodern and non-Western cultures, despite an awareness of the range of possible variations in human sexual behavior, refuse to individuate human beings at the level of sexual preference and assume, instead, that we all share the same fundamental set of sexual appetites, the same "sexuality." For most of the world's inhabitants, in other words, "sexuality" is no more a "fact of life" than "dieticity." Far from being a necessary or intrinsic constituent of human life, "sexuality" seems indeed to be a uniquely modern, Western, even bourgeois production—one of those cultural fictions which in every society give human beings access to themselves as meaningful actors in their world, and which are thereby objectivated.

If there is a lesson that we should draw from this picture of ancient sexual attitudes and behaviors, it is that we need to de-center *sexuality* from the focus of the cultural interpretation of sexual experience—and not only ancient varieties of sexual experience. Just because modern bourgeois Westerners are so obsessed with sexuality, so convinced that it holds the key to the hermeneutics of the self (and hence to social psychology as an object of historical study), we ought not therefore to conclude that everyone has always considered sexuality a basic and irreducible element in, or a central feature of, human life. Indeed, there are even sectors of our own societies to which the ideology of "sexuality" has failed to penetrate. A socio-sexual system that coincides with the Greek system, insofar as it features a rigid hierarchy of sexual roles based on a set of socially articulated power-relations, has been documented in contemporary America by Jack Abbott, in one of his infamous letters written to Norman Mailer from a federal penitentiary; because the text is now quite inaccessible (it was not reprinted in Abbott's book), and stunningly apropos, I have decided to quote it here at length.

> It really was years, many years, before I began to actually realize that the women in my life—the prostitutes as well as the soft, pretty girls who giggled and teased me so much, my several wives and those of my friends—it was years before I realized that they were not women, but men; years before I assimilated the notion that this was unnatural. I still only know this intellectually, for the most part—but for the small part that remains to my ken, I know it is like a hammer blow to my temple and the shame I feel is profound. Not because of the thing itself, the sexual love I have enjoyed with these women (some so devoted it aches to recall it), but because of shame—and anger—that the world could so intimately betray me; so profoundly touch and move me—and then laugh at me and accuse my soul of a sickness, when that sickness has rescued me from mental derangement and despairs so black as to cast this night that surrounds us in prison into day. I do not mean to say I never knew the physical difference—no one but an imbecile could make such a claim. I took it, without reflection or the slightest doubt, that this was a natural sex that emerged within the society of men, with attributes that naturally complemented masculine attributes. I thought it was a natural phenomenon in the society of women as well. The attributes were feminine and so there seemed no gross misrepresentation of facts to call them (among us men) "women." . . . Many of my "women" had merely the appearance of handsome, extremely neat, and polite young men. I

have learned, analyzing my feelings today, that those attributes I called feminine a moment ago were not feminine in any way as it appears in the real female sex. These attributes seem now merely a tendency to need, to depend on another man; to need never to become a rival or to compete with other men in the pursuits men, among themselves, engage in. It was, it occurs to me now, almost boyish—not really feminine at all.

This is the way it always was, even in the State Industrial School for Boys—a penal institution for juvenile delinquents—where I served five years, from age twelve to age seventeen. They were the possession and sign of manhood and it never occurred to any of us that this was strange and unnatural. It is how I grew up—a natural part of my life in prison.

It was difficult for me to grasp the definition of the clinical term "homosexual"—and when I finally did it devastated me, as I said.[45]

Abbott's society surpasses classical Athenian society in the extent to which power relations are gendered. Instead of the Greek system which preserves the distinction between males and females but overrides it when articulating categories of the desirable and undesirable in favor of a distinction between dominant and submissive persons, the system described by Abbott wholly assimilates categories of socio-sexual identity to categories of gender identity—in order, no doubt, to preserve the association in Abbott's world between "masculinity" and the love of "women." What determines gender, for Abbott, is not anatomical sex but social status and personal style. "Men" are defined as those who "compete with other men in the pursuits men, among themselves, engage in," whereas "women" are characterized by the possession of "attributes that naturally complement masculine attributes"—namely, a "tendency to need, to depend on another man" for the various benefits won by the victors in "male" competition. In this way "a natural sex emerges within the society of men" and qualifies, by virtue of its exclusion from the domain of "male" precedence and autonomy, as a legitimate target of "male" desire.

The salient features of Abbott's society are uncannily reminiscent of those features of classical Athenian society with which we are already familiar. Most notable is the division of the society into superordinate and subordinate groups and *the production of desire* for members of the subordinate group in members of the superordinate one. Desire is sparked in this system, as in classical Athens, only when it arcs across the political divide, only when it traverses the boundary that marks out the limits of intramural competition among the elite and that thereby distinguishes subjects from objects of sexual desire. Sex between "men"—and, therefore, "homosexuality"—remains unthinkable in Abbott's society (even though sex between anatomical males is an accepted and intrinsic part of the system), just as sex between citizens, between members of the empowered social caste, is practically inconceivable in classical Athenian society.

Similarly, sex between "men" and "women" in Abbott's world is not a private experience in which social identities are lost or submerged; rather, in Abbott's society as in classical Athens, the act of sex—instead of implicating both sexual partners in a common "sexuality"—helps to articulate, to define, and to actualize the differences in status between them.

To discover and to write the history of sexuality has long seemed to many a sufficiently radical undertaking in itself, inasmuch as its effect (if not always the intention behind it) is to call into question the very naturalness of what we currently take to be essential to our individual natures. But in the course of implementing that ostensibly radical project many historians of sexuality seem to have reversed—perhaps unwittingly—its radical design: by preserving "sexuality" as a stable category of historical analysis not only have they not denaturalized it but, on the contrary, they have newly idealized it.[46] To the extent, in fact, that histories of "sexuality" succeed in concerning themselves with *sexuality*, to just that extent are they doomed to fail as *histories* (Foucault himself taught us that much), unless they also include as an essential part of their proper enterprise the task of demonstrating the historicity, conditions of emergence, modes of construction, and ideological contingencies of the very categories of analysis that undergird their own practice.[47] Instead of concentrating our attention specifically on the history of sexuality, then, we need to define and refine a new, and radical, historical sociology of psychology, an intellectual discipline designed to analyze the cultural poetics of desire, by which I mean the processes whereby sexual desires are constructed, mass-produced, and distributed among the various members of human living-groups.[48] We must train ourselves to recognize conventions of feeling as well as conventions of behavior and to interpret the intricate texture of personal life as an artifact, as the determinate outcome, of a complex and arbitrary constellation of cultural processes. We must, in short, be willing to admit that what seem to be our most inward, authentic, and private experiences are actually, in Adrienne Rich's admirable phrase, "shared, unnecessary and political."[49]

A little less than fifty years ago W. H. Auden asked, in the opening lines of a canzone, "When shall we learn, what should be clear as day, We cannot choose what we are free to love?"[50] It is a characteristically judicious formulation: love, if it is to be love, must be a free act, but it is also inscribed within a larger circle of constraint, within conditions that make possible the exercise of that "freedom." The task of distinguishing freedom from constraint in love, of learning to trace the shifting and uncertain boundaries between the self and the world, is a dizzying and, indeed, an endless undertaking. If I have not significantly advanced this project here, I hope at least to have encouraged others not to abandon it.

NOTES

1. Or, if it does, that history is a matter for the evolutionary biologist, not for the historian; see Lynn Margulis and Dorion Sagan, *The Origins of Sex* (New Haven, CT: Yale University Press, 1985).

2. I adapt this formulation from a passage in Louis Adrian Montrose, "'Shaping Fantasies': Figurations of Gender and Power in Elizabethan Culture," *Representations* 2 (1983): 61–94 (passage on p. 62), which describes in turn the concept of the "sex/gender system" introduced by Gayle Rubin, "The Traffic in Women: Notes on the 'Political Economy' of Sex." In *Toward an Anthropology of Women*, ed. Rayna R. Reiter (New York, 1975), pp. 157–210.

3. Volumes Two and Three of Foucault's *History of Sexuality*, published shortly before his death, depart significantly from the theoretical orientation of his earlier work in favor of a more concrete interpretative practice; see my remarks in "No Views of Greek Love: Harald Patzer and Michel Foucault," *One Hundred Years of Homosexuality*, pp. 62–71, esp. p. 64.

4. Michel Foucault, *The History of Sexuality, Volume I: An Introduction*, trans. Robert Hurley (New York, 1978), p. 127. See Teresa de Lauretis, *Technologies of Gender: Essays on Theory, Film, and Fiction* (Bloomington: Indiana University Press, 1987), pp. 1–30, esp. p. 3, who extends Foucault's critique of sexuality to gender.

5. Foucault, *The History of Sexuality*, pp. 105–106.

6. Of special relevance are: Robert A. Padgug, "Sexual Matters: On Conceptualizing Sexuality in History," *Radical History Review* 20 (1979): 3–23; George Chauncey Jr., "From Sexual Inversion to Homosexuality: Medicine and the Changing Conceptualization of Female Deviance," in *Homosexuality: Sacrilege, Vision, Politics*, ed. Robert Boyers and George Steiner, *Salmagundi* 58–59 (1982–1983): 114–46; Arnold I. Davidson, "Sex and the Emergence of Sexuality," *Critical Inquiry* 14 (1987–1988): 16–48. See also *The Cultural Construction of Sexuality*, ed. Pat Caplan (London, 1987); T. Dunbar Moodie, "Migrancy and Male Sexuality on the South African Gold Mines," *Journal of Southern African Studies* 14 (1987–1988): 228–56; George Chauncey Jr., "Christian Brotherhood or Sexual Perversion? Homosexual Identities and the Construction of Sexual Boundaries in the World War One Era," *Journal of Social History* 19 (1985–1986): 189–211.

7. E.g., Michel Foucault, *The Use of Pleasure. The History of Sexuality*, vol. 2, trans. Robert Hurley (New York, 1985), pp. 92, 253.

8. In applying the term "ideological" to sexual experience, I have been influenced by the formulation of Stuart Hall, "Culture, the Media, and the 'Ideological Effect,'" in *Mass Communication and Society*, ed. James Curran, Michael Gurevitch, Janet Woolacott, et al. (London, 1977), pp. 315–48, esp. p. 330: "ideology as *a social practice* consists of the 'subject' positioning himself in the specific complex, the objectivated field of discourses and codes which are available to him in language and culture at a particular historical conjuncture" (quoted by Ken Tucker and Andrew Treno, "The Culture of Narcissism and the Critical Tradition: An Interpretative Essay," *Berkeley Journal of Sociology* 25 [1980]: 341–55 [quotation on p. 351]); see also Hall's trenchant discussion of the constitutive role

510   PHILOSOPHY AND SEX

of ideology in "Deviance, Politics, and the Media," in *Deviance and Social Control*, ed. Paul Rock and Mary McIntosh, Explorations in Sociology 3 (London, 1974), pp. 261–305.

9. Padgug, "Sexual Matters," p. 16.

10. I say "phallus" rather than "penis" because (1) what qualifies as a phallus in this discursive system does not always turn out to be a penis (see note 29, below) and (2) even when phallus and penis have the same extension, or reference, they still do not have the same intension, or meaning: "phallus" betokens not a specific item of the male anatomy *simpliciter* but that same item *taken under the description* of a cultural signifier; (3) hence, the meaning of "phallus" is ultimately determined by its function in the larger sociosexual discourse; i.e., it is that which penetrates, that which enables its possessor to play an "active" sexual role, and so forth: see Rubin, "The Traffic in Women," pp. 190–92.

11. Foucault, *The Use of Pleasure*, p. 215, puts it very well: "sexual relations—always conceived in terms of the model act of penetration, assuming a polarity that opposed activity and passivity—were seen as being of the same type as the relationship between a superior and a subordinate, an individual who dominates and one who is dominated, one who commands and one who complies, one who vanquishes and one who is vanquished."

12. In order to avoid misunderstanding, I should emphasize that by calling all persons belonging to these four groups "statutory minors," I do not wish either to suggest that they enjoyed the *same* status as one another or to obscure the many differences in status that could obtain between members of a single group—e.g., between a wife and a courtesan—differences that may not have been perfectly isomorphic with the legitimate modes of their sexual use. Nonetheless, what is striking about Athenian social usage is the tendency to collapse such distinctions as did indeed obtain between different categories of social subordinates and to create a simple opposition between them all, *en masse*, and the class of adult male citizens: on this point, see Mark Golden, "*Pais*, 'Child' and 'Slave,'" *L'Antiquité classique* 54 (1985): 91–104, esp. pp. 101 and 102, n. 38.

13. I have borrowed this analogy from Arno Schmitt, who uses it to convey what the modern sexual categories would look like from a traditional Islamic perspective: see Gianni De Martino and Arno Schmitt, *Kleine Schriften zu zwischenmännlicher Sexualität und Erotik in der muslimischen Gesellschaft* (Berlin, 1985), p. 19. Note that even the category of anatomical sex, defined in such a way as to include both men and women, seems to be absent from Greek thought for similar reasons: the complementarity of men and women as sexual partners implies to the Greeks a polarity, a difference in species, too extreme to be bridged by a single sexual concept equally applicable to each. In Greek medical writings, therefore, "the notion of sex never gets formalized as a functional identity of male and female, but is expressed solely through the representation of asymmetry and of complementarity between male and female, indicated constantly by abstract adjectives (*to thêly* ['the feminine'], *to arren* ['the masculine'])," according to Paola Manuli, "Donne mascoline, femmine sterili, vergini perpetue: La ginecologia greca tra Ippocrate e Sorano," in Silvia Campese, Paola Manuli, and Giulia Sissa, *Madre materia: Sociologia e biologia della donna greca* (Turin, 1983), pp. 147–92, esp. pp. 151 and 201n.

14. Maurice Godelier, "The Origins of Male Domination," *New Left Review* 127 (May/June 1981): 3–17 (quotation on p. 17); cf. Maurice Godelier, "Le sexe comme fondement ultime de l'ordre social et cosmique chez les Baruya de Nouvelle—Guinée.

Mythe et realite," in *Sexualité et pouvoir*, ed. Armando Verdiglione (Paris, 1976), pp. 268–306, esp. pp. 295–96.

15. I am indebted for this observation to Professor Peter M. Smith of the University of North Carolina at Chapel Hill, who notes that Sappho and Plato are the chief exceptions to this general rule.

16. See John J. Winkler, "Unnatural Acts: Erotic Protocols in Artemidoros' *Dream Analysis*," *Constraints of Desire: The Anthropology of Sex and Gender in Ancient Greece* (New York, 1989), pp. 17–44, 221–24.

17. S. R. F. Price, "The Future of Dreams: From Freud to Artemidorus," *Past and Present* 113 (November 1986): 3–37, abridged in *Before Sexuality: The Construction of Erotic Experience in the Ancient Greek World*, ed. David M. Halperin, John J. Winkler, and Froma I. Zeitlin (Princeton, NJ: Princeton University Press, 1990), pp. 365–87; see also Michel Foucault, *The Care of the Self, The History of Sexuality*, vol. 3, trans. Robert Hurley (New York, 1986), pp. 3–36, esp. pp. 26–34.

18. See Waud H. Kracke, "Dreaming in Kagwahiv: Dream Beliefs and Their Psychic Uses in an Amazonian Indian Culture," *Psychoanalytic Study of Society* 8 (1979): 119–71, esp. pp. 130–32, 163 (on the predictive value of dreams) and pp. 130–31, 142–45, 163–64, 168 (on the reversal of the Freudian direction of signification—which Kracke takes to be a culturally constituted defense mechanism and which he accordingly undervalues); Thomas Gregor, "'Far, Far Away My Shadow Wandered . . .': The Dream Symbolism and Dream Theories of the Mehinaku Indians of Brazil," *American Ethnologist* 8 (1981): 709–20, esp. pp. 712–13 (on predictive value) and 714 (on the reversal of signification), largely recapitulated in Thomas Gregor, *Anxious Pleasures: The Sexual Lives of an Amazonian People* (Chicago, 1985), pp. 152–61, esp. p. 153. Foucault's comments on Artemidorus, in *The Care of the Self*, pp. 35–36, are relevant here: "The movement of analysis and the procedures of valuation do not go from the act to a domain such as sexuality or the flesh, a domain whose divine, civil, or natural laws would delineate the permitted forms; they go from the subject as a sexual actor to the other areas of life in which he pursues his [familial, social, and economic] activity. And it is in the relationship between these different forms of activity that the principles of evaluation of a sexual behavior are essentially, but not exclusively, situated."

19. Note that even the human genitals themselves do not necessarily figure as sexual signifiers in all cultural or representational contexts: for example, Caroline Walker Bynum, "The Body of Christ in the Later Middle Ages: A Reply to Leo Steinberg," *Renaissance Quarterly* 39 (1986): 399–439, argues in considerable detail that there is "reason to think that medieval people saw Christ's penis not primarily as a sexual organ but as the object of circumcision and therefore as the wounded, bleeding flesh with which it was associated in painting and in text" (p. 407).

20. Padgug, "Sexual Matters," p. 8.

21. Paul Veyne, in "La famille et l'amour sous le Haut-Empire romain," *Annales* (E. S. C.) 33 (1978): 35–63, remarks (p. 50) that Seneca's *Phaedra* is the earliest text to associate homosexual inclinations with a distinct type of subjectivity. The question is more complex than that, however, and a thorough exploration of it would require scrutinizing more closely the ancient figure of the *kinaidos*, a now-defunct sexual life-form:

for details, see Maud W. Gleason, "The Semiotics of Gender: Physiognomy and Self-Fashioning in the Second Century C.E.," in *Before Sexuality*, pp. 389–415; John J. Winkler, "Laying Down the Law: The Oversight of Men's Sexual Behavior in Classical Athens," *Constraints of Desire*, pp. 45–70, 224–26.

22. See Padgug, "Sexual Matters," 3, who mistakenly ascribes Athenaeus's comment to Alexis of Samos (Jacoby, *Fragmente der griechischen Historiker* 539, fr. 2).

23. See K. J. Dover, *Greek Homosexuality* (London, 1978), pp. 63–67, for an extensive, but admittedly partial, list; also, Robert Parker, *Miasma: Pollution and Purification in Early Greek Religion* (Oxford, 1983), p. 94. For some Roman examples, see T. Wade Richardson, "Homosexuality in the Satyricon," *Classica et Mediaevalia* 35 (1984): 105–27, esp. p. 111.

24. I wish to emphasize that I am *not* claiming that all Greek men must have felt such indifference: on the contrary, plenty of ancient evidence testifies to the strength of individual preferences for a sexual object of one sex rather than another (see note 42, below). But many ancient documents bear witness to a certain constitutional reluctance on the part of the Greeks to predict, in any given instance, the sex of another man's beloved merely on the basis of that man's past sexual behavior or previous pattern of sexual object-choice.

25. *P. Tebtunis* I 104, translated by A. S. Hunt and C. C. Edgar, in *Women's Life in Greece and Rome*, ed. Mary Lefkowitz and Maureen B. Fant (Baltimore, 1982), pp. 59–60; another translation is provided, along with a helpful discussion of the document and its typicality, by Sarah B. Pomeroy, *Women in Hellenistic Egypt from Alexander to Cleopatra* (New York, 1984), pp. 87–89.

26. "Une bisexualité de sabrage": Veyne, 50–55; see the critique by Ramsay Mac-Mullen, "Roman Attitudes to Greek Love," *Historia* 32 (1983): 484–502, esp. pp. 491–97. Other scholars who describe the ancient behavioral phenomenon as "bisexuality" include Luc Brisson, "Bisexualité et mediation en Grèce ancienne," *Nouvelle revue de psychoanalyse* 7 (1973): 27–48; Alain Schnapp, "Une autre image de l'homosexualité en Grèce ancienne," *Débat* 10 (1981): 107–17, esp. pp. 116–17: Lawrence Stone, "Sex in the West," *New Republic* (July 8, 1985): 25–37, esp. pp. 30–32 (with doubts). Contra, Padgug, "Sexual Matters," p. 13: "to speak, as is common, of the Greeks as 'bisexual' is illegitimate as well, since that merely adds a new, intermediate category, whereas it was precisely the categories themselves which had no meaning in antiquity."

27. T. M. Robinson, [Review of Dover's *Greek Homosexuality*], *Phoenix* 35 (1981): 160–63, esp. p. 162: "the reason why a heterosexual majority might have looked with a tolerant eye on 'active' homosexual practice among the minority, and even in some measure within their own group [!], . . . is predictably a sexist one: to the heterosexual majority, to whom (in a man's universe) the 'good' woman is *kata physin* [i.e., naturally] passive, obedient, and submissive, the 'role' of the 'active' homosexual will be tolerable precisely because his goings-on can, without too much difficulty, be equated with the 'role' of the male heterosexual, i.e., to dominate and subdue; what the two have in common is greater than what divides them." But this seems to me to beg the very question that the distinction between heterosexuality and homosexuality is supposedly designed to solve.

28. An excellent analysis of the contemporary Mediterranean version of this ethos

has been provided by David Gilmore, "Introduction: The Shame of Dishonor," in *Honor and Shame and the Unity of the Mediterranean,* ed. Gilmore, Special Publication of the American Anthropological Association, 22 (Washington, DC, 1987), pp. 2–21, esp. pp. 8–16.

29. By "phallus" I mean a culturally constructed signifier of social power: for the terminology, see note 10, above. I call Greek sexual discourse phallic because (1) sexual contacts are polarized around phallic action—i.e., they are defined by who has the phallus and by what is done with it; (2) sexual pleasures other than phallic pleasures do not count in categorizing sexual contacts; (3) in order for a contact to qualify as sexual, one—and no more than one—of the two partners is required to have a phallus (boys are treated in pederastic contexts as essentially unphallused) (see Martial, 11.22; but cf. *Palatine Anthology* 12.3, 7, 197, 207, 216, 222, 242) and tend to be assimilated to women; in the case of sex between women, one partner—the "tribad"—is assumed to possess a phallus-equivalent (an overdeveloped clitoris) and to penetrate the other: sources for the ancient conceptualization of the tribad—no complete modern study of this fascinating and long-lived fictional type, which survived into the early decades of the twentieth century, is known to me—have been assembled by Friedrich Karl Forberg, *Manual of Classical Erotology,* trans. Julian Smithson (Manchester, 1884; repr. New York, 1966), pp. 11, 108–67; Paul Brandt [pseud. "Hans Licht"], *Sexual Life in Ancient Greece,* trans. J. H. Freese, ed. Lawrence H. Dawson (London, 1932), pp. 316–28; Gaston Vorberg, *Glossarium eroticum* [Hanau, 1965], pp. 654–55; and Werner A. Krenkel, "Masturbation in der Antike," *Wissenschaftliche Zeitschrift der WilhelmPieck-Universität Rostock* 28 (1979), pp. 159–78, esp. p. 171. For a recent discussion, see Judith P. Hallett, "Female Homoeroticism and the Denial of Roman Reality in Latin Literature," *Yale Journal of Criticism* 3.1 (1989).

30. Exceptions include Vern L. Bullough, *Homosexuality: A History* (New York, 1979), pp. 3–5, and John Boswell, *Christianity, Social Tolerance, and Homosexuality: Gay People in Western Europe from the Beginning of the Christian Era to the Fourteenth Century* (Chicago, 1980), pp. 53n., 75n.

31. For an earlier use of *mollis* in this almost technical sense, see Juvenal, 9.38.

32. See P. H. Schrijvers, *Eine medizinische Erklärung der männlichen Homosexualität aus der Antike* (*Caelius Aurelianus De Morbis Chronicis* IV 9) (Amsterdam, 1985), p. 11.

33. I have borrowed this entire argument from Schrijvers, *Eine medizinische Erklarung,* pp. 7–8; the same point about the passage from *De morbis acutis* had been made earlier—unbeknownst to Schrijvers, apparently—by Boswell, *Christianity, Social Tolerance, and Homosexuality,* p. 53, n. 33; p. 75, n. 67.

34. Translation (with my emphasis and amplification) by I. F. Drabkin, ed. and trans., *Caelius Aurelianus On Acute Diseases and On Chronic Diseases* (Chicago, 1950), p. 413.

35. As his chapter title, "De mollibus sive subactis," implies.

36. See especially the pseudo-Aristotelian *Problemata* 4.26, well discussed by Dover, *Greek Homosexuality,* pp. 168–70, and by Winkler, "Laying Down the Law," pp. 67–69; generally, Boswell, *Christianity, Social Tolerance, and Homosexuality,* p. 53; Foucault, *The Use of Pleasure,* pp. 204–14.

37. The Latin phrase *quod utramque Venerem exerceant* is so interpreted by both

Drabkin, *Caelius Aurelianus*, p. 901n., and Schrijvers, *Eine medizinische Erklärung*, pp. 32–33, who secures this reading by citing Ovid, *Metamorphoses* 3.323, where Teiresias, who had been both a man and a woman, is described as being learned in the field of *Venus utraque*; Compare Petronius, *Satyricon* 43.8: *omnis minervae homo.*

38. I follow, once again, the insightful commentary by Schrijvers, *Eine medizinische Erklärung*, p. 15.

39. I quote from the translation by Drabkin, *Caelius Aurelianus*, p. 905, which is based on his plausible, but nonetheless speculative, reconstruction (accepted by Schrijvers, *Eine medizinische Erklärung*, p. 50) of a desperately corrupt text. For the notion expressed in it, compare Marcel Proust, *À la recherche du temps perdu*, ed. Pierre Clatac and Andre Ferri (Paris, 1954), III: 204, 212; *Remembrance of Things Past*, trans. C. K. Scott Moncrieff and Terence Kilmartin (New York, 1981), III: 203, 209; discussion by Eve Kosofsky Sedgwick, "Epistemology of the Closet (II)," *Raritan* 8 (Summer 1988): 102–30.

40. Anonymous, *De physiognomonia* 85 (vol. ii, p. 114.5–.14, Förster); Vettius Valens, 2.16 (p. 76.3–.8, Kroll); Clement of Alexandria, *Paedagogus* 3.21.3; Firmicus Maternus, *Mathesis* 6.30.15–.16 and 7.25.3–.23 (esp. 7.25.5).

41. See Foucault, *The History of Sexuality*, p. 43: "As defined by the ancient civil or canonical codes, sodomy was a category of forbidden acts; their perpetrator was nothing more than the juridical subject of them. The nineteenth-century homosexual became a personage, a past, a case history, and a childhood, in addition to being a type of life, a life form, and a morphology, with an indiscreet anatomy and possibly a mysterious physiology. Nothing that went into his total composition was unaffected by his sexuality. It was everywhere present in him: at the root of all his actions because it was their insidious and indefinitely active principle; written immodestly on his face and body because it was a secret that always gave itself away. It was consubstantial with him, less as a habitual sin than as a singular nature." See also Randolph Trumbach, "London's Sodomites: Homosexual Behavior and Western Culture in the 18th Century," *Journal of Social History* 11 (1977): 1–33, esp. p. 9; Richard Sennett, *The Fall of Public Man* (New York, 1977), pp. 6–8; Padgug, "Sexual Matters," pp. 13–14; Jean-Claude Feray, "Une histoire critique du mot homosexuality [IV]," *Arcadie* 28, no. 328 (1981): 246–58, esp. pp. 246–47; Schnapp (note 26, above), p. 116 (speaking of Attic vase-paintings): "One does not paint acts that characterize persons so much as behaviors that distinguish groups"; Pierre J. Payer, *Sex and the Penitentials: The Development of a Sexual Code 550–1150* (Toronto, 1984), pp. 40–44, esp. pp. 40–41: "there is no word in general usage in the penitentials for homosexuality as a category. . . . Furthermore, the distinction between homosexual acts and people who might be called homosexuals does not seem to be operative in these manuals" (also, pp. 14–15, 140–53); Bynum, "The Body of Christ," p. 406.

42. For attestations to the strength of individual preferences (even to the point of exclusivity) on the part of Greek males for a sexual partner of one sex rather than another, see Theognis, 1367–68; Euripides, *Cyclops*, 583–84; Xenophon, *Anabasis* 7.4.7–.8; Aeschines, 1.41, 195; the *Life of Zeno* by Antigonus of Carystus, cited by Athenaeus, 13.563e; the fragment of Seleucus quoted by Athenaeus, 15.697de (*Collectanea Alexandrina*, ed. J. U. Powell [Oxford, 1925], p. 176); an anonymous dramatic fragment cited by Plutarch, *Moralia*, pp. 766f–767a (*Tragicorum Graecorum Fragmenta*, ed. August Nauck,

2nd ed. [Leipzig, 1926], p. 906, #355; also in Theodor Kock, *Comicorum Atticorum Fragmenta* [Leipzig, 1880–1888], III: 467, #360); Athenaeus, 12.540e, 13.60le and ff.; Achilles Tatius, 2.35.2–.3; pseudo-Lucian, *Erôtes* 9–10; Firmicus Maternus, *Mathesis* 7.15.1–.2; and a number of epigrams by various hands contained in the *Palatine Anthology* 5.19, 65, 116, 208, 277, 278; 11.216; 12.7, 17, 41, 87, 145, 192, 198, and *passim* (cf. P. G. Maxwell-Stuart, "Strato and the Musa Puerilis," *Hermes* 100 [1972]: 215–40). See, generally, Dover, *Greek Homosexuality*, pp. 62–63; John Boswell, "Revolutions, Universals and Sexual Categories," in *Homosexuality: Sacrilege, Vision, Politics* (note 6, above), pp. 89–113, esp. pp. 98–101; Winkler, "Laying Down the Law"; and, for a list of passages, Claude Courouve, *Tableau synoptique de references a l'amour masculin: Auteurs grecs et latins* (Paris, 1986).

43. Hilary Putnam, in *Reason, Truth, and History* (Cambridge, UK, 1981), pp. 150–55, in the course of analyzing the various criteria by which we judge matters of taste to be "subjective," implies that we are right to consider sexual preferences more thoroughly constitutive of the human personality than dietary preferences, but his argument remains circumscribed, as Putnam himself points out, by highly culture-specific assumptions about sex, food, and personhood.

44. Foucault, *The Use of Pleasure*, pp. 51–52, remarks that it would be interesting to determine exactly when in the evolving course of Western cultural history sex became more morally problematic than eating; he seems to think that sex won out only at the turn of the eighteenth century, after a long period of relative equilibrium during the middle ages: see also *The Use of Pleasure*, p. 10; *The Care of the Self*, p. 143; "On the Genealogy of Ethics: An Overview of Work in Progress," in Hubert L. Dreyfus and Paul Rabinow, *Michel Foucault: Beyond Structuralism and Hermeneutics*, 2nd ed. (Chicago, 1983), pp. 229–52, esp. p. 229. The evidence lately assembled by Stephen Nissenbaum in *Sex, Diet, and Debility in Jacksonian America: Sylvester Graham and Health Reform*, Contributions in Medical History, 4 (Westport, CT, 1980); and by Caroline Walker Bynum, *Holy Feast and Holy Fast: The Religious Significance of Food to Medieval Women* (Berkeley, 1987), suggests that moral evolution may not have been quite such a continuously linear affair as Foucault appears to imagine.

45. Jack H. Abbott, "On 'Women,'" *New York Review of Books* 28, no. 10 (June 11, 1981): 17. It should perhaps be pointed out that this lyrical confession is somewhat at odds with the more gritty account contained in the edited excerpts from Abbott's letters that were published a year earlier in the *New York Review of Books* 27, no. 11 (June 26, 1980): 34–37. (One might compare Abbott's statement with some remarks uttered by Bernard Boursicot in a similarly apologetic context and quoted by Richard Bernstein, "France Jails Two in a Bizarre Case of Espionage," *New York Times* [May 11, 1986]: "I was shattered to learn that he [Boursicot's lover of twenty years] is a man, but my conviction remains unshakable that for me at that time he was really a woman and was the first love of my life.")

46. See Davidson (note 6, above), p. 16.

47. I wish to thank Kostas Demelis for helping me with this formulation. Compare Padgug, "Sexual Matters," p. 5: "In any approach that takes as predetermined and universal the categories of sexuality, real history disappears."

48. Stephen Greenblatt, "Fiction and Friction," in *Reconstructing Individualism:*

516   PHILOSOPHY AND SEX

Autonomy, Individuality, and the Self in Western Thought, ed. Thomas C. Heller, Morton Sosna, and David E. Wellbery, with Arnold I. Davidson, Ann Swidler, and Ian Watt (Stanford, 1986), pp. 30–52, 329–32, esp. p. 34, makes a similar point; arguing that "a culture's sexual discourse plays a critical role in shaping individuality," he goes on to say, "It does so by helping to implant in each person an internalized set of dispositions and orientations that governs individual improvisations." See also Padgug, "Sexual Matters"; generally, Julian Henriques, Wendy Holloway, Cathy Urwin, Venn Couze, and Valerie Walkerdine, *Changing the Subject: Psychology, Social Regulation and Subjectivity* (London, 1984).

49. "Translations" (1972), lines 32–33, in Adrienne Rich, *Diving into the Wreck: Poems 1971–1972* (New York, 1973), pp. 40–41 (quotation on p. 41).

50. "Canzone" (1942), lines 1–2, in W. H. Auden, *Collected Poems*, ed. Edward Mendelson (New York, 1976), pp. 256–57 (quotation on p. 256).

LIST OF CONTRIBUTORS

THOMAS AQUINAS (1225–1274), Italian/French religious philosopher, taught at the University of Paris.

AUGUSTINE (November 13, 354–August 28, 430), Bishop of Hippo, philosopher and theologian.

ROBERT B. BAKER is Williams D. Williams Professor of Philosophy at Union College (NY) and Director of the Union Graduate College Mount Sinai School of Medicine Bioethics Program.

JEREMY BENTHAM (1748–1832), English jurist and philosopher, taught at the University of London.

SHULAMITH BLACKSTONE is a founder of the radical feminist movement in the United States and author of *The Dialectic of Sex*.

EVELYN BLACKWOOD teaches anthropology at Purdue University.

SUSAN J. BRISON teaches philosophy at Dartmouth College.

HÉLÈNE CIXOUS is a philosopher and linguist at the Centre National de la Recherche Scientifique, Paris.

MILTON DIAMOND teaches at the Department of Anatomy and Reproductive Biology, Pacific Center for Sex and Society, University of Hawai`i at Manoa.

ALICE DOMURAT DREGER is Associate Professor of Clinical Medical Humanities and Bioethics in the Medical Humanities and Bioethics Program at the Feinberg School of Medicine of Northwestern University, Chicago.

ANNE FAUSTO-STERLING is Professor of Biology and Gender Studies in the Department of Molecular and Cell Biology and Biochemistry at Brown University.

BETH GOLDBLATT is Senior Research Officer, Gender Research Project, Centre for Applied Legal Studies, University of the Witwatersrand.

JOHN SCOTT GRAY teaches in the Department of Humanities, Ferris State University, Big Rapids, Michigan.

KIM Q. HALL teaches philosophy at Appalachian State University.

DAVID M. HALPERIN teaches in the Department of Sociology, Culture, and Communication at the University of New South Wales.

LUCE IRIGARAY teaches at the University de Paris, the Sorbonne, and the University de Bordeaux.

ROBERT JENSEN teaches communications at the University of Texas at Austin.

JEFF JORDAN teaches philosophy at the University of Delaware.

FRANCES MYRNA KAMM is Littauer Professor of Philosophy and Public Policy, Kennedy School, Harvard.

KENNETH KIPNIS teaches in the Department of Philosophy, University of Hawai`i at Manoa.

MICHAEL LEVIN teaches in the philosophy program at CUNY Graduate School and University Center.

MIKE W. MARTIN teaches philosophy at Chapman University in Orange County, California.

LARRY MAY teaches philosophy at Washington University in St. Louis, Missouri.

SUSAN MENDUS teaches political philosophy at the University of York, England.

THOMAS NAGEL teaches philosophy at New York University.

ALICIA OUELLETTE is an Associate Professor at Albany Law School and Professor of Bioethics at Union Graduate College-Mt. Sinai School of Medicine Bioethics Program.

POPE PAUL VI (1897–1978) reigned as the pope from 1963 to 1978.

ALAN SOBLE retired from the University of New Orleans in 2006 (after Hurricane Katrina) and now teaches philosophy in the Philadelphia area and virtually, online, in Nevada.

ROBERT C. SOLOMON (1942–2007) taught philosophy at the University of Texas at Austin.

ROBERT STRIKWERDA teaches philosophy at Indiana University in Kokomo.

JUDITH JARVIS THOMSON teaches in the Department of Linguistics and Philosophy at the Massachusetts Institute of Technology.

JOYCE TREBILCOT (1933–2009) was Emerita, Associate Professor of Philosophy and Women's Studies, University of California at Santa Barbara.

ARCHBISHOP DESMOND TUTU is the South African Anglican Archbishop Emeritus of Cape Town.

RICHARD WASSERSTROM is Emeritus Professor of Philosophy at Phil Board/Cowell College, the University of California, Santa Cruz.

KATHLEEN J. WININGER teaches philosophy as well as Women and Gender Studies at the University of Southern Maine at Portland.